Epidemiology
for Athletic Trainers

Integrating Evidence-Based Practice

Epidemiology for Athletic Trainers

Integrating Evidence-Based Practice

Melanie Adams, PhD, CSCS, AT-Ret
Assistant Professor
Physical Education Department
Keene State College
Keene, New Hampshire

Wanda Swiger, EdD, ATC, CES
Associate Professor
Athletic Training Program Director
Physical Education Department
Keene State College
Keene, New Hampshire

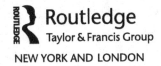
Routledge
Taylor & Francis Group

NEW YORK AND LONDON

Epidemiology for Athletic Trainers: Integrating Evidence-Based Practice includes ancillary materials specifically available for faculty use. Please visit www.routledge.com/9781617119163 to obtain access.

First published in 2016 by SLACK Incorporated

Published 2024 by Routledge
605 Third Avenue, New York, NY 10158

and by Routledge
4 Park Square, Milton Park, Abingdon, Oxon OX14 4RN

Routledge is an imprint of the Taylor & Francis Group, an informa business

© 2016 Taylor & Francis Group

Library of Congress Cataloging-in-Publication Data

Names: Adams, Melanie, 1970- , editor. | Swiger, Wanda, 1970- , editor.
Title: Epidemiology for athletic trainers : integrating evidence-based
  practice / editors, Melanie Adams, Wanda Swiger.
Description: Thorofare, NJ : SLACK Incorporated, [2015] | Includes
  bibliographical references and index.
Identifiers: LCCN 2015038346 | ISBN 9781617119163 (alk. paper)
Subjects: | MESH: Athletic Injuries--epidemiology. | Athletic
  Injuries--prevention and control. | Evidence-Based Practice.
Classification: LCC RD97 | NLM QT 261 | DDC 617.1/027--dc23 LC record available at http://lccn.loc.gov/2015038346

ISBN: 9781617119163 (pbk)
ISBN: 9781003523994 (ebk)

DOI: 10.4324/9781003523994

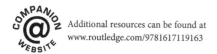

Additional resources can be found at
www.routledge.com/9781617119163

DEDICATION

We would like to thank SLACK Incorporated for giving us the opportunity to bring our vision to the athletic training community.

We are thankful for our dedicated and diligent contributing authors. Their patience during the editing process and willingness to be accommodating made for a smooth and fulfilling process.

Finally, we are most appreciative to our families for their understanding and patience through long hours of research, writing, and editing to create this work.

Melanie Adams, PhD, CSCS, AT-Ret

Wanda Swiger, EdD, ATC, CES

CONTENTS

Dedication. . . . . *v*

About the Authors . . . . *ix*

Contributing Authors . . . . *xi*

Foreword by Herbert K. Amato, DA, ATC . . . . *xiii*

Introduction. . . . . *xv*

Section I   Introduction to Epidemiology 1

Chapter 1   Epidemiology and the Leading Causes of Death 3
             Melanie Adams, PhD, CSCS, AT-Ret

Chapter 2   Epidemiology and Physical Activity 21
             Jeffrey Timmer, PhD, CEP

Chapter 3   Statistics for Clinical Epidemiology 41
             Ashley S. Long, PhD, LAT, ATC and Melanie Adams, PhD, CSCS, AT-Ret

Chapter 4   Injury Surveillance Systems. 65
             Wanda Swiger, EdD, ATC, CES

Chapter 5   Evidence-Based Practice 83
             Thomas Cappaert, PhD, ATC, CSCS

Section II   Sport-Related Epidemiology 103

Chapter 6   Sport-Related Concussion 105
             Johna K. Register-Mihalik, PhD, LAT, ATC

Chapter 7   Sudden Death in Sport 119
             Brendon P. McDermott, PhD, ATC and William M. Adams, MS, ATC

Chapter 8   Musculoskeletal Injuries in Sport 137
             Ashley S. Long, PhD, LAT, ATC

Chapter 9   Mental Health 167
             Melanie Adams, PhD, CSCS, AT-Ret

Section III Screening and Prevention of Sport-Related Injury. 205

Chapter 10   Pre-Activity Screening. 207
             Wanda Swiger, EdD, ATC, CES and Melanie Adams, PhD, CSCS, AT-Ret

Chapter 11   Prevention Methods. 241
                      Wanda Swiger, EdD, ATC, CES and Scot A. Ward, MS, ATC

Financial Disclosures. *269*
Index *271*

Epidemiology for Athletic Trainers: Integrating Evidence-Based Practice includes ancillary materials specifically available for faculty use. Please visit www.routledge.com/9781617119163 to obtain access.

ABOUT THE AUTHORS

Melanie Adams, PhD, CSCS, AT-Ret has been an Assistant Professor at Keene State College since 2012. She teaches courses in Exercise Science and Athletic Training. Prior to completing a doctorate degree in Kinesiology, Dr. Adams was a certified athletic trainer for 15 years at the National Collegiate Athletic Association Division I and III levels. She brings a variety of experiences to her teaching and scholarship. Although the health and performance of competitive athletes were her early focuses, she is currently more interested in promoting physical activity across the lifespan. She emphasizes evidence-based practice in Athletic Training and Exercise Science courses and helps students develop the skills needed to understand and apply scientific literature.

Originally from Tennessee, Dr. Adams's education and career have taken her up and down the East Coast. She is a graduate of Keene State College, the University of Virginia, and the University of North Carolina at Greensboro. Dr. Adams was the Coordinator for Sports Medicine and an Instructor of Physical Education at Hood College in Frederick, Maryland, before pursuing her PhD. While at the University of North Carolina at Greensboro, she was selected as a research mentee for the National Institutes of Health Center of Excellence for Health Disparities, housed in the School of Nursing. It was here where she developed her research skills and strong interest in epidemiology.

Her own research focuses on increasing physical activity and reducing sedentary behavior in populations at risk for chronic disease. In addition, she collaborates with students in the Athletic Training Education Program on their senior research projects. Dr. Adams has published articles on physical activity's link to quality of life and on strategies to decrease sedentary behavior in overweight adults. She has presented her work at the annual meetings of the North American Society for Sport and Physical Activity, American Society for Metabolic and Bariatric Surgery, the Association of Applied Sport Psychologists, and at New England chapter of the American College of Sports Medicine.

Wanda Swiger, EdD, ATC, CES is the Program Director of Athletic Training and an Associate Professor at Keene State College, where she teaches courses in Athletic Training, Physical Education, and Exercise Science. A native of Tionesta, Pennsylvania, Dr. Swiger earned her undergraduate and doctoral degrees from West Virginia University and her master's degree from Shippensburg University of Pennsylvania.

Dr. Swiger has been a practicing athletic trainer for more than 20 years, with experience at the National Collegiate Athletic Association Collegiate and National Association of Intercollegiate Athletics Collegiate and interscholastic levels of sport and has practiced in multiple states in an outpatient setting. She has had the opportunity to work in alternative settings. Dr. Swiger has been teaching in higher education since 2000 and has been a program director since 2005. Dr. Swiger's passion is developing curricula that focus on a bottom-up philosophy and are grounded in the natural sciences. Her assessment work has focused on academic standards within athletic training and has led her to serve as Chair of the Academic Standards Committee approving academic admissions standards. Dr. Swiger served on the Academic Overview Committee reviewing the quality of educational programs at Keene State College.

Her teaching has fostered undergraduate research in many areas, such as evaluation, rehabilitation, pharmacology, and general medical conditions. With her background in Special Education and Adapted Physical Education, Dr. Swiger has focused her service activities around physical disabilities and sport participation. While at her previous institution, she was the coordinator for an adaptive sports program that provided multiple sports activities for youth. Since 2008, Dr. Swiger has been part of the medical teams covering the Boston Marathon. She served as co-medical director for the 2013 USA Deaflympic games after being a member of the medical staffs for USA Track and Field and Deaflympics beginning in 2009. Dr. Swiger has presented locally and nationally on the needs of deaf athletes and on emergency preparedness and management of large athletic events.

CONTRIBUTING AUTHORS

William M. Adams, MS, ATC (Chapter 7)
Director of Sport Safety Policy Initiatives
Korey Stringer Institute
Department of Kinesiology
University of Connecticut
Storrs, Connecticut

Thomas Cappaert, PhD, ATC, CSCS (Chapter 5)
Professor of Biostatistics
Director of Student Research
Rocky Mountain University of Health
    Professions
Provo, Utah

Ashley S. Long, PhD, LAT, ATC (Chapters 3
    and 8)
Research Consultant
Carolinas Healthcare System
Department of Family Medicine
Department of Sports Medicine and Special
    Events
Charlotte, North Carolina

Brendon P. McDermott, PhD, ATC (Chapter 7)
Assistant Professor of Athletic Training
Department of Health, Human Performance
    and Recreation
University of Arkansas
Fayetteville, Arkansas

Johna K. Register-Mihalik, PhD, LAT, ATC
    (Chapter 6)
Assistant Professor of Exercise and Sport
    Science
Research Scientist, Injury Prevention Research
    Center
Faculty, Matthew Gfeller Sport-Related TBI
    Research Center
University of North Carolina at Chapel Hill
Chapel Hill, North Carolina

Jeffrey Timmer, PhD, CEP (Chapter 2)
Associate Professor
Physical Education/Exercise Science
Keene State College
Keene, New Hampshire

Scot A. Ward, MS, ATC (Chapter 11)
Assistant Clinical Professor
Coordinator of Clinical Education
Keene State College
Keene, New Hampshire

FOREWORD

As a former Athletic Training Program Director for 22 years, I see the need for this textbook and how it can be used in educating athletic training students. I was glad to be part of the initial conversations around an athletic training–specific text for epidemiology. The authors and I talked on numerous occasions from the start to the finish of this book. These conversations dealt with who should publish the book, who the best contributors were, what contents should be included, and who would read the evidence-based practice (EBP). We all agreed that this emphasis would fill a gap that many other athletic training books miss.

Epidemiology for Athletic Trainers: Integrating Evidence-Based Practice is designed to help instructors and students address the multiple Commission on Accreditation of Athletic Training Education Learning Outcomes related to EBP and prevention and health promotion (PHP). The majority of the book focuses on the EBP and PHP outcomes; however, other content areas of the Athletic Training Educational Competencies are scattered throughout the book. The 9 contributing authors, through their education and professional experience, all play key roles in the quality of each chapter. Jointly, they bring a strong but diverse background that gives this book a good overview of the impact that epidemiology has had on medicine, public health, and exercise science.

Section I of this book introduces the reader to the history of epidemiology and how sports epidemiology can be beneficial to entry-level athletic trainers and the most experienced clinicians in our field. This section highlights how to collect data and use results. Chapter 3, titled, "Statistics for Clinical Epidemiology," gives the reader a basic understanding of statistics, predicting risk, and avoiding sample bias. In addition to the EBP, injury data collection, and epidemiology focus of this book, current topics related to concussion, screening for anterior cruciate ligament risk factors, psychological concerns, and preventing sudden death in athletes are covered in Sections II and III. In my experience doing workshops to help students prepare for the Board of Certification examination, a common question is, "Where can I find information regarding policies and rules related to equipment?" The final chapter of this book helps to answer this question. In current textbooks, there is little information regarding policies, rules, and protective equipment used by athletic training educators.

This book is much more than dry facts associated with epidemiology. It takes patterns, causes, and effects related to sports medicine injury, conditions, and illnesses and demonstrates how they are relevant to an athletic trainer's day-to-day responsibilities. The application questions in the chapter review sections, "Bringing It Together," tie the book material to real-life athletic training scenarios. The true value of this book is that it introduces athletic training students to skills that will help them become lifelong learners. Knowing where to find reliable information and the ability to critically process it is the link they need between data collection and day-to-day professional practice.

Herbert K. Amato, DA, ATC
Associate Vice Provost for University Programs
James Madison University
Harrisonburg, Virginia

INTRODUCTION

As Athletic Training advances as an allied-health care profession, it is critical for athletic trainers to have a similar understanding of epidemiology and evidence-based practice as other medical practitioners. Athletic training education programs have been asked to increase their focus on epidemiology, injury data collection, and evidenced-based practice. A large number of the CAATE learning outcomes focus on knowledge and skill in the areas of Prevention and Health Promotion and Evidenced-Based Practice.

The idea for *Epidemiology for Athletic Trainers: Integrating Evidence-Based Practice* was developed after a revision in our curriculum and the planning of a new course for the pre-professional athletic training major. The course we envisioned at Keene State College focused on incidence and risk factors for sport-related injury, the evaluation of common screenings, prevention strategies, and understanding the steps of evidence-based practice. Dr. Swiger and I were struck by the lack of athletic training specific textbooks on these topics. After a semester of piecing together readings from nursing, physical therapy, and public health, we knew we could create a better option. We drew on the expertise of colleagues across the country. The collaboration produced much greater breadth than we could have provided on our own. There are many more topics we would like to pursue and hope that the textbook will grow with each edition. While this textbook was written specifically for pre-professional athletic training students, post-professional programs may find value in developing courses that focus on sport epidemiology and the integration of applied evidence-based practice.

Epidemiology originated when infectious diseases were the leading causes of death. The careful study of personal and environmental characteristics during outbreaks of cholera, smallpox, and polio uncovered carriers and agents that then could be eradicated through improved sanitation and eventually through vaccination. In the last half century, epidemiologists have played a key role in determining risk factors for everything from cancer to addiction. Epidemiological data provide targets for interventions. A target that athletic training students are familiar with is the need to increase physical activity. The link between physical activity and health is used in Chapter 1 to demonstrate the impact epidemiology has had in the fields of medicine, public health, and exercise science. Sports epidemiology is a relatively new specialty. While athletic trainers have been at the forefront for data collection (especially at the NCAA level), our research has lacked the lengthy longitudinal cohort studies needed to establish risk factors. Physical activity epidemiology illustrates how the results of longitudinal studies were used to develop the national physical activity guidelines. We believe this model is important for future athletic training researchers as they investigate changes to pre-participation screening, physical conditioning, equipment, rules, and return-to-play guidelines.

Students at Keene State College have enjoyed this approach and begin to see themselves as part of the larger health care system, rather than singularly focused practitioners. Illustrating the basic concepts of incidence, risk, and surveillance through the lens of general health helps students understand why physical activity is health promoting and how chronic exposure to sports increases certain risks. Core research methods that are embedded in epidemiology are discussed to help students read, appraise, and contribute to the literature. Injury surveillance methods help future clinicians understand the critical role athletic trainers play in the data collection process. The hot topics of concussion, screening for ACL risk, and preventing sudden death in athletes are covered in a way that makes the evidence understandable and practical.

Our aim was to make the literature accessible, connect commonly used clinical strategies to evidence, and inspire a fun classroom experience. To facilitate this, each chapter has a list of classroom activities including debates, games, and research activities. Once a student learns to find, read, and critically appraise evidence, there is no limit to where he or she can draw knowledge from. We are most proud when students cross disciplines, from oncology to psychology, to find the best evidence. While originally intended for a traditional classroom, this text is also an excellent resource to current clinicians interested in improving their evidence-based practice skills. In particular, the chapters on statistics and evidence-based practice will give anyone the confidence to read original research. The chapter on injury surveillance allows the practicing clinician the opportunity to become an active participant in data collection.

How to Use This Textbook

We believe that *Epidemiology for Athletic Trainers: Integrating Evidence-Based Practice* will be a valuable resource for both pre- and post-professional clinicians. The text is divided into 3 sections. The first section provides an introduction to epidemiology and develops students' knowledge of incidence, risk factors, and measurement of risk.

- Chapter 1 focuses on the history of epidemiology with its roots in public health and disease, while Chapter 2 connects those concepts to physical activity.

- Chapter 3 describes the statistics most commonly used in epidemiology and encourages students to think critically about the statistical significance and the difference between correlational and causal research.

- Chapter 4 details the goals and current methods of injury surveillance systems. The chapter identifies the need for athletic trainers to be actively involved in the data collection process.

- Chapter 5 leads the students through the steps of evidence-based practice and gives them a practical model to follow.

Section II takes an epidemiological view of sport-related injury and highlights current trends in sport injury, practice and what evidence is needed to improve athlete care. Rather than just reporting on occurrence and risk, these chapters review the key evidence and etiology and suggest areas for future research.

- Chapters 6 through 8 focus on content that athletic trainers would typically be exposed to in the sport setting.

- Chapter 9 is a comprehensive look at the topic of mental health.

Section III focuses students on the application of the first two sections. Once students understand epidemiology, research, and sport-related injury, they can now be asked to apply evidence-based strategies to critically assess the use of screenings, stretching, or strengthening programs for injury prevention and for rule and equipment changes in sport.

- Chapter 10 discusses the currently accepted screening protocols and emerging ideas in the areas of pre-participation and functional movement.

- Chapter 11 demonstrates how rules and equipment have changed as our knowledge of injury mechanisms improved. This chapter further identifies prevention strategies that have demonstrated effectiveness.

Instructor's Materials

The information in the text is best paired with classroom activities and assignments that require students to practice evidence retrieval, appraisal, and decision making. Important research skills such as developing answerable questions, database searches, and determining the strength of the evidence are enhanced when students take ownership over a clinical question. The instructor's online manual outlines classroom activities and provides additional resources. Each chapter ends with suggested activities or review questions to help students integrate key material with clinical practice. Out-of-class assignments don't have to be full critically appraised papers or critically appraised topics. Case studies where students work in groups to find the best plan of care for a patient and debates that create discussion about policies, rules, or screening methods work well. Students enjoy creating knowledge and many of the topics discussed in the text lend to both academic and popular web searches. Web links have been provided in the Bringing It Together section of each chapter and online. These are excellent resources for both students and instructors. The review questions can be used as quiz material or as a study guide for students.

While intended for a singular course at Keene State, educators may use this textbook across the curriculum. Students should be encouraged to keep this text throughout their program and into their early years in the profession. The CAATE learning outcomes that *Epidemiology for Athletic Trainers: Integrating Evidence-Based Practice* fulfills are as follows:

- Evidenced Based Practice, 1-10, 12, and 14
- Prevention and Health Promotion, 1-6, 8, 9, 17(a,c,d,f,h,i), 20, 22, 25-27, 29, 33, 43, 45-47
- Clinical Examination, 8, 10, 23
- Acute Care, 36a-e
- Psychosocial Strategies and Referral, 11, 13-15, 17
- Health Care Administration, 23

After reading this textbook, it is our hope that students make the important connections between epidemiology, injury surveillance, and evidence-based practice and feel more confident using these skills as an allied health care provider. The text serves as a bridge from student athletic trainers to active health care providers. However, we highly recommend that the reader keep abreast of current updates to sport epidemiology to provide best practices in athletic health care.

Melanie Adams, PhD, CSCS, AT-Ret
Wanda Swiger, EdD, ATC, CES

I

Introduction to Epidemiology

1

Epidemiology and the Leading Causes of Death

Melanie Adams, PhD, CSCS, AT-Ret

CHAPTER OBJECTIVES

- Define the following terms: *epidemiology, risk factor, prevalence,* and *incidence.*
- Identify risk factors associated with chronic disease and recognize that racial/ethnic disparities exist in disease prevalence in the United States.
- Describe the basic etiologies of the most common chronic diseases in the United States.
- Recognize the relationship between low amounts of physical activity and multiple chronic diseases.

INTRODUCTION

Epidemiology is the study of disease or injury within populations of people. The most basic form of epidemiology is tracking how many people in a community, region, or nation have a disease or injury. This descriptive type of study, called *surveillance*, reports the number of cases as a condition's *incidence* or *prevalence*. Incidence tells you the number of new cases that have occurred within a certain time (usually 1 year). The prevalence includes the new cases and those that continue to live with the disease or injury. More than just counting who has what, epidemiologists observe populations to determine what puts people at risk for certain diseases or injuries.[1] This type of study analyzes the relationship between exposure and acquiring the disease or injury. All types of medical concerns can be studied using epidemiology, from infectious diseases, such as measles, to mental health diagnoses, such as depression, to sports injuries, such as concussions. Epidemiological studies provide the evidence used by physicians, public health professionals, and athletic trainers to develop prevention strategies and treatment plans.

Adams M, Swiger W.
*Epidemiology for Athletic Trainers: Integrating
Evidence-Based Practice (pp 3-19).*
© 2016 Taylor & Francis Group.

History of Epidemiology

Epidemiology has its roots in public health. The first epidemiologists studied outbreaks of infectious diseases in Europe, such as smallpox and cholera, in the 1700s and 1800s. American epidemiologists began their work in the mid-1800s when yellow fever, typhoid fever, and influenza were problematic in large cities. These early researchers were usually physicians who were curious about why some people were more susceptible than others. They were the first to consider the role of inoculation, sanitation, and disease carriers. After reports in the late 1700s that dairy maids appeared to be immune to smallpox, an English physician, Edward Jenner, recognized that the maids were exposed to cowpox and that this dose of disease protected them. He developed a vaccine using the premise that the body would build an immunity if exposed to a small amount of a bacteria.[2]

Cases of infectious diseases often cluster in neighborhoods or sections of cities before spreading. In 1854, John Snow plotted the home and work locations of cholera cases in a section of London and identified a single water pump as the source of the contamination.[3] The story of Typhoid Mary provides a similar example. Outbreaks of typhoid fever in New York and New Jersey in the early 1900s were concerning because the known cause, poor sanitation, was thought to be fixed. An astute sanitation engineer traced the new cases to a single carrier, Mary Mallon. Mallon had worked as a cook in several homes where typhoid cases appeared, but she, herself, never got sick.[4]

Eventually, the record keeping that helped early epidemiologists make these connections was taken over by city health departments created to track disease and monitor conditions that led to outbreaks. The American Public Health Association was founded in 1872, and a permanent national Public Health Service was established in 1912.[5] Records of births and deaths allowed health workers to find common causes of death and consider ways to reduce citizens' risks of dying. Mortality data continue to be a large part of epidemiology. The major threats are no longer from the spread of bacteria or viruses, but from noninfectious diseases and accidents. Noninfectious diseases have no single cause, but they are related to lifestyle factors, such as tobacco use, physical inactivity, diet, or stress. In the past 50 years, epidemiology has advanced the knowledge of factors related to heart disease, diabetes mellitus, cancer, depression, and Alzheimer's disease. Identifying common factors and knowing who is at risk of disease or injury is the first step in being able to reduce the number of people who develop illnesses or are injured each year.

Risk Factors and Statistics

A basic premise of epidemiology is that exposure to a disease agent increases the chances of getting the disease. The exposure idea is most obvious for infectious diseases (eg, influenza). The more contact one has with people that have the virus, the more likely one is to get sick. Exposure to a disease can also come from behaviors, the environment, or personal characteristics. Epidemiologists use statistics to quantify how much a disease or injury is related to behavioral, social, environmental, or personal characteristics. These links to disease and injury are called *risk factors*. Risk factors are conditions that increase the chances of being diagnosed with a disease or having a particular injury. They can be physiological, genetic, or inherited traits; health-related behaviors; or related to the physical surroundings.[1] However, risk factors are not causes of disease; they simply have a connection to the disease. Based on the presence or absence of a particular risk factor, epidemiologists can calculate the probability, or risk, of developing a specific disease or injury. Several statistics are used to describe risk, such as relative risk, odds ratio, or population attributable risk. Also, life expectancy and disability-adjusted life years are statistics used by epidemiologists to show the impact of disease on longevity and quality of life. Chapter 3 explains many common epidemiology statistics in detail.

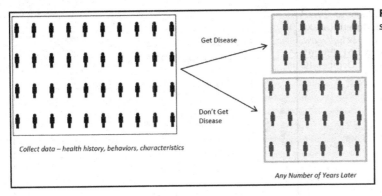

Figure 1-1. Longitudinal cohort study.

Environments

How strongly a risk factor relates to the onset of a disease or injury has a lot to do with the environment in which a person lives. Differences in health between groups of people are called *health disparities*. It is important to consider how known risk factors for disease are made worse by situations that are outside of an individual's control. Some risk factors are changeable and are referred to as modifiable. However, for some people, there may be limits to how modifiable these risk factors are. Epidemiology helps make health care providers and policy makers aware of who needs the most help to change their risk factors. For example, smoking tobacco is a behavior that greatly increases the risk of heart disease and cancer. Smoking is more prevalent in minority populations and in those with lower levels of socioeconomic status. This knowledge has allowed health professionals to start smoking-prevention programs in elementary schools and has convinced lawmakers to increase taxes on cigarettes to make smoking less affordable. In terms of sports, differences in injury rates between genders, positions, and in different sports are risk factors that are made better or worse by larger circumstances, such as rules, playing conditions, and access to protective equipment.

Sports Epidemiology

Sports epidemiology is relatively new. Sports injuries were typically categorized as accidents by general physicians and epidemiologists 20 years ago. However, a need for more evidence on risk factors, prevention, and treatment methods in athletes motivated clinicians and researchers to use epidemiology methods when studying athletes. The key study that was missing from sports medicine research was the longitudinal cohort study. This is when a researcher measures the characteristics of a large sample of people and then waits to see how many are diagnosed with different diseases (Figure 1-1). Some epidemiology studies follow thousands of participants for 15 or more years to collect this type of data. Prior to 2000, there were few such studies in American sports. Because athletic careers are relatively short, longitudinal studies in sports epidemiology may only last for 1 to 2 years. However, similar to public health epidemiology, sports injury researchers examine patterns between the characteristics of the athlete and his or her sport and the likelihood that he or she will sustain a specific injury. For example, Badgeley et al[6] examined 10,000 high school football injuries by position, mechanism of injury, athlete's activity when injured, and whether the injury occurred during a game or practice, all of which helps identify who is more likely to get hurt and under what conditions. Sports epidemiologists also test the effect of changes to risk factors on the incidence of injury. After high school girl's lacrosse required players to wear an eye shield, Lincoln et al[7] saw that facial injuries decreased but the number of concussions increased.

As mentioned previously, public health and medicine have successfully used epidemiology to make evidence-based decisions and have provided a path for sports injury specialists to reduce

Figure 1-2. US life expectancy 2006 to 2011.[9] (Reprinted with permission from Hoyert DL, Xu J. Deaths: preliminary data for 2011. http://www.cdc.gov/nchs/data/nvsr/nvsr61/nvsr61_06.pdf. Published October 10, 2012. Accessed October 15, 2015.)

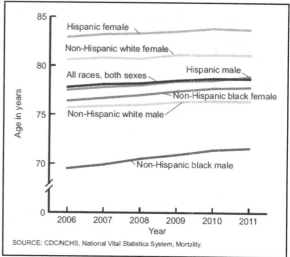

SOURCE: CDC/NCHS, National Vital Statistics System, Mortality.

injuries. There are 3 key steps. First, describe the scope of the problem and identify common factors through careful documentation. Next, examine the effect of reducing a single disease factor. Last, find the best approach to reduce that factor, realizing that a solution may require multiple tries.

To better understand the type of information that epidemiology provides, the next section reviews the authors' current knowledge of the leading causes of death. In Chapter 2, this knowledge is connected to the role of physical activity in reducing disease incidence and decreasing the number of people with risk factors.

Prevalence and Leading Causes of Death in the United States

Life expectancy among Americans continues to rise. Children born in 2011 will live on average 78.7 years.[8] This is improved from 76.86 years in 2001.[9] Since the Centers for Disease Control and Prevention (CDC) began tracking life expectancy in 1902, there has been a steady increase in years until death (Figure 1-2). This is not surprising given the advancements in sanitation and medicine since the Industrial Revolution. What may be surprising is the fact that the United States lags behind other nations in life expectancy. Data collected by the United Nations found that the United States ranked 51st overall.[10] Other large industrial nations similar to the United States have greater life expectancies. Japan's average was 83.91 years, followed by Australia at 81.9 and Canada at 81.48.[10]

Life expectancy also differs by race and gender. For example, Black males have considerable lower life expectancies than White males. Black females tend to live longer than all males but are significantly lower than White females.[11] Several behavioral, social, and environmental factors are related to these disparities, such as access to health care, education, access to healthy food, neighborhood safety, and employment opportunities.[12]

Although life expectancy continues to increase, there has been relatively little change to the leading causes of death for Americans in the past 60 years.[7] The top 10 leading causes of death are shown in Table 1-1. Five of the top 10 have a common risk factor. Heart disease, some cancers, cerebrovascular disease, Alzheimer's disease, and type 2 diabetes mellitus (T2DM) occur less frequently among people who are physically active.[13,14] Incorporating physical activity into the treatment of these diseases improves the outcomes in 6 of the top 10, including heart disease,

	CAUSE OF DEATH	DEATHS	RATE*	AGE-ADJUSTED RATE*
	TABLE 1-1 **TOP 10 CAUSES OF DEATH IN 2011[8]**			
1	Heart disease	596,339	191.4	173.7
2	Cancer	575,313	184.6	168.6
3	Chronic lower respiratory disease	143,382	46	42.7
4	Cerebrovascular disease	126,931	41.4	37.9
5	Accidents	122,777	39.4	38
6	Alzheimer's disease	84,691	27.2	24.6
7	Diabetes mellitus	73,282	23.5	21.5
8	Influenza and pneumonia	53,667	17.2	15.7
9	Kidney disease	45,731	14.7	13.4
10	Suicide	38,285	12.3	12
	All-causes	2,512,873	806.5	740.6

*per 100,000.

some cancers, cerebrovascular disease, Alzheimer's disease, T2DM, and chronic respiratory infections.[15-17]

Cardiovascular Disease

Heart disease has been the leading cause of death in the United States since the 1920s, although the number of deaths has been steadily declining since 1960 (Figure 1-3).[18] Heart disease includes coronary heart disease (CHD), arrhythmia (irregular heart beat), congestive heart failure (ineffective heart contractions), heart infections, and congenital heart defects (birth defects).[19,20] The term *cardiovascular disease* (CVD) is commonly used in place of heart disease, but it is a broader term that includes hypertension (high blood pressure) and stroke.[20]

More than 1 in 3 adults in the United States have one or more CVDs (approximately 83.6 million people).[20] Older adults are affected at a higher rate than those younger than 40 years. Seventy percent of those aged 60 to 79 years have at least one CVD. The most common CVD is hypertension. An estimated 77.9 million (30%) Americans have high blood pressure. The second most common condition is CHD, with 15.4 million (approximately 6%) living with the disease.[21] However, CHD has the highest rate of death. It has accounted for 49% of CVD deaths in 2009.[20] There are significant differences in mortality between genders and races. Females develop CVD an average of 7 to 10 years later than males[22] and survive for longer.[23] However, Blacks have a higher mortality rate than Whites.[24]

Optimal function of the cardiovascular system depends on the health of the heart muscle, the lungs, the blood vessels, and the blood. If one segment of the system is not healthy, the others must work harder to make up for the deficit. The risk factors that are common to all CVDs have a negative impact on the function of the heart, lungs, blood, and blood vessels. These include a lack of regular physical activity, cigarette smoking, obesity, family history of CVD, diabetes mellitus, and high cholesterol.[20] The links between cardiovascular risk factors and the development of the disease are strong. For example, blood vessels become rigid and inflexible due to the development of plague within their walls. Excess cholesterol in the blood stream starts the process by which those plagues form. The thicker, less flexible vessel walls then contribute to hypertension. The

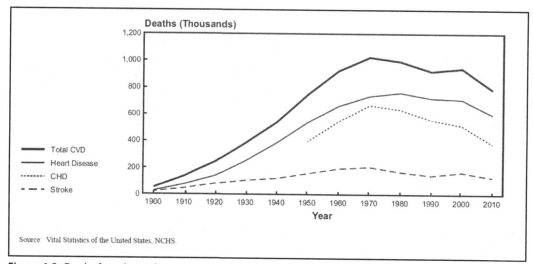

Figure 1-3. Deaths from heart disease 1900 to 2010. (Reprinted with permission from National Heart, Lung, and Blood Institute. Diease statistics. http://www.nhlbi.nih.gov/about/documents/factbook/2012/chapter4#4_1. Accessed October 14, 2015.)

role of physical activity in reducing cholesterol and blood pressure is discussed in Chapter 2. The study of how a disease begins and the steps it takes as it progresses is called *etiology*. When disease processes are well understood from years of research, the risk factors are closely tied to their etiologies.

Atherosclerosis

CVD originates with physical changes to blood vessels, whether in the heart (coronary arteries), brain (stroke), or arms and legs (peripheral artery disease). The opening through which blood flows is called the *lumen*. Healthy blood vessels have a smooth layer of epithelial cells that line the lumen. When there are high levels of low-density lipoproteins (LDLs) in the blood, some of the LDL molecules cross the lining into the area just above the muscle layer of the vessel wall called the *intima*. The LDLs irritate the endothelium and trigger an inflammatory response that brings white blood cells (monocytes) to the intima (Figure 1-4).[25] The LDLs are treated as foreign invaders by the monocytes. Once a monocyte engulfs the LDL molecule, it transforms into a foam cell that hardens over time. This progress is continual so that a build-up of hardened foam cells creates atherosclerotic plaques inside the walls of arteries. Initially, the artery remodels and pushes the plaque outward away from the lumen. This allows the vessel to maintain its normal diameter. The surface of the lumen changes because of the plaque below becoming thinner.[26] This fibrous cap is weaker and less flexible than the undamaged epithelium and is more likely to rupture.

When a rupture occurs, an even greater inflammatory response occurs, and the site is packed with platelets and macrophages trying to seal the break in the intima. This clot is called a *thrombus* and can slow or block blood flow through the artery. Rather than completely occluding an artery, a thrombus will heal as a scar on the inside of the lumen and slowly encroach on blood flow. The cells that get oxygen and nutrients from that blood vessel will die if they cannot get adequate blood flow. When those cells are heart muscle cells, the damage makes it harder for the heart to contract normally. If enough cells die, the heart will not be able to produce normal contractions, and the risk of a heart attack is high.[27] Over time, if the plaque buildup in the vessel walls gets to be great, the artery will not be able to remodel the external wall of the vessel anymore, and the diameter of the lumen will shrink (see Figure 1-4) and restrict blood flow.[26]

Treatment for atherosclerosis includes medications for hypertension (beta blockers) and high cholesterol (statins). Changes in diet and physical activity are also suggested. Increasing

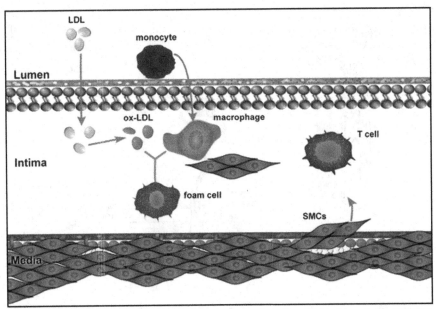

Figure 1-4. Atherosclerosis. (Reprinted with permission from Hao W, Friedman A. The LDL-HDL profile determines the risk of atherosclerosis: a mathematical model. *PLoS One.* 2014;9(3):e90497.)

physical activity can reduce blood pressure,[14] heart rate,[14] and chronic inflammation.[28] Dietary recommendations include reducing the intake of saturated fats and salt.[29] If a coronary artery is nearly blocked by plaque or occluded, surgery is typically done. An angioplasty is a procedure in which a narrow tube with a balloon is placed in the artery and the balloon is expanded to push the plaque against the wall of the artery so that a larger opening is made.[30] A stent is a small mechanical device that can be inserted into the artery to hold it open. A coronary bypass is another surgical option in which a section of healthy blood vessel is taken from another part of the body and connected to the heart so that the blood flow to the heart can be improved. Fortunately, the number of Americans having surgery for heart disease has been declining. Between 2007 and 2008, there were approximately 216,500 surgeries performed, down from 239,145 in 2005 and 2006.[31]

Cerebrovascular Disease

These conditions are characterized by a disruption in blood flow to brain cells. Stroke is the most common type of cerebrovascular disease. Stroke was also listed as a CVD because cerebrovascular accidents, another term for stroke, have the same etiology and risk factors as heart disease. Blood vessels in the brain become rigid and clogged by plaque the same way they do in the heart. This reduces or stops blood flow to brain cells. Approximately 16.8 million strokes occur each year in the United States, and stroke accounts for 6.4% of all CVD deaths.[20] In 2010, cerebrovascular disease was the fourth leading cause of death.[7]

There are 2 types of stroke, ischemic and hemorrhagic. Ischemic strokes (Figure 1-5) are more common and are due to atherosclerosis. Symptoms, such as difficulty speaking, walking, or impaired vision, are the result of tissue death in the brain centers that control those functions. Signs of stroke also include severe headache and mental confusion.[33] In the case of a hemorrhagic stroke, the blood vessel has ruptured or is so weakened that blood leaks out into the brain (Figure 1-6). Brain cells are damaged by the pressure that builds up inside the skull.

Another cerebrovascular disease is a transient ischemic attack (TIA), sometimes referred to as a mini-stroke.[33] The symptoms of TIA are the same as a stroke and only last for a few minutes. They resolve when the blockage in the blood vessel is resolved naturally. A third of those diagnosed

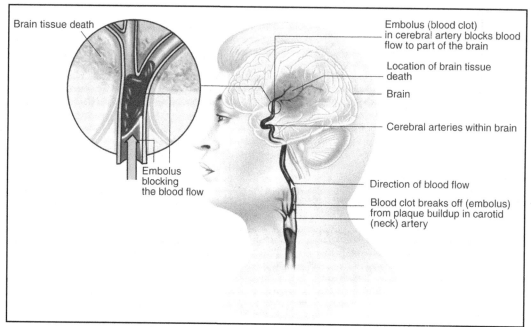

Figure 1-5. Ischemic stroke.

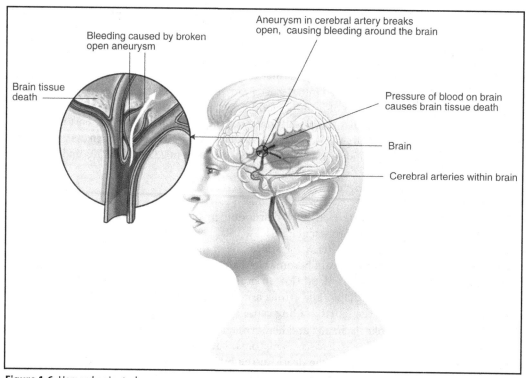

Figure 1-6. Hemorrhagic stroke.

with TIA have a stroke within 1 year.[34] The true incidence of TIA is hard to know because so many people never report their symptoms. The American Stroke Association estimates that between 200,000 and 500,000 people experience a TIA each year.[34]

The risk factors for stroke and TIA are identical to those for heart disease. Hypertension is a key factor and should be controlled with a combination of physical activity, diet, and medication. Other risk factors for stroke are smoking, obesity, high cholesterol, and family history. Also similar to heart disease are the racial disparities for stroke. Blacks are nearly twice as likely to have a stroke than Whites.[35]

Diabetes Mellitus

In 2010, approximately 1.9 million Americans aged 20 and older were diagnosed with diabetes mellitus.[36] When one considers diagnosed and undiagnosed cases, 8.3% of the population has diabetes mellitus. Diabetes mellitus is a chronic disease, meaning that once it has been diagnosed, it requires lifelong treatment. Those with the disease lack the ability to absorb carbohydrates from their bloodstream. Normally, carbohydrates, in the form of glucose, are assisted across cell membranes by the hormone insulin. Diabetics either do not produce enough insulin or their cells are not sensitive to the insulin they produce. Without this mechanism (called insulin-mediated glucose transport), glucose levels in the bloodstream increase, and cells that need energy are not able to function.

There are 2 forms of the disease, including type 1 (T1DM) and T2DM. In T1DM, the pancreas cannot produce enough insulin to move the glucose into the cells. This form of the disease is most often diagnosed in childhood. T1DM has a strong genetic link.[37] T2DM is related to obesity and health behaviors, such as physical activity and diet, as well as family history.[36] The key difference between the diseases is that in T2DM, the pancreas produces sufficient insulin but the cells are not sensitive to the hormone and require more and more insulin to move smaller amounts of glucose across the membranes. T2DM was previously known as adult-onset diabetes mellitus because its etiology was only seen in those older than 20 years. That trend has reversed because people between ages 10 and 19 years are frequently diagnosed with T2DM.[36]

From 1996 to 2008, there was a steady increase in the number of new cases of diabetes mellitus each year in the United States (Figure 1-7).[38] As many as 95% of these cases have T2DM.[37] Due to insulin resistance, those with T2DM have high levels of circulating glucose and insulin. These 2 substances have a negative effect on the health of blood vessels and nerve tissue. When the disease is not well controlled, there are serious complications, including kidney disease, blindness, loss of sensation in limbs, heart disease, and stroke.[36] Diabetes mellitus is the seventh leading cause of death.[8]

Risk factors for T2DM include central obesity, lack of physical activity, impaired glucose tolerance, family history of diabetes mellitus, or history of gestational diabetes mellitus.[39] The risk of diabetes mellitus increases with age. Fifty-five percent of new diagnoses are for people between the ages of 45 and 65 years.[36] Having an ethnic background is also a risk factor. Diabetes mellitus is 2 to 4 times more prevalent among Blacks, Hispanics, Asians, and Native Americans than it is for Whites.[40]

Chronic Respiratory Infections

Since 2008, the third leading cause of death is due to a collection of lung diseases (asthma, chronic bronchitis, and emphysema) referred to as lower respiratory infections. Chronic bronchitis and emphysema are grouped together into chronic obstructive pulmonary disease (COPD), which accounts for the largest portion of lower respiratory infections.[8] These are progressive conditions that limit oxygen exchange intake and leave patients with high levels of disability. Despite the severity of COPD, accurate data on its prevalence are not kept by all 50 states. The CDC's best estimate is that 6.3% of American adults are living with chronic bronchitis or emphysema.[41] That is approximately 15 million people who report having been diagnosed. An additional 12 million potentially have COPD but have not yet been diagnosed.[42]

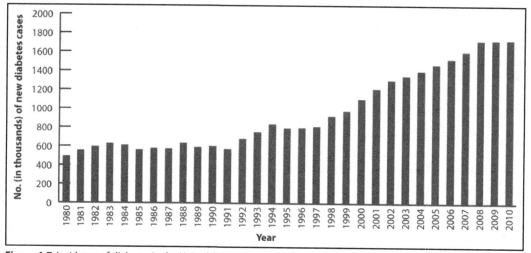

Figure 1-7. Incidence of diabetes in the United States since 1980. (Reprinted with permission from Centers for Disease Control and Prevention. Diabetes report card 2012. http://images.slideplayer.com/1/220735/slides/slide_11.jpg. Published 2012. Accessed October 14, 2015.)

Exposure to airborne irritants, such as tobacco smoke, chemical fumes, or dust from manufacturing, are the main risk factors for developing COPD. Prevalence is higher in those older than 55 years, which indicates that long-term exposure is a key aspect of the disease.[41] Initially, symptoms, such as coughing with mucus and shortness of breath with physical activity, are mild. Over time, they become more pronounced, and wheezing or rapid breathing occur. COPD reduces lung volume. In chronic bronchitis, the lining of the bronchioles is inflamed and mucus is produced, which narrows the passageways for air. The smaller diameter of the bronchioles increases the resistance to air flow, making it harder for someone to take a full breath. In emphysema, damage from fumes and irritants has caused some of the alveoli, or air sacks at the end of the bronchioles, to deflate. Without functioning alveoli, there are fewer places for oxygen and carbon dioxide to be exchanged, which results in lower oxygen content in the blood.[33]

A common comorbidity of COPD is hypertension and CVD. A comorbidity is a disease that occurs with another disease.[1] Because the lungs are less efficient at moving air and exchanging oxygen for carbon dioxide, the body compensates by increasing heart rate and blood pressure so that the oxygen needs of the cells are met. Those with severe COPD find even light physical activity to be difficult because of the poor oxygenation of their blood. Once diagnosed, it is important for those with mild to moderate cases of COPD to stay physically active. Lung volumes, inflammation, and mucus buildup are improved by regular physical activity, such as walking or household chores. Patients who reported at least some physical activity had a lower risk of death and less likelihood of hospitalization for their symptoms.[43]

Some disparities exist between gender, ethnic, economic groups, and by geographic region. Women have higher rates of COPD than men until age 75, when both genders are nearly equal in prevalence.[44] Women aged 65 to 71 years have the highest prevalence at 10.4%, whereas 8.3% of similar aged men are living with COPD. Puerto Rican and White Americans account for more cases of COPD than Black or Hispanic Americans (Figure 1-8). Prevalence[44] and disability[45] are also inversely related to income. This is likely due to the environmental hazards found in less well-paying jobs and the greater number of smokers in low-income populations.[46] States in the central south (Kentucky, Tennessee, Alabama, and Mississippi) have the highest rate of COPD at 7.5%, whereas the Pacific Coast states (Washington, Oregon, California, and Hawaii) have the lowest rate at 3.9%.[44] Although more women are diagnosed with COPD, men die from the disease at

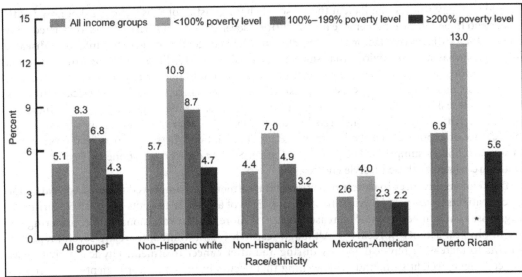

Figure 1-8. US Prevalence of COPD by race/ethnicity and income.[43] (Reprinted with permission from Akinbami LJ, Liu X. Chronic obstructive pulmonary disease among adults aged 18 and over in the United States, 1998-2009. *NCHS Data Brief.* 2011;[63]:1-8.)

TABLE 1-2			
CANCER INCIDENCE BY GENDER AND ANNUAL DEATHS FROM CANCER[47]			
	NUMBER	**% MALE**	**% FEMALE**	**DEATHS**
Breast	235,030	1	99	40,430
Prostate	233,000	100		29,480
Lung	224,210	52	48	159,260
Colon	96,830	50	50	50,310
Skin	81,220	57	43	12,980

higher rates. According to data from 2007, 70 men per every 100,000 died from COPD compared to 50 per 100,000 women.[44]

Cancer

Cancer is the second leading cause of death in the United States.[8] According to Surveillance, Epidemiology and End Result data, 12,549,000 Americans were living with the disease in 2009.[47] Cancer is a disease in which dysfunctional cells are reproduced at a high rate. These cells cluster together in growths called *tumors.* Not all tumors are malignant, or cancerous. Because the body is constantly replicating cells from the DNA of older cells, some mistakes are to be expected. Normally, these mistake cells are identified and removed by the immune system before they overproduce. If not eliminated, these cells develop over time into larger masses that interfere with the processes of the organ or tissue in which they are situated. Diagnoses are specific to the structure or body system that has been disrupted. The most prevalent forms of cancer are breast, prostate, lung, colon, and skin.[48] Table 1-2 shows that although lung cancer ranks third in diagnosis, it results in the greatest numbers of deaths.

Epidemiology studies that look at the personal characteristics of those who are diagnosed with cancer and those who are cancer free have identified several modifiable risk factors associated with cancer. A modifiable risk factor is changeable, unlike age, gender, or genetic links to a disease. Although it may appear obvious that smoking is a risk factor for lung cancer or sunburns are a risk factor for skin cancer, there are risk factors that overlap multiple types of cancer. For example, tobacco use also increases one's risk of prostate[49] and liver cancer.[50] Lack of physical activity is a modifiable risk factor for breast, colon, and lung cancers.[51] An average of 30 to 60 minutes of physical activity a day reduces one's risk by 20% to 24%.[52,53] Other modifiable risk factors include tobacco use or exposure, obesity, low fruit and vegetable intake, diets high in animal protein and fat, and alcohol consumption. The American Cancer Society estimates that one-third of all cancer deaths are related to these lifestyle choices.[54]

Tremendous advances in cancer detection and treatment have improved the life expectancy for cancer patients in the past 50 years. In 1950, only 35% of all cancer patients survived 5 years post-diagnosis. That number has now increased to 69%.[47] More health professionals are considering the role of physical activity in recovery. Although research is still limited, there are several reported benefits to increasing physical activity during and after cancer treatment. Physical activity may reduce fatigue, weight gain, and arm swelling that occurs in breast cancer patients.[55,56] Women who participated in even small amounts of physical activity had better survival rates than those who reported no physical activity.[57] This was also true of men with prostate cancer.[58]

Alzheimer's Disease

Over the next 30 years, the number of Americans older than 65 years will more than double.[59] An estimated 79 million will be living in the United States by 2040, making older adults more than one-third of the adult population.[60] This shift will have a tremendous impact on the health care system. More citizens will require more services because the prevalence of chronic disease increases with age. In particular, Alzheimer's disease will present challenges because treatment options are limited and the burden to family members is high.

Alzheimer's disease is a progressive neurogenerative disorder of the brain that results in a severe loss of cognitive ability. It is the most common cause of dementia in older adults.[61] More than memory loss, Alzheimer's disease causes a complete disruption in the way nerves send messages to each other, making even self-care activities almost impossible.[62] In 2010, an estimated 4.7 million adults were living with the disease.[63] Early symptoms of Alzheimer's disease include problems planning money, finding the right words, getting lost in familiar places, or displaying poor judgment in decision making. As the disease progresses, these lapses become more frequent and make normal daily tasks difficult. Mood and personality changes are also noted. It is at this stage that Alzheimer's disease is usually diagnosed.[62]

The decline in cognitive function and physical health is rapid. The average survival time after the diagnosis of Alzheimer's disease is 8 to 12 years.[64,65] It is the sixth leading cause of death in the United States.[8] The brains of patients with Alzheimer's disease have 3 signs of damage. The first is an accumulation of a protein called beta-amyloid, which forms plaques in the spaces between neurons (Figure 1-9). The second is the development of neurofibrillary tangles inside the neurons that stop communication with other neurons (see Figure 1-9). Lastly, the presence of the plaques and tangles is believed to cause the neurons to degenerate and die. This results in atrophy of the brain; the mass of the brain decreases dramatically (Figure 1-10). Brain cells are highly specialized and conduct messages for thoughts, memories, motor skills, and emotional control. Persons with Alzheimer's disease do not regenerate nerve cells at a high enough rate to maintain this complex network and experience more and more symptoms as time passes.

There are 2 forms of the disease, including early and late onset. Early-onset occurs before age 60 and is rare.[66] This form is strongly linked to a family history of Alzheimer's disease and mutations of a chromosomes that have a role in developing the precursor to beta-amyloid.[61] Much

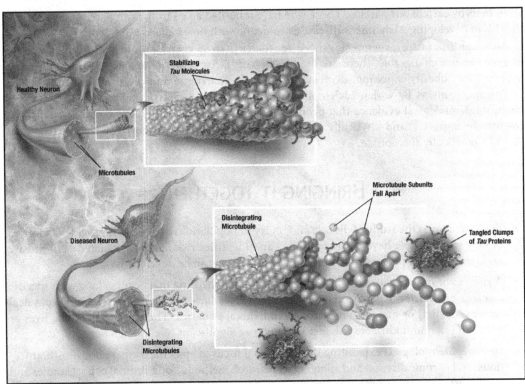

Figure 1-9. Beta-amyloid and tau protein tangles. (Reprinted with permission from the National Institute of Health. http://commons.wikimedia.org/wiki/File:TANGLES_HIGH.jpg.)

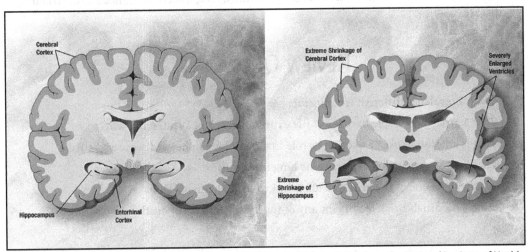

Figure 1-10. Brain atrophy from Alzheimer's disease. (Reprinted with permission from the National Institute of Health. http://commons.wikimedia.org/wiki/File:Alzheimer's_disease_brain_comparison.jpg.)

more common is the late-onset form, which accounts for 95% of all cases.[62] Genetics also play a part in late-onset but are thought to be influenced by environment and lifestyle, including one's amount of physical activity.[66] There is an increased risk for those who have a variation of a gene called *apolipoprotein E* (APOE). The form of APOE that is most related to late-onset Alzheimer's disease is the e4 allele. Roughly 40% of those with late-onset have the APOE e4 gene. One allele is given to us by each of our parents. Those who have inherited an e4 from both parents have 8 times the risk of developing Alzheimer's disease as someone with no e4 alleles.[66,67]

Although risk factors, such as advanced age (older than 85 years), family history, or the APOE e4 gene are not changeable, there are modifiable risk factors for Alzheimer's disease, including hypertension, obesity, smoking, depression, cognitive inactivity, and physical inactivity.[68] The precise mechanisms by which each risk factor impacts brain cells is not known, but there is strong epidemiological evidence that people who had less CVD[69] at mid-life remain socially and cognitively engaged[70] and physically active[71,72] as older adults experience less dementia even if they are genetically susceptible.[73]

Bringing It Together

- Epidemiology is the study of disease and injury in populations of people. It provides estimates of how many people have what conditions and identifies risk factors associated with disease and injury so that prevention and treatment strategies can be developed.

- A risk factor is not a cause of illness or injury but is something that occurs along with specific diseases or injuries. Risk factors can be modifiable, such as a behavior (smoking, physical activity, or diet) or may be outside of an individual's control. The environment one lives or works in is a nonmodifiable risk factor but plays a significant role in one's health.

- Sports epidemiology is expanding the traditional focus of epidemiology (public health, infectious, and chronic disease) and applying its research methods (longitudinal cohort studies and risk statistics) to sport-related injuries.

- In 5 of the top 10 leading causes of death, lack of physical activity is a risk factor. These include heart and cerebrovascular disease, diabetes mellitus, lung infections, cancer, and Alzheimer's disease.

Review Questions

1. How is prevalence different from incidence?
2. What 3 groups of people have lower life expectancies than Whites and why?
3. What is atherosclerosis? Describe its role in the etiology in heart disease and stroke.
4. What diseases are included in chronic lung infections?
5. What is the name of the gene and allele linked to Alzheimer's Disease?
6. Name 3 modifiable risk factors for any of the leading causes of death.

Learning Activities

1. Calculate the incidence and prevalence of common illnesses and injuries among your friends and classmates. For example, ask how many of them have had the flu in the past year. Use the basic equations for incidence and prevalence:
   - Incidence = new cases ÷ population number
   - Prevalence = new and old cases ÷ population number

Suggested injuries include ankle sprain, concussion, and delayed muscle soreness. The time frame can be expanded to include multiple years or a lifetime history.

2. Sort the risk factors of several diseases or injuries into 3 groups: behavioral, genetic, or environmental. Which ones could fit into multiple categories? Highlight which risk factors are modifiable. Possible diseases/injuries to use are the following:

   - Stroke

   - Type 2 diabetes mellitus

   - Alzheimer's disease

   - COPD

3. Smoking is the greatest risk factor for lung cancer, but it is also linked to mortality from many other diseases. Create a list of diseases that would have reduced mortality if the smoking rates in the United States continue to decline. Use the following article as a resource: www.cdc.gov/pcd/issues/2012/11_0295.htm. How do attributable risk statistics improve our understanding of what health behaviors need to change.

REFERENCES

1. Bonita R, Beaglehole R, Kjellström T. *Basic Epidemiology.* 2nd ed. Geneva, Switzerland: World Health Organization; 2006.
2. Jenner E. An inquiry to the causes and effects of the variolae vaccine. In: Buck C, Llopis A, Najera E, Terris M, eds. *The Challenge of Epidemiology: Issues and Selected Readings.* Washington, DC: World Health Organization; 1988:31-32.
3. Snow J. On the mode of communication of cholera. In: Buck C, Llopis A, Najera E, Terris M, eds. *The Challenge of Epidemiology: Issues and Selected Readings.* Washington, DC: World Health Organization; 1988:42-45.
4. Health News. *Medical Milestone: Mary Mallon, Typhoid Mary, November 1968.* New York, NY: New York Department of Health; 1968.
5. US Department of Health & Human Services. Commissioned Corps of the US Public Health Service. http://www.usphs.gov/aboutus/history.aspx. Accessed November 20, 2015.
6. Badgeley MA, McIlvain NM, Yard EE, Fields SK, Comstock RD. Epidemiology of 10,000 high school football injuries: patterns of injury by position played. *J Phys Act Health.* 2013;10(2):160-169.
7. Lincoln AE, Caswell SV, Almquist JL, et al. Effectiveness of the women's lacrosse protective eyewear mandate in the reduction of eye injuries. *Am J Sports Med.* 2012;40(3):611-614.
8. Hoyert DL, Xu J. Deaths: preliminary data for 2011. http://www.cdc.gov/nchs/data/nvsr/nvsr61/nvsr61_06.pdf. Published October 10, 2012. Accessed October 13, 2015.
9. Arias E, Curtin L, Wei R, Anderson R. *U.S. Decennial Life Tables for 1999-2001, United States Life Tables.* Hyattsville, MD: National Center for Health Statistics; 2008.
10. United Nations. Table 2a: life expectancy. Social Indicators. http://unstats.un.org/unsd/demographic/products/socind/. Published 2012. Accessed October 21, 2013.
11. CDC. *Life Expectancy at Birth, by Sex and Black or White Race—National Vital Statistics System, United States, 2000–2011.* Atlanta, GA: National Center for Health Statistics; 2013.
12. Braveman PA, Cubbin C, Egerter S, Williams DR, Pamuk E. Socioeconomic disparities in health in the United States: what the patterns tell us. *Am J Public Health.* 2010;100(suppl 1):S186-S196.
13. Haskell W, Lee IM, Pate RR, et al. Physical activity and public health: updated recommendation for adults from the American College of Sports Medicine and the American Heart Association. *Circulation.* 2007;116(9):1081-1093.
14. Warburton DE, Nicol CW, Bredin SS. Health benefits of physical activity: the evidence. *CMAJ.* 2006;174(6):801-809.
15. Naci H, Ioannidis JP. Comparative effectiveness of exercise and drug interventions on mortality outcomes: metaepidemiological study. *BMJ.* 2013;347.
16. Penedo FJ, Dahn JR. Exercise and well-being: a review of mental and physical health benefits associated with physical activity. *Curr Opin Psychiatry.* 2005;18(2):189-193.
17. Nelson ME, Rejeski WJ, Blair SN, et al. Physical activity and public health in older adults: recommendation from the American College of Sports Medicine and the American Heart Association. *Med Sci Sports Exerc.* 2007;39(8):1435-1445.

18. Centers for Disease Control and Prevention (CDC). Decline in deaths from heart disease and stroke--United States, 1900-1999. *MMWR Morb Mortal Wkly Rep.* 1999;48(30):649-656.

19. Mayo Clinic. Heart disease: definition. http://www.mayoclinic.com/health/heart-disease/DS01120. Accessed October 17, 2013.

20. Go AS, Mozaffarian D, Roger VL, et al. Heart disease and stroke statistics--2013 update: a report from the American Heart Association. *Circulation.* 2013;127(1):e6-e245.

21. Centers for Disease Control and Prevention (CDC). Prevalence of coronary heart disease--United States, 2006-2010. *MMWR Morb Mortal Wkly Rep.* 2011;60(40):1377-1381.

22. Maas AH, Appelman YE. Gender differences in coronary heart disease. *Neth Heart J.* 2010;18(12):598-602.

23. Crimmins EM, Hayward MD, Ueda H, Saito Y, Kim JK. Life with and without heart disease among women and men over 50. *J Women Aging.* 2008;20(1-2):5-19.

24. Mensah GA, Mokdad AH, Ford ES, Greenlund KJ, Croft JB. State of disparities in cardiovascular health in the United States. *Circulation.* 2005;111(10):1233-1241.

25. Hao W, Friedman A. The LDL-HDL profile determines the risk of atherosclerosis: a mathematical model. *PLoS One.* 2014;9(3):e90497.

26. Tabas I. Macrophage death and defective inflammation resolution in atherosclerosis. *Nat Rev Immunol.* 2010;10(1):36-46.

27. Libby P, Ridker PM, Hansson GK; Leducq Transatlantic Network on Atherothrombosis. Inflammation in atherosclerosis: from pathophysiology to practice. *J Am Coll Cardiol.* 2009;54(23):2129-2138.

28. Chung HY, Kim HJ, Kim JW, Yu BP. The inflammation hypothesis of aging: molecular modulation by calorie restriction. *Ann N Y Acad Sci.* 2001;928:327-335.

29. American Heart Association Nutrition Committee, Lichtenstein AH, Appel LJ, et al. Diet and lifestyle recommendations revision 2006: a scientific statement from the American Heart Association Nutrition Committee. *Circulation.* 2006;114(1):82-96.

30. National Heart, Lung, and Blood Institute. What Is coronary angioplasty? https://www.nhlbi.nih.gov/health/health-topics/topics/ca. Published March 2, 2012. Accessed March 27, 2014.

31. Epstein AJ, Polsky D, Yang F, Yang L, Groeneveld PW. Coronary revascularization trends in the United States, 2001-2008. *JAMA.* 2011;305(17):1769-1776.

32. Murphy SL, Xu J, Kochanek KD; Division of Vital Statistics. Deaths: final data for 2010. In: Volume 61, Number 4. Hyattsville, MD: Centers for Disease Control and Prevention, US Dept of Health and Human Services; 2013:1-118.

33. National Heart, Lung, and Blood Institute. What are the signs and symptoms of a stroke? http://www.nhlbi.nih.gov/health/health-topics/topics/stroke/signs.html. Accessed November 7, 2013.

34. Easton JD, Saver JL, Albers GW, et al. Definition and evaluation of transient ischemic attack: a scientific statement for healthcare professionals from the American Heart Association/American Stroke Association Stroke Council; Council on Cardiovascular Surgery and Anesthesia; Council on Cardiovascular Radiology and Intervention; Council on Cardiovascular Nursing; and the Interdisciplinary Council on Peripheral Vascular Disease. The American Academy of Neurology affirms the value of this statement as an educational tool for neurologists. *Stroke.* 2009;40(6):2276-2293.

35. Roger VL, Go AS, Lloyd-Jones DM, et al. Heart disease and stroke statistics--2012 update: a report from the American Heart Association. *Circulation.* 2012;125(1):e2-e220.

36. Centers for Disease Control and Prevention. National Diabetes Fact Sheet: National Estimates and General Information on Diabetes and Prediabetes in the United States. Atlanta, GA: Centers for Disease Control and Prevention, US Dept of Health and Human Services; 2011.

37. American Diabetes Association. Diagnosis and classification of diabetes mellitus. *Diabetes Care.* 2011;34(suppl 1):S62-S69.

38. Centers for Disease Control and Prevention. *Diabetes Report Card 2012.* Atlanta, GA: Centers for Disease Control and Prevention, US Dept of Health and Human Services; 2012.

39. National Institute of Diabetes and Digestive and Kidney Diseases. *Am I at Risk for Type 2 Diabetes? Taking Steps to Lower Your Risk of Getting Diabetes.* Bethesda, MD: National Institutes of Health; 2012.

40. Chow EA, Foster H, Gonzalez V, McIver L. The disparate impact of diabetes on racial/ethnic minority populations. *Clin Diabetes.* 2012;30(3):130-133.

41. Centers for Disease Control and Prevention (CDC). Chronic obstructive pulmonary disease among adults--United States, 2011. *MMWR Morb Mortal Wkly Rep.* 2012;61(46):938-943.

42. National Heart, Lung, and Blood Institute. *COPD Learn More Breathe Better.* Bethesda, MA: National Institutes of Health; 2013.

43. Garcia-Aymerich J, Lange P, Benet M, Schnohr P, Antó JM. Regular physical activity reduces hospital admission and mortality in chronic obstructive pulmonary disease: a population based cohort study. *Thorax.* 2006;61(9):772-778.

44. Akinbami LJ, Liu X. Chronic obstructive pulmonary disease among adults aged 18 and over in the United States, 1998-2009. *NCHS Data Brief.* 2011;(63):1-8.

45. Eisner MD, Blanc PD, Omachi TA, et al. Socioeconomic status, race and COPD health outcomes. *J Epidemiol Community Health.* 2011;65(1):26-34.

46. Centers for Disease Control and Prevention (CDC). Current cigarette smoking among adults - United States, 2011. *MMWR Morb Mortal Wkly Rep.* 2012;61(44):889-894.

47. Howlader N, Noone AM, Krapcho M, et al. *SEER Cancer Statistics Review, 1975-2009 (Vintage 2009 Populations).* Bethesda, MD: National Cancer Institute; 2012.

48. American Cancer Society. *Cancer Facts and Figures 2014.* Atlanta, GA: American Cancer Society; 2014.

49. Zu K, Giovannucci E. Smoking and aggressive prostate cancer: a review of the epidemiologic evidence. *Cancer Causes Control.* 2009;20(10):1799-1810.

50. Trichopoulos D, Bamia C, Lagiou P, et al. Hepatocellular carcinoma risk factors and disease burden in a European cohort: a nested case-control study. *J Natl Cancer Inst.* 2011;103(22):1686-1695.

51. Stein CJ, Colditz GA. Modifiable risk factors for cancer. *Br J Cancer.* 2004;90(2):299-303.

52. Lee IM, Oguma Y. Physical activity. In: Schottenfeld D, Fraumeni JF, eds. *Cancer Epidemiology and Prevention.* 3rd ed. New York, NY: Oxford Univeristy Press; 2006:449-467.

53. Wolin KY, Yan Y, Colditz GA, Lee IM. Physical activity and colon cancer prevention: a meta-analysis. *Br J Cancer.* 2009;100(4):611-616.

54. American Cancer Society. Diet and physical activity: what's the cancer connection? http://www.cancer.org/cancer/cancercauses/dietandphysicalactivity/diet-and-physical-activity. Accessed April 14, 2014.

55. Speck RM, Courneya KS, Mâsse LC, Duval S, Schmitz KH. An update of controlled physical activity trials in cancer survivors: a systematic review and meta-analysis. *J Cancer Surviv.* 2010;4(2):87-100.

56. Schmitz KH, Ahmed RL, Troxel A, et al. Weight lifting in women with breast-cancer-related lymphedema. *N Engl J Med.* 2009;361(7):664-673.

57. Meyerhardt JA, Giovannucci EL, Holmes MD, et al. Physical activity and survival after colorectal cancer diagnosis. *J Clin Oncol.* 2006;24(22):3527-3534.

58. Kenfield SA, Stampfer MJ, Giovannucci E, Chan JM. Physical activity and survival after prostate cancer diagnosis in the health professionals follow-up study. *J Clin Oncol.* 2011;29(6):726-732.

59. Centers for Disease Control and Prevention. *The State of Aging and Health in America 2013.* Atlanta, GA: Centers for Disease Control and Prevention, US Dept of Health and Human Services; 2013.

60. United States Census Bureau. Population and housing unit estimates. http://www.census.gov/popest/index.html. Accessed February 20, 2014.

61. Gandy S. The role of cerebral amyloid beta accumulation in common forms of Alzheimer disease. *J Clin Invest.* 2005;115(5):1121-1129.

62. National Institute on Aging. Alzheimer's disease fact sheet. http://www.nia.nih.gov/alzheimers/publication/alzheimers-disease-fact-sheet. Accessed February 20, 2014.

63. Hebert LE, Weuve J, Scherr PA, Evans DA. Alzheimer disease in the United States (2010-2050) estimated using the 2010 census. *Neurology.* 2013;80(19):1778-1783.

64. Dal Forno G, Carson KA, Brookmeyer R, Troncoso J, Kawas CH, Brandt J. APOE genotype and survival in men and women with Alzheimer's disease. *Neurology.* 2002;58(7):1045-1050.

65. Brookmeyer R, Corrada MM, Curriero FC, Kawas C. Survival following a diagnosis of Alzheimer disease. *Arch Neurol.* 2002;59(11):1764-1767.

66. National Institute on Aging. Alzheimer's disease genetics fact sheet. http://www.nia.nih.gov/alzheimers/publication/alzheimers-disease-genetics-fact-sheet. Accessed February 21, 2004.

67. National Institute on Aging. *Alzheimer's Disease Progress Report: Intensifying the Research Effort.* Bethesda, MD: Department of Health and Human Services; 2012.

68. Barnes DE, Yaffe K. The projected effect of risk factor reduction on Alzheimer's disease prevalence. *Lancet Neurol.* 2011;10(9):819-828.

69. Tolppanen AM, Solomon A, Soininen H, Kivipelto M. Midlife vascular risk factors and Alzheimer's disease: evidence from epidemiological studies. *J Alzheimers Dis.* 2012;32(3):531-540.

70. Wilson RS, Mendes De Leon CF, Barnes LL, et al. Participation in cognitively stimulating activities and risk of incident Alzheimer disease. *JAMA.* 2002;287(6):742-748.

71. Lee Y, Back JH, Kim J, et al. Systematic review of health behavioral risks and cognitive health in older adults. *Int Psychogeriatr.* 2010;22(2):174-187.

72. Erickson KI, Weinstein AM, Lopez OL. Physical activity, brain plasticity, and Alzheimer's disease. *Arch Med Res.* 2012;43(8):615-621.

73. Luck T, Riedel-Heller SG, Luppa M, et al. Apolipoprotein E epsilon 4 genotype and a physically active lifestyle in late life: analysis of gene-environment interaction for the risk of dementia and Alzheimer's disease dementia. *Psychol Med.* 2014;44(6):1319-1329.

2

Epidemiology and Physical Activity

Jeffrey Timmer, PhD, CEP

CHAPTER OBJECTIVES

- Define the following terms: *physical activity, exercise,* and *physical fitness.*
- Explain the physiological responses to physical activity that are responsible for the health benefits.
- Understand what research has led to the national guidelines for physical activity.
- Consider barriers to physical activity, and suggest strategies to promote physical activity.

INTRODUCTION

Most people recognize that physical activity and exercise are good for one's health. The benefits of physical activity (decreased risk of cardiovascular disease [CVD], diabetes mellitus, obesity, depression, and Alzheimer's disease) are widely shared in the media and taught in schools. Despite this knowledge, the majority of Americans do not get enough physical activity.[1] Epidemiologists played a critical role in establishing that physical activity is health promoting. They used statistics to link a cause of death or the onset of a disease to lifestyle behaviors, such as physical activity, smoking, and diet. Before exploring the health benefits and their mechanisms, it is important to clearly define what is meant by the terms *physical activity, exercise,* and *physical fitness.*

Defining Physical Activity, Exercise, and Physical Fitness

Physical activity includes all movements produced by the contraction of skeletal muscle. It includes a range of activities, from casual walking to vigorous sports. All of these movements substantially increase energy expenditure compared to sitting or lying down.[2] Physical activities

Adams M, Swiger W.
*Epidemiology for Athletic Trainers: Integrating
Evidence-Based Practice (pp 21-40).*
© 2016 Taylor & Francis Group.

are generally categorized as occupational or leisure time.[3] Exercise is a specific type of leisure-time physical activity that maintains or improves physical fitness. To qualify as exercise, a physical activity has to be sustained long enough or be demanding enough to cause the body to improve how it makes energy and delivers oxygen.[4] Leisure-time physical activity can be further divided into lifestyle physical activity and active transportation. Daily tasks that require movement, such as shopping, house cleaning, and yardwork, make up lifestyle physical activity.[5] Commuting places by walking or biking are examples of active transport.[6] Sports are another type of leisure-time physical activity. Sports are more competitive than exercise, and the amount of physical activity required varies greatly depending on the sport and the level of play.[7] In general, athletes are considered highly physically active.

Activities of daily living (ADLs) include lifestyle physical activity and basic self-care, such as bathing and cooking.[8] Ability to do these daily physical tasks without assistance is a measure of one's physical function. Higher levels of physical function are related to greater amounts of physical activity,[9] and for older adults, physical function is associated with greater independence.[10] A step beyond physical function is physical fitness. Being physically fit means that one can complete his or her "daily tasks with vigor and alertness, without undue fatigue and ample energy…"[11] Physical fitness includes naturally occurring and acquired abilities.[2] Exercise training can improve physical fitness, especially the health-related components.[12]

Components of Physical Fitness

Rather than a single item, physical fitness comprises several components that combine to make performing physical activities easier. These components are divided into the following 2 categories: skill and health related. The skill-related components include qualities that are important in sports performance, such as agility or reaction time. The health-related components are needed by athletes and the general population to reduce the risk of injury and chronic disease. The 5 components of health-related physical fitness are cardiorespiratory endurance, muscular strength, muscular endurance, flexibility, and body composition. Each is measurable and can be improved with exercise training.

Cardiorespiratory endurance is the ability of the heart, lungs, and metabolic pathways to provide oxygen to active muscles and resist fatigue so that physical activity can continue over a period of time.[13] Aerobic exercise improves cardiorespiratory endurance by increasing one's heart rate (HR) and oxygen consumption for extended amounts of time. Physical activity research has long focused on cardiorespiratory endurance and continuous aerobic exercise as being the key to reducing the risk of chronic disease. More recent studies[14] suggest that shorter bursts of strenuous activities, such as sprinting, can also improve the risk factors for CVD.

Muscular strength is the ability to create enough force to move a heavy object once. Muscular endurance is the ability to perform multiple contractions one after another. Exercises that improve muscle strength and endurance are important for maintaining health and physical function. The pull of the muscles on bone, particularly those at the pelvis and spine, encourages the regeneration of bony tissue that prevents osteoporosis.[15] Muscles respond to exercise by increasing the number and size of their fibers. This adaptation helps reduce the loss of muscle tissue in older adults. The loss of muscle with age has negative effects on force production and balance; the risk of falling is greater in older adults who do not exercise.[16]

Flexibility is the ability to move one's joints through normal ranges of motion (ROMs) without pain or limitation.[17] An individual's flexibility is based on several factors, such as age,[18] gender,[19] types and volume of physical activity,[20] and history of injury.[16] Each joint has a specific ROM that is determined by the bony structures and musculature of the joint. Changes in the collagen fibers of the tendons and joint inflammation occur with age and account for some of the losses experienced over time. Repetitive use or disuse of muscles may also cause muscles to lengthen or shorten excessively. For example, sitting at a computer with head and shoulders slouched forward can limit one's neck, back, and shoulder ROM (Figure 2-1).[21]

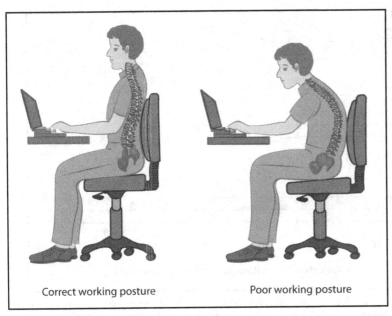

Figure 2-1. Sitting postures.

Correct working posture   Poor working posture

The mix of fat to nonfat tissues in the body is called *body composition*. Nonfat, or lean, tissues include the muscles, bones, and organs. There are multiple measures for body composition. It can be measured as a ratio of height to weight, called the *body mass index* (BMI), as the percentage of fat relative to the whole body, or by the taking the circumference of the abdomen. Obesity is defined as having a BMI greater than 30[22] or having a body fat greater than 25% for men and 32% for women.[23] The risk for chronic disease is greater in obese persons than those with normal body masses.[24] However, the risk for overweight and obese people who are physically fit is similar to those of normal weight.[25]

HEALTH BENEFITS OF PHYSICAL ACTIVITY

The amount of physical activity and one's level of fitness have been linked to a reduced risk for chronic disease and mortality. Pioneering epidemiologists, such as Jeremy Morris, Ralph Paffenbarger, and Steven Blair, opened the door to studying physical activity as a way to enhance health and longevity. In particular, their studies assessing the risk of CVD among those with different levels of physical activity and physical fitness provided the evidence for the addition of physical inactivity as a risk factor for heart disease in 1996.[26] Since then, a lack of physical activity has been associated with a higher risk of hypertension,[27] type 2 diabetes mellitus (T2DM),[28] stroke,[29] obesity,[30] Alzheimer's disease,[31] depression,[32] osteoporosis,[15] and some cancers,[33] whereas people who are physically active have better stress management,[34] a higher quality of life,[35] and greater levels of independence as older adults.[10] Being physically active is not just about living longer; it is about living better. As the saying goes, "It's not how many years are in your life but how much life is in your years."[36]

Health benefits from physical activity are well established in the literature; however, understanding how best to obtain those benefits continues to grow as new exercise prescription models are developed. Briefly, to improve health and fitness, one should engage in physical activities that overload the body above baseline abilities. This overload places stress on the body, causing the body to adapt and respond to those stressors. For aerobic exercise, the body must improve the delivery of blood, oxygen, and nutrients to the active muscles. An overload in resistance exercises

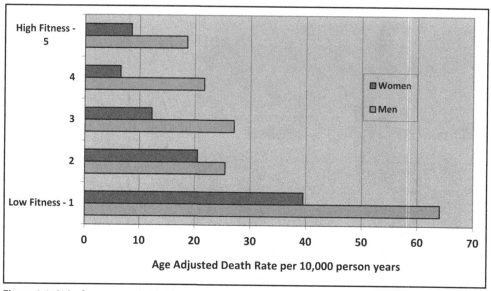

Figure 2-2. Risk of premature death. Fitness was assessed using total time on the treadmill during a maximal test. (Adapted from Blair SN, Kohl HW III, Paffenbarger RS Jr, Clark DG, Cooper KH, Gibbons LW. Physical fitness and all-cause mortality. A prospective study of healthy men and women. *JAMA*. 1989;262(17):2395-2401.)

results in adaptations in muscle size and strength and bone density. Using overload and proper progressions, every individual can show improvement in the 5 health-related fitness components.

It is the job of exercise and health care professionals to ensure that physical activity programs are individualized and match the starting abilities of participants. For example, jogging for 20 minutes at 5 miles/hour may represent 20% of a well-trained athlete's maximal ability (measured as maximal oxygen consumption [VO_2max]) but may be 80% of the capacity for a sedentary individual who is just starting an exercise program. Although all components of a quality physical activity program are important (intensity, duration, and frequency), research has shown that the amount of physical activity may be the most important aspect of gaining overall health benefits. Research has indicated that the type of exercise does not matter; what matters is engaging in physical activity that raises the HR and puts stress on the body for an extended period of time. Looking at the risk reduction for premature death (Figure 2-2), the group with the greatest decrease in risk is not trained individuals who increase their training volume; rather, it is in those who move from being sedentary to participating in a slightly active lifestyle.[37]

The Physical Activity Guidelines for Americans (Table 2-1) were written as broad recommendations for a variety of people, from young adults to those older than 65 years.[38,39] All have different levels of fitness and experience with physical activity. According to the Physical Activity Guidelines for Americans, every adult should accumulate 150 minutes/week of moderate-intensity activity or 75 minutes/week of vigorous activity. It is recommended for the activities to be spread out over an entire week. Also, each adult should strive to perform muscle-strengthening exercises of moderate to vigorous intensity for all major muscle groups twice a week. Individuals also need to know that some of the health benefits may require years of participation in a proper physical activity program, whereas other benefits can be seen in a several weeks to a few months.

Adaptations to Physical Activity

Understanding the benefits of physical activity is imperative to cause behavior change. To truly understand the benefits, it is important to study the possible physiological mechanisms responsible for the protective effect of physical activity on health. During aerobic exercise, the body must

TABLE 2-1
NATIONAL PHYSICAL ACTIVITY GUIDELINES

2011 ACSM/AHA PHYSICAL ACTIVITY GUIDELINES

Cardiovascular/ aerobic exercise	Duration	Intensity	Frequency	Total
	> 30 min/day, can be broken into 3 10-min bouts	Moderate	> 5 days/ wk	150 min moderate PA/ wk
	or			
	> 20 min/day	Vigorous	> 3 days/wk	75 min vigorous PA/wk
	or			
	Combination of moderate and vigorous activity to achieve > 500 to 1000 MET/min/wk			
Resistance exercise	2 to 3 days/wk, exercise each major muscle group			
Flexibility exercise	60 sec each exercise, > 2 days/wk			
Neuromotor exercise	> 20 to 30 min	Not determined	> 2 to 3 days/wk	Exercises to improve balance, agility, gait, and coordination

2008 PHYSICAL ACTIVITY GUIDELINES FOR AMERICANS

Aerobic exercise	Adults should perform at least 150 min/wk of moderate-intensity or 75 min/wk of vigorous-intensity or equivalent combination of moderate and vigorous physical activity in bouts of at least 10 min
	For greater health benefits, adults should perform 300 min/wk of moderate-intensity or 150 min/wk of vigorous-intensity PA or equivalent combination of moderate and vigorous activity
Muscle strengthening exercise	Moderate- to high-intensity exercises involving all major muscle groups > 2 days/wk

Abbreviations: MET, metabolic equivalent of task; PA, physical activity.

become more efficient at delivering oxygen and nutrients to the muscles. On average, previously untrained individuals will show a 16% increase in the ability to uptake oxygen (VO$_2$max).[40] Increases in stroke volume (SV) and cardiac output (Q) are the major reasons for the rise in VO$_2$max. Also, resting and exercise HR decline with training. Using the formula, Q = HR × SV; at-rest Q will not change. Therefore, based on the formula, as SV increases, HR will decrease. This change reduces the overall metabolic demands on the heart. The ability to increase VO$_2$ allows the body to become more efficient at using fats and carbohydrates for energy while decreasing the buildup of lactic acid in the muscle cells. Studies have also shown improvements in blood pressure (BP) with endurance training[41] and coronary blood vessel wall function with regular aerobic exercise. Individuals with coronary heart disease can increase coronary blood flow and increase plaque stability.[42] The combination of these adaptations is only the beginning to understanding the protective effect exercise has on cardiac function. At the cell level, adaptations include an increase in the size and number of mitochondria, an increase in oxidative enzyme capacity, and an increase in the capillary density of muscle. These adaptations allow each muscle fiber to increase work performance and resist fatigue. These adaptations further reduce the myocardial demand during exercise and for ADLs.

Other adaptations from regular physical activity are a reduction in triglyceride levels and low-density lipoprotein cholesterol while increasing high-density lipoprotein cholesterol (HDL-C). LDL and triglyceride levels are associated with an increase in atherosclerosis and plaque formation. HDL has been shown to reduce, maintain, and stabilize plaque formation. With greater amounts of weekly physical activity, all blood cholesterol levels improve, which may help reduce the risk of coronary artery disease.[43]

If an individual performs resistance exercise, further adaptations can be realized within the muscle fibers. Resistance training alters muscle function and size, ultimately leading to an increase in muscular strength and endurance. The most noticeable adaptation due to a properly designed resistance training program is muscle fiber hypertrophy. When working at intensities significant enough to induce overload and cause muscular cell damage, the body responds through cell repair and remodeling. Common theories on fiber hypertrophy include an increase in structural proteins, including myofibrils, and an increase in contractile proteins, myosin, actin, and sarcomeres.[44] Increases in the protein content of the fiber ultimately cause the increase in muscle size. Other muscular adaptations due to resistance training include neural, neuroendocrine, and enzymatic adaptations. Within a few weeks of starting a resistance training program, an increase in strength occurs, with no changes in the cross-sectional area of muscle or change in limb size. This initial increase in strength is not because of hypertrophy, but rather, because of neural adaptations, such as the synchronization of motor unit recruitment; decrease in the coactivation of agonist and antagonist muscle; decrease in protective mechanisms of muscle, such as the Golgi tendon organ response; and possible changes in the neuromuscular junction.[45,46] The neuromuscular changes are exciting because strength can increase without gains in muscle mass. The strength gains decrease the work needed to accomplish daily tasks and decrease the myocardial load. Studies show that resistance training decreases the resting HR and possibly BP and decreases the rate-pressure product, which is a good estimate of cardiac work and oxygen consumption.[47,48] Additional strength gains and regular resistance training further reduce the risk of all-cause mortality, the risk of functional limitations, and the likelihood of future CVD events.[49,50]

Other-health related adaptations from regular resistance exercise include improved body composition (decrease in fat mass, increase in lean mass), reduction in blood glucose levels, and improvement in insulin sensitivity.[51,52] The combined benefits to the cardiovascular system and for the use of glucose and insulin are called *cardiometabolic*. All types of physical activity or muscle contraction reduce blood glucose levels, increase insulin sensitivity, and decrease the risk of T2DM.[51,53,54] Exercise promotes glucose uptake into the muscle cells for energy that is noninsulin dependent. This movement mechanism plays a significant role in the maintenance of serum glucose levels throughout the day. In theory, the more active one is throughout the day, the more stable his or her blood glucose levels will be. This decreases the need for insulin and helps maintain insulin sensitivity in the cell.[55,56]

PHYSICAL ACTIVITY GUIDELINES

In 1975, the American Heart Association began to recognize the need for more Americans to become physically active. The American Heart Association recommended 3 to 4 days/week of aerobic activity at 70% to 85% of the HR_{max} for 20 to 30 minutes. With those guidelines established, the American College of Sports Medicine (ACSM) presented their first recommendation in 1978 with a similar prescription that included 3 to 5 days a week at 50% to 80% VO_2max (60% to 90% HR_{max}), for a duration of 20 to 60 minutes. Over the next 30 years, the activity guidelines evolved based on the available epidemiological evidence. In 1995, the ACSM lowered the intensity recommendation to 40% to 85% of the VO_2max, suggesting that Americans could exercise at a lower intensity and receive a similar health benefit. In 1996, the Surgeon General's Report on Physical Activity attempted to explain what type of exercise represented moderate intensity. For instance, the report stated that the average person who engaged in brisk walking for 30 minutes or dancing for 30 minutes would use approximately 150 kcal/session, with the added suggestion of being active most days of the week, suggesting that everyone expend 1000 kcal/week. Based on brisk walking, that is roughly 210 minutes/week of moderate physical activity. Current ACSM guidelines from 2011 state that one should perform at least 150 minutes/week of moderate physical activity, performing 30 to 60 minutes 5 days/week, or 20 to 60 minutes of vigorous exercise 3 days/week (see Table 2-1). So, how much physical activity is truly needed to gain the health benefits? A historical view of the guidelines shows an evolution on the best available evidence. Although the epidemiological evidence is clear that physical activity has a dose-response relationship with health, it is less clear as to what specific intensity and volume is best. As researchers continue to gather information, guidelines are being written more clearly and practically than ever before.

The next section reviews some key studies used in developing the current physical activity guidelines. Each new study shaped the messages that physicians, public health professionals, educators, coaches, and athletic trainers provided on the health benefits of exercise. Two consistent themes can be seen regardless of the specific disease studied. The first is that more physical activity is associated with less risk of disease. The second is that many forms and intensities of physical activity can provide health benefits. However, the physical activity guidelines of 150 minutes/week of moderate physical activity provides each individual with a starting framework to participate in enough physical activity to confidently assume an improvement in overall health.

Exercise and All-Cause Mortality

Physical activity has a clear inverse association with all-cause mortality. In 2010, heart and cerebrovascular disease, cancer, and diabetes mellitus represented more than 50% of all deaths in the United States. Each disease is a related to low levels of physical activity. Lee et al[33] reported that there would a 9.9% reduction in all-cause mortality in the United States if physical activity levels increased as little as 25%. The following section begins with the relationship of physical activity with all-cause mortality and then reviews individual disease's links to physical activity. Physical activity benefits do not just impact the incidence of disease but, rather, life as a whole.

Research on physical activity and all-cause mortality has a long history. Epidemiologists used longitudinal cohort studies with large numbers of participants and followed them over the courses of their lives to establish links between the amount of physical activity participants reported and their life expectancies. Starting in 1976, the Nurse's Health study enrolled female registered nurses aged 30 to 55 years. Participants completed a baseline questionnaire regarding their medical histories and physical activity and were sent follow-up questionnaires every 2 years. Between 1982 and 1996, 4746 of the 80,348 women had died. Physical activity was inversely related to all-cause mortality. The most active women had the lowest risk. However, moderate physical activity showed approximately the same risk reduction as more vigorous activity, and the sharpest decrease in mortality was for those who participated in 1 to 1.9 hours/week of physical activity compared to those who had less than 1 hour/week of physical activity. The relationship was strongest with respiratory disease and CVD.[57]

One of the most important research studies on physical activity and risk of disease was the Harvard Alumni Health Study published in 1986. Paffenbarger et al[58] followed roughly 17,000 men for 12 to 16 years until 1978, during which time 1413 men died. They assessed physical activity using questionnaires, and the self-reported data were converted by the researchers into kcal expended per week. The age-adjusted death rates showed a steady decrease as energy expenditure increased. Those who expended the least energy (< 500 kcal/week) had the highest death rate (94/10,000 person-years), and those who expended > 2000 kcal/week had the lowest death rate (54/10,000 person-years; P < .0001).

In 1998, The Cardiovascular Health Study was published, with a cohort of 5201 men and 628 women. Physical activity was assessed using the Minnesota Leisure Time Activity Questionnaire that evaluated the frequency and duration of participation in 15 leisure-time activities. This information was then converted to energy expended in kcal/week. After 5 years, 646 deaths were reported. Many variables were considered, but physical activity was shown to lower the risk of all-cause mortality by 30% in the men and women who expended between 980 and 1890 kcal/week. Those who expended more than 1980 kcal/week had nearly half the risk of death from all causes.[59] Also, in 1998, a study of 3331 adult Japanese men showed that those who participated in regular physical activity (> 3 days/week) had the fewest coronary risk factors; however, those who engaged in physical activity once a week had fewer risk factors compared to the sedentary group.[60]

A 2008 report presented by an expert panel appointed by the federal government concluded that the evidence from 73 studies showed a significant inverse relationship between physical activity and all-cause mortality in 67 of those studies.[38] The median risk reduction was 31% for those who were the most active compared to those who were the least active, and the inverse association was shown for all ages. The panel also suggested the Physical Activity Guidelines for Americans based on its research.[38] One year later, a meta-analysis of 38 studies reported findings of a 22% risk reduction in men who were highly active compared to low-active men and a 31% risk reduction in highly active women.[61]

The Aerobics Center Longitudinal Study is an ongoing cohort study. In 2011, Lee et al[62] reported 31,818 men and 10,555 women who received a medical examination between 1978 and 2002. The subjects were followed until December 2003. During that time, 1492 men and 230 women died. Again, physical activity had a significant inverse association with mortality. More importantly, the researchers also presented data that showed a stronger relationship between cardiorespiratory fitness and mortality. Although physical activity was proven to be helpful, this research suggests that improving an unfit person's cardiorespiratory fitness would have the greatest impact on the risk of all-cause mortality. Participants who did not reach 500 metabolic equivalent of task (MET) minutes/week (approximately 150 minutes/week) but were cardiovascularly fit and those who met the MET cut-off and were fit had a significantly lower risk those who did not meet the guidelines and were unfit. A MET minute represents the amount of time in an activity multiplied by the MET intensity of that activity. For example, a moderate-intensity activity has a MET range between 3 and 5.9 METs, and performing it for 30 minutes would yield between 90 and 177 MET minutes of activity. Also, 150 minutes/week of a 3.3-MET activity would equal 500 MET minutes. In the study above, the 2 fit groups showed no difference in their mortality risk. Meeting the physical activity guideline was not as important as being cardiovascularly fit.[62]

Exercise and Cardiovascular Disease

As noted in Chapter 1, CVD continues to be the number one cause of death in men and women in the United States. Although CVD is prevalent in all populations, a reduction in smoking and better medication for hypertension and cholesterol seemed to have reduced mortality numbers. Physical activity can also play a beneficial role in reducing the risk of CVD. Maybe the real question becomes not how to completely prevent CVD but, rather, how much physical activity is necessary to award the human body a protective effect against this common disease.

A cohort of 12,516 men from the Harvard Alumni Health Study reported 2135 cases of coronary heart disease (CHD). There was a significant inverse association with physical activity and risk of developing CHD. Those who expended less than 500 kcal/week showed the highest risk, and those expending between 1000 and 2999 kcal/week showed similar risk for CHD. A dose-response of physical activity was seen at the 1000-kcal/week level. The term *dose-response* refers to the level of the treatment needed to get a positive result. Here, it appears that getting at least 1000 kcal/week of physical activity was the dose needed to show a benefit. This study also reported a significant inverse association with vigorous activity, sport, and recreational activities and developing CHD.[63]

Swain and Franklin[64] showed that the benefits from vigorous activity provided a significantly greater cardioprotective benefit than moderate exercise. They examined more than 500 scientific reports concerning exercise, physical activity, risk reduction, and cardiovascular changes and concluded that vigorous physical activity (> 6 MET) compared to moderate physical activity (3 to 5.9 MET) produced a more favorable risk profile. Vigorous physical activity at a level greater than 60% of the person's aerobic capacity improved diastolic BP, glucose control, and aerobic capacity compared to moderate intensities. There was no difference between vigorous and moderate physical activity in terms of systolic BP (SBP), improvements in lipid profile, or body fat loss.[64]

Volume of Physical Activity

The total amount of time spent in physical activity is an important element of the guidelines. The combination of duration (time) and intensity is known as volume. The weekly volume needed to achieve health benefits results in a calorie expenditure of at least 1000 kcal. The Nurses' Health Study included 72,488 women. At the 8-year follow-up, 645 nonfatal heart attacks or deaths were reported. Physical activity was calculated using MET-hours/week through a questionnaire. There was a strong inverse association between total energy expenditure and CHD risk. Women who had a significantly lower risk of CHD were physically active in equivalent to 3 hours of brisk walking each week or 1.5 hours of vigorous exercise each week.[65]

Another study from the Women's Health Study used a cohort of 38,987 disease-free women and followed them for a mean of 10.9 years. In that time, 948 cases of CHD were reported. The authors found that a normal-weight person showed no significant reduction in risk by expending 1000 kcal/week or more; however, there was a significant reduction in risk of CHD in women classified as overweight and obese. Both groups showed a significant reduction in risk of CHD by expending greater than 1000 kcal/week. Also, the data showed a dose-gradient increase in risk, starting with the women who were completely sedentary and ending with those who were active for more than 4 hours/week. The greatest or most significant reduction in risk could be seen between the groups who were active for more than 1 hour/week compared to the sedentary group and women who participated in less than 1 hour/week of physical activity. The risk reduction did not end there because it was shown that the walking speed also had a significant inverse trend in risk, with a faster walking pace having the lowest risk of developing CHD (Figure 2-3).[66]

Longer durations are not required for health benefits. The ACSM suggests that a minimum time of 10 minutes is effective as long as a total of 150 minutes is accumulated over a week. An article published in 1997 that used patients from the Multiple Risk Factor Intervention Trial reported that men in the least active (< 5 minutes/day) had a 22% higher CHD death rate than those who were only slightly more active. This study suggested that exercising longer than 20 minutes/day is associated with no additional reduction in the risk of dying from CHD.[67]

In a meta-analysis published in 2011, the researchers sought to validate the current guidelines for physical activity of 150 and 300 minutes/week for additional benefits. Although physical activity contains different levels of intensity and volume, the researchers focused their efforts on the duration of physical activity that best matched the current guidelines. Therefore, focusing on the duration recommended, the authors found 33 studies that met their initial criteria for inclusion. The risk reduction in all studies that measured leisure time physical activity showed a 26% reduction in CHD in those who were active compared to those who were sedentary. The individuals who met the minimum criteria of 150 minutes/week had a 14% decrease in risk of CHD compared to those with no activity, and those who received 300 minutes/week showed a

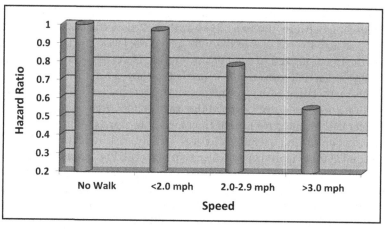

Figure 2-3. Relationship between walking pace and coronary heart disease. (Adapted from Weinstein AR, Sesso HD, Lee IM, et al. The joint effects of physical activity and body mass index on coronary heart disease risk in women. *Arch Intern Med.* 2008;168(8):884-890.)

20% decrease in CHD risk. The authors also showed that individuals who were active below the minimum guidelines still showed a significant decrease in risk compared to individuals who were inactive, supporting the notion that any physical activity is better than no physical activity.[68] The DREW trial showed a significant increase in cardiovascular fitness (4.2%) in sedentary, overweight, postmenopausal women who performed 4 kcal/kg/week, equivalent to about 72 minutes/week of moderate physical activity.[69]

Resistance Training and Risk

Although aerobic exercise has been the focus of most large epidemiological studies, there is support for resistance training to reduce the risk of CVD. The Aerobics Center Longitudinal Study also measured muscular strength in a cohort of men to determine its impact on CVD, cancer, and all-cause mortality. Following more than 10,000 men with 501 deaths, it was clear that those in the lowest-strength groups had the highest risk for all-cause mortality and a higher risk of death from CVD. Even when the data were adjusted for cardiorespiratory fitness, it was clear that muscular strength has a relationship with CVD and all-cause mortality.[49] Age was also controlled for, and the inverse relationship between strength and CVD remained. The benefits of resistance training not only reduce all-cause mortality and CVD, but also increase functional capacity, increase ability to perform ADLs, and overall improve one's quality of life.

Exercise and Cancer

Cancer is the second leading cause of death in America, and the numbers are continuing to increase. Although a cure or better treatment is medicine's ultimate goal, the link between physical inactivity and certain types of cancers offers hope for prevention. The most recent reports estimate that one-third of cancer deaths each year are attributed to poor diet and an inactive lifestyle.[70] The mechanisms for physical activity's effect on cancer are not yet well understood, but this should not take away from the epidemiological evidence showing lower risk for regular exercisers.

Data from the Aerobics Longitude Study from the Cooper Institute (N = 10,265) were used to examine the relationship between muscular strength, CVD, and cancer. This is one of the few strength studies that used a more practical measure of upper and lower body strength, the one repetition maximum. Prior strength studies measured hand-grip strength, which does not indicate full-body strength. In this all-male cohort, 145 died from CVD and 199 died from cancer. Subjects were split into the following 3 strength groups: high, medium, and low. The upper 2 groups showed a significant reduction in risk of death from CVD and a significant reduction in risk of death from cancer compared to the low group. The risk of death from all causes and cancer remained significant even when the data were adjusted for differences in cardiovascular fitness and body weight. The risk of death from cancer was 1.45 times greater for the low strength group compared to those in the medium group and was 1.24 times greater when compared to the high-strength group.[71]

In 2005, a cohort from the Nurses' Health Study was used to determine the risk of breast cancer relative to levels of physical activity. The study included 2987 female nurses diagnosed with breast cancer between 1984 and 1998, and they were followed until 2002 or death. The risk of death from breast cancer was 20% to 30% higher in women who had less than 9 MET hours/week of physical activity. Nine MET hours is equivalent to 540 MET minutes, which is roughly 150 minutes/week of moderate physical activity. Women who engaged in 9 or more MET hours/week reduced their mortality rate by 6% compared to the group with the fewest MET hours. However, the researchers concluded that the greatest benefit was seen in women who walked 3 to 5 hours/week compared to the group that got less than 3 hours/week of activity.[72]

In 2009, a review article reported a link between physical activity and colon cancer risk reduction.[73] Several studies were reviewed, and the researchers concluded that regular physical activity reduced the risk of colon cancer in men and women. According to the review, 7 hours/week of activity had the greatest impact and lowered the risk by 40%. However, a reduction in tumor formation was seen for any duration greater than 1 hour/week. Also, a higher rate of survival after diagnosis was seen in those who were physically active for more than 4 hours/week, lowering overall mortality by 39% and disease-specific mortality by 51%.[74]

Exercise and Hypertension

The ACSM position statement on aerobic exercise and hypertension states that exercise causes a reduction in BP, but the magnitude of the reduction is complicated by many other factors. First, BP changes occur more significantly among the group that is hypertensive at baseline compared to normotensive subjects. Furthermore, during a training period, exercise intensity seems to have little effect on the magnitude of the BP reduction. As for the effect of resistance exercise on BP, the evidence is less clear and somewhat conflicting. Therefore, resistance exercise should be seen as a supplement to aerobic exercise for the reduction of hypertension.[74]

A female cohort (N = 4884) from the Aerobics Center Longitudinal Study that had normal BP was given a maximal treadmill test to assess cardiovascular fitness. The women completed a health survey approximately 5 years after the treadmill test, at which time 157 women were diagnosed with hypertension. The researchers reported that for each 1-MET increase in treadmill performance, there was a 19% reduction in the likelihood of becoming hypertensive. Higher levels of fitness were also associated with a reduction in hypertension in normal-weight and overweight women.[75]

In 2007, a randomized, controlled trial of 464 sedentary overweight or obese women with elevated BP looked at the effect of exercise training on fitness levels and BP. Although the researchers reported a dose-response relationship between the amount of physical activity and fitness, the researchers found no significant changes in SBP or diastolic BP from baseline to the 6-month measurement. Participants did not significantly reduce weight or improve serum cholesterol. The expected benefits of physical activity were not realized by 6 months. The lack of difference between the exercising group and the control group could be due to in part to an unstable control group. The participants with the most activity (12 kcal/kg) showed a reduction in SBP. However, it was not significant when compared to the control group, which also had lower SBP even though they performed no physical activity.[69] As stated in the ACSM position statement, many factors are involved in the reduction of BP, and the role of weight loss, fat metabolism, and gender needs further study.

Exercise and Diabetes Mellitus

Although physical activity and diabetes mellitus are linked, diabetes mellitus is a multifaceted disease that cannot be predicted by one variable. Physical activity and diabetes mellitus have a strong relationship with each other, but so do BMI, central obesity, diet, and family history. All of these factors are important in any discussion about diabetes mellitus. The next section focuses on what is known about physical activity and T2DM.

From the Nurse's Health Study, it was clear that even a single bout of vigorous physical activity/ a week lowered the risk of T2DM.[76] Another cohort from the Nurse's Health Study showed that when participants were divided into quintile physical activity groups, the highest quintile group had a 46% reduction in risk compared to the lowest physical activity group. Here, the physical activity did not have to be vigorous exercise to be effective; it just had to be greater than none. The low-quintile activity group (2.1 to 4.6 MET hours/week) showed a significant reduction in risk of 23% when compared to the sedentary group (< 2 MET hours/week).[51] At levels less than the recommended guidelines, some risk reduction was evident in the low-quintile physical activity group. This illustrates the idea of a dose gradient. The benefits of physical activity increase with the amount or dose received. The MONICA/KORA study also showed a risk reduction in men and women with increasing levels of physical activity, with the highest activity group (> 2 hours/week) showing the least incidence rate compared to all other levels. The moderate group represented participants who regularly participated in 1 hour/week of physical activity.[77] The moderate-to-high levels in this study hover just around the recommended physical activity guidelines, and with a risk reduction in diabetes mellitus, there is a risk reduction in heart disease. The Women's Health Study looked at 37,878 women; 1361 developed T2DM in the 6.9-mean-year follow-up. Of that group, 12,936 women were considered active based on expending 1000 kcal/week. Of the women who were considered active, they showed a 15% decrease in diabetes mellitus risk. Also, 5 groups were formed based on time spent walking. Even in the group performing less than 1 hour/week of walking, there was a reduction in the risk of developing diabetes mellitus. However, the greatest reduction in risk was shown in the group that walked between 2 and 3 hours/week, which is in line with the Physical Activity Guidelines for Americans.[78] In a large prospective study on 23,444 men, men who were physically active compared to sedentary were associated with decreased risk of diabetes mellitus. The men were separated into groups by the activity in which they participated or were placed in the sedentary group. The walking, jogging, running group and those who participated in sports/fitness activities had 56% and 40% reductions, respectively, in the risk of developing diabetes mellitus compared to the sedentary group. Also, when separated by fitness levels, the low-fitness group (bottom 20% of subjects) regardless of type of physical activity performed showed a 6-fold higher risk of diabetes mellitus compared to the high-fitness group (upper 40% of subjects).[79] Although it is clear that physical activity reduces risk of developing diabetes mellitus, it also seems clear that higher fitness levels, regardless of type of physical activity performed, can reduce diabetes mellitus risk.

Exercise and Hyperlipidemia

Research supports that higher HDL-C reduces the risk of CHD.[80] The reason for a focus on HDL-C levels is based on the idea that CVD risk can be reduced by incorporating lifestyle changes, such as regular physical activity and a diet high in fruits and vegetables. Large-population studies have shown HDL-C to be positively associated with physical activity.[81,82]

The Lipid Research Clinics Coronary Primary Prevention Trial took more than 7000 men who had hyperlipidemia and categorized them by amount of physical activity they received in and out of work and the frequency of exercise or physical labor. Once they were rated on their physical work and leisure-time physical activities, they were placed into 3 activity groups (low, moderate, and high). Results indicated that physical activity levels were a significant predictor of HDL-C and triglyceride levels, even after controlling for smoking, alcohol use, and total cholesterol.[43]

A single 30-minute exercise session/week proved to be helpful in lowering subcutaneous fat and triglycerides and increasing HDL-C in a study of Japanese men.[60] The greatest benefit was observed in the most active group (30 minutes for >3 days/week), but compared to the sedentary group that did not exercise, it was clear that even minimal activity can positively impact CVD risk factors.[60] Although some evidence was found regarding the effectiveness of physical activity on cholesterol levels, more epidemiological research regarding the best intensity and duration needed to change HDL-C and triglyceride levels would help solidify the physical activity recommendation.

Exercise and Weight Loss

The ACSM guidelines offered an extraordinary amount of health benefits, but they were not established to cause a large amount of weight loss. Instead, the 150 minutes/week of moderate physical activity might be enough activity to prevent weight gain. The reason for this is that the health benefits of physical activity are independent of weight loss, meaning that one does not have to lose weight to lower the risk of chronic disease. One has to be physically active. The media presents a picture of physical activity and weight loss that is sometimes exaggerated. Magazine articles, fitness websites, exercise equipment, infomercials, and common gym talk give people the idea that the purpose of exercise is to lose weight. The message should be that physical activity will help keep and improve health.

Although exercise is seen by many as the pathway to weight loss, it can be argued that this expectation is part of the physical inactivity problem because many people become discouraged by unsuccessful attempts to lose weight by increasing exercise. These same people are discouraged to continue with daily exercise because it is not accomplishing their goal for beginning physical activity. Evidence shows that as many as 50% of those who begin an exercise program will drop their exercise routine within 6 months.[83] To receive the most protection from physical activity, regular sessions throughout the lifespan are needed. However, if a majority of people believe that a physical activity program will make them lose weight, they will likely be discouraged and stop before realizing the health benefits. With a narrow focus on weight loss, an individual can lose sight of the more significant and true benefits presented in this chapter.

People seeking weight loss through physical activity need to understand that fitness may have a greater impact on their health. A study of older adults (N = 2603, >60 years old) investigated the effects of cardiovascular fitness and central obesity on mortality. Researchers separated participants into 5 fitness groups based on their performance on a maximal exercise test. As expected, fitness was inversely related to mortality. The lowest fitness group had the highest death rate. The researchers found that when the data were adjusted for BMI and central obesity, fitness levels were still a significant predictor of mortality regardless of a person's weight.[84]

More recently, 44,674 men participated in part of the Cooper Center Longitudinal Study that examined the association of cardiorespiratory fitness, BMI, and heart failure mortality. The men were free of CVD at the start of the study and were placed in the fit or unfit group based on a treadmill test. At the follow-up (average of 19.8 years later), 153 had died from heart failure. Fitness and BMI had a significant impact on heart failure mortality. When the data were adjusted for BMI, the fit group had a lower risk of mortality regardless of normal or overweight status.[85] This research underscores the impact of fitness and that increased physical activity is needed to become fit rather than lose weight. Physical activity should be undertaken at a level that overloads the body to improve one's cardiorespiratory fitness to receive the most benefit.

IMPACT OF EPIDEMIOLOGICAL RESEARCH

Based on these and many other large prospective studies with diverse populations, physical activity that expends approximately 1000 kcal/week or 150 minutes/week of moderate-intensity physical activity lowers the risk of all-cause mortality. The recommendation can be met from a combination of moderate and vigorous activity or by accumulating the 150 minutes through multiple 10-minute sessions through the day. The guidelines for resistance training are 2 whole-body training sessions/week working all major muscle groups of the body.

Although the majority of the literature supports the established guidelines, several studies suggest less physical activity is beneficial. At least 3 studies have found that half the recommended volume (500 kcal/week) may reduce the risk of premature death.[63,69,86] It seems clear to suggest that more physical activity is better than some and some is better than none. Each individual will have slightly different outcomes based on personal factors, including baseline physical fitness, current health, and genetic makeup. Multiple studies report that the most benefit or greatest reduction in health risk occurs in the movement of sedentary individuals into the slightly active category (see Figure 2-2).[38]

National statistics paint a grim picture concerning American's lack of physical activity. The evidence for physical activity is overwhelming, and the statistical estimates for its impact on disease worldwide are startling. According to Lee et al,[87] physical inactivity directly causes 6% of all heart disease, 7% of T2DM, and 10% of breast and colon cancer. If inactivity was reduced by 25%, more than 1 million deaths could be postponed every year, and there would be an increase in life expectancy worldwide.[87] In the United States, approximately 56% of adults do not meet the recommendations for physical activity of 150 minutes/week at moderate intensity.[88] One study of adolescents and adults showed that Americans averaged 8 hours of sedentary behavior a day and more than 35% of US adults spend no time participating in leisure-time physical activity.[89] The estimate for health care costs associated with physical inactivity is now more than $100 billion/year.[90] Only 34% of individuals reported receiving any exercise or physical activity recommendations from their health care provider during their last medical visit.[91]

Although there are 5 components of health-related physical fitness, cardiovascular fitness could be argued as the most important component. Physical activity and cardiovascular fitness reduce the risk of all-cause mortality. It is vital that aerobic activity be the foundation of individual exercise programs for overall health and that resistance exercise be included for increases in muscular strength and bone density. In a society that craves a magic pill for all health problems, physical activity is the closest option. With the ability to affect health in so many different ways and in so many different systems of the body, it is hard to believe that the population is becoming increasingly sedentary.

Epidemiology has laid the foundation for change. The evidence is overwhelming from years of dedication to research of the link between physical activity and health. It is time that the passion for research overlaps with a passion for lifestyle and behavior change. Without change soon, as a society, there will be a crisis in the health care system and an ever-declining quality of life. Future medical advances in drug therapy and technology may prolong life, but at the cost of decades of disease management, dependency on medication, diminished physical function, and reduced independence in daily tasks. This is how society will realize the true impact of the knowledge gained from epidemiology. How can we change our physical activity habits?

Physical Activity Promotion

There is no single answer. In the age of technology, fast food, and quick solutions, the battle is growing increasingly difficult. Schools are cutting physical education classes and eliminating or reducing recess so that children experience less physical activity than ever before. Without this structure, they lack the skills to participate and do not develop a sense of pleasure or satisfaction from physical activity. The habit of being sedentary continues into adulthood. Breaking this trend is increasingly difficult considering the low rates of physical activity in adults from whose examples children learn. As more experts consider physical inactivity to be an epidemic, a multifaceted approach is needed to change the tide. From governments to school districts, insurance companies to doctors, and parents to children, physical activity needs to be made a priority in all aspects of life.

Perhaps a change in focus is needed to improve physical activity levels. Beyond the physical benefits associated with physical activity, the mental benefits are also great. Studies show exercising at the recommended levels reduces depression in a dose-response manner.[92,93] Chapter 9 details how physical activity impacts depression and stress. Self-efficacy is another important mental benefit. It is the confidence one has to complete tasks or engage in certain activities. Single bouts of exercise and long-term exercise programs have been shown to increase self-efficacy,[94,95] and improved self-efficacy is a predictor of exercise adherence and increasing the amount of physical activity one completes.[96,97]

More success with physical activity is needed. The physical activity guidelines are clear; one needs to achieve 150 minutes/week of moderate physical activity. This goal can be accomplished through planning, habit formation, receiving social support, recognizing success, and feeling the confidence that comes with success. Rather than reaching for a 100-lb loss in 2 months, one needs to start small, achieve success, and feel better about one's self and one's ability to perform the activities. Also, more people need to understand that performing high-intensity training is unnecessary for health benefits but, rather, one can climb a few more stairs, sit an hour less in a day, walk the dog, mow the lawn, wash the car, etc, to better accomplish one's physical activity for a day or a week. Lastly, research points to the importance of social support and having friends and family who have similar goals or are encouraging of the behavior change. Multiple types of social support were shown to increase physical activity levels in middle-aged adults.[98] The benefits of success are evident and better than any pill could ever provide.

BRINGING IT TOGETHER

Physical activity beyond normal daily living is critical to the health of the human body. Many physiological adaptations occur in the body due to the added physical stress from activity and exercise. These adaptations are critical to combating chronic diseases that have plagued society for generations. The 2008 Physical Activity Guidelines and the ACSM's 2011 Guidelines for Physical Activity are based on a wealth of historical and current epidemiological evidence. The research findings paint a significant picture of the health benefits afforded by physical activity, which cannot be explained by chance or coincidence. The overwhelming significant evidence shown in a variety of populations concerning physical activity and a reduction in the risk of CHD, certain types of cancer, hypertension, hyperlipidemia, depression, and overall mortality should be enough to convince every American to improve his or her physical activity profile. Although the guidelines were established to encourage Americans to achieve the minimum amount of physical activity necessary to receive many health benefits, the evidence also shows that moderate physical activity greater than 300 minutes/week is related to greater benefits in a dose-response effect not completely understood. The guidelines of 150 minutes/week were established to provide Americans with the knowledge and understanding of the impact moderate physical activity can have on their overall health. As researchers continue to gather information regarding the benefits of physical activity on health, it is important to recognize and understand the vital role that epidemiological research plays in the development of professional and/or general public guidelines and policies. Without the strong work of the researchers and committees on gathering quality information over long periods of time, we may not have a full understanding of the benefits of physical activity on health.

However, with this knowledge and understanding of physical activity comes the responsibility of all health professionals to help the American population become more physically active.

REVIEW QUESTIONS

1. What are the 5 components of health-related physical fitness? Which is the most important to improve to reduce the risk of disease?

2. What is the difference between a dose response and a dose gradient?

3. What is the percentage of max HR that has to be achieved for a physical activity to be considered moderately intense?

4. List the adaptations that come from aerobic and resistance exercise.

5. Describe 2 ways researchers measure the amount of physical activity participants perform.

6. How does improved self-efficacy impact the promotion of physical activity?

7. In your own words, describe how the epidemiological evidence impacted the current Physical Activity Guidelines for Americans.

LEARNING ACTIVITIES

1. Calculate your target HR for moderate physical activity using the HR_{max} formula: $208 - (.7 \times .60)$. What speed of walking or jogging do you think you would have to do to reach that HR? Do that pace for 10 minutes and record your 5- and 10-minute HRs. Were you correct about how intense moderate physical activity really is? How might what counts as moderate for different people change based on age, fitness, and experience with a particular exercise?

2. The American College of Cardiology recently developed a CVD risk calculator. Enter your data to determine your 10-year risk of a cardiac event. The tool is not valid for those younger than 40 years, but it will help you see what risk factors are important. You can find the calculator at, www.cvriskcalculator.com and an article on the debate of its use at, www.health.harvard.edu/blog/cholesterol-guidelines-update-controversy-over-heart-risk-calculator-201311196886.

3. Use self-report questionnaires to find out the average amount of physical activity your friends and classmates are getting. There are several valid surveys available on the Internet, including the Godin Leisure-time Physical Activity Questionnaire, the International Physical Activity Questionnaire, and the Global Physical Activity Questionnaire. Be sure to carefully read the directions on how to transform these data into MET minutes/week.

4. How can you increase your daily physical activity considering your busy schedule? What barriers do you face? What strategies do you think those who are more physically active are using?

5. Based on the information in this chapter, briefly describe an epidemiological research study that you would begin in hopes of improving or adding to the information we have regarding physical activity and health.

REFERENCES

1. Troiano RP, Berrigan D, Dodd KW, Masse LC, Tilert T, McDowell M. Physical activity in the United States measured by accelerometer. *Med Sci Sports Exerc.* 2008;40(1):181-188.

2. Caspersen CJ, Powell KE, Christenson GM. Physical activity, exercise, and physical fitness: definitions and distinctions for health-related research. *Public Health Reports (Washington, D.C.: 1974).* 1985;100(2):126-131.

3. Howley ET. Type of activity: resistance, aerobic and leisure versus occupational physical activity. *Med Sci Sports Exerc.* 2001;33(6 Suppl):S364-S369.

4. Swain RA, Harris AB, Wiener EC, et al. Prolonged exercise induces angiogenesis and increases cerebral blood volume in primary motor cortex of the rat. *Neuroscience.* 2003;117(4):1037-1046.

5. Dunn AL, Andersen RE, Jakicic JM. Lifestyle physical activity interventions. History, short- and long-term effects, and recommendations. *Am J Prev Med.* 1998;15(4):398-412.

6. Sallis JF, Frank LD, Saelens BE, Kraft MK. Active transportation and physical activity: opportunities for collaboration on transportation and public health research. *Transportation Research Part A: Policy and Practice.* 2004;38(4):249-268.

7. Ainsworth BE, Haskell WL, Whitt MC, et al. Compendium of physical activities: an update of activity codes and MET intensities. *Med Sci Sports Exerc.* 2000;32(9):S498-S516.

8. Wiener, JM, Hanley, RJ, Clark, R, Van Nostrandu, JF. Measuring the activities of daily living: comparisons across national surveys. *J Gerontol.* 1990; 45(6) S229-237.

9. Garber C, Greaney M, Riebe D, Nigg C, Burbank P, Clark P. Physical and mental health-related correlates of physical function in community dwelling older adults: a cross sectional study. *BMC Geriatrics.* 2010;10(1):6.

10. Huang Y, Macera CA, Blair SN, Brill PA, Kohl HW, Kronenfeld JJ. Physical fitness, physical activity, and functional limitation in adults aged 40 and older. *Med Sci Sports Exerc.* 1998;30(9):1430-1435.

11. Clark HH. Basic understanding of physical fitness. Sport President's Council on Physical Fitness and Sport. *Physical Fitness Research Digest.* Vol 1. Washington, DC. 1971.

12. Haskell WL, Montoye HJ, Orenstein D. Physical activity and exercise to achieve health-related physical fitness components. *Public Health Reports.* Washington, D.C. 1985;100(2):202-212.

13. Pate R, Kriska A. Physiological basis of the sex difference in cardiorespiratory endurance. *Sports Med.* 1984;1(2):87-89.

14. Gibala MJ, Little JP, MacDonald MJ, Hawley JA. Physiological adaptations to low-volume, high-intensity interval training in health and disease. *Physiology.* 2012;590(5):1077-1084.

15. Suominen H. Physical activity and health: Musculoskeletal issues. *Adv Physiotherapy.* 2007;9(2):65-75.

16. LaStayo PC, Ewy GA, Pierotti DD, Johns RK, Lindstedt S. The positive effects of negative work: increased muscle strength and decreased fall risk in a frail elderly population. *Bio Sci Med Sci.* 2003;58(5):M419-M424.

17. *ACSM's Resources for the Personal Trainer.* In: Thompson W, ed. 3rd ed. Baltimore, MD: Lippincott Williams & Wilkins; 2010.

18. Holland GJ, Tanaka, K., Shigematsu, R., & Nakagaichi, M. Flexibility and physical functions of older adults: a review. *J Aging Phys Activity.* 2002;10(2):169-206.

19. Youdas JW, Krause DA, Hollman JH, Harmsen WS, Laskowski E. The influence of gender and age on hamstring muscle length in healthy adults. *JOSPT.* 2005;35(4):246-252.

20. Hahn T, Foldspang A, Vestergaard E, Ingemann-Hansen T. Active knee joint flexibility and sports activity. *Scan J Med Sci Sports.* 1999;9(2):74-80.

21. Fowler K, Kravitz L. The perils of poor posture. *IDEA Fitness.* 2011;8(4):45-51.

22. CDC. About BMI for Adults. http://www.cdc.gov/healthyweight/assessing/bmi/adult_bmi/. Accessed December, 5, 2013.

23. American Council on Exercise(ACE). Percent Body Fat Norms for Men and Women. http://www.acefitness.org/acefit/healthy_living_tools_content.aspx?id=2. Accessed December, 5, 2013.

24. Poirier P, Giles TD, Bray GA, et al. Obesity and cardiovascular disease: pathophysiology, evaluation, and effect of weight loss: an update of the 1997 american heart association scientific statement on obesity and heart disease from the obesity committee of the council on nutrition, physical activity, and metabolism. *Circulation.* February 14, 2006 2006;113(6):898-918.

25. Katzmarzyk PT, Church TS, Janssen I, Ross R, Blair SN. Metabolic syndrome, obesity, and mortality: impact of cardiorespiratory fitness. *Diabetes Care.* 2005;28(2):391-397.

26. Physical Activity and Health: A report of the Surgeon General. U.S. Department of Health and Human Services, National Center for Chronic Disease Prevention and Health Promotion. Atlanta, GA. 1996.

27. Hu G, Barengo NC, Tuomilehto J, Lakka TA, Nissinen A, Jousilahti P. Relationship of physical activity and body mass index to the risk of hypertension: a prospective study in finland. *Hypertension.* 2004;43(1):25-30.

28. Colberg SR, Albright AL, Blissmer BJ, et al. Exercise and type 2 diabetes: American College of Sports Medicine and the American Diabetes Association: joint position statement. Exercise and type 2 diabetes. *Med Sci Sport Exer.* 2010;42(12):2282-2303.

29. Lee CD, Folsom AR, Blair SN. Physical activity and stroke risk: a meta-analysis. *Stroke*. October 1, 2003 2003;34(10):2475-2481.

30. Ball K, Owen N, Salmon J, Bauman A, Gore C. Associations of physical activity with body weight and fat in men and women. *Inter J Obes Metabol*. 2001;25:914-919.

31. Rovio S, Kåreholt I, Helkala E-L, et al. Leisure-time physical activity at midlife and the risk of dementia and Alzheimer's disease. *Lancet Neuro*. 2005;4(11):705-711.

32. Martinsen EW. Physical activity in the prevention and treatment of anxiety and depression. *Nordic J Psychiat*. 2008;62 Suppl 47:25-29.

33. Lee IM, Shiroma EJ, Lobelo F, et al. Effect of physical inactivity on major non-communicable diseases worldwide: an analysis of burden of disease and life expectancy. *Lancet*. 2012;380(9838):219-229.

34. Nguyen-Michel ST, Unger JB, Hamilton J, Spruijt-Metz D. Associations between physical activity and perceived stress/hassles in college students. *Stress & Health*. 2006;22(3):179-188.

35. Thompson WW, Zack MM, Krahn GL, Andresen EM, Barile JP. Health-related quality of life among older adults with and without functional limitations. *Am J Public Health*. 2012;102(3):496-502.

36. Stieglitz EJ. *The Second Forty Years*. Philadelphia, PA: Lippincott; 1946.

37. Blair SN, Kohl HW, Paffenbarger RS Jr, Clark DG, Cooper KH, Gibbons LW. Physical fitness and all-cause mortality. A prospective study of healthy men and women. *JAMA*. 1989;262(17):2395-2401.

38. Physical Activity Guidelines Advisory Committee. Physical Activity Guidelines Advisory Committee Report, 2008. Washington, DC: U.S. Department of Health and Human Services, 2008.

39. Garber CE, Blissmer B, Deschenes MR, et al. American College of Sports Medicine position stand. Quantity and quality of exercise for developing and maintaining cardiorespiratory, musculoskeletal, and neuromotor fitness in apparently healthy adults: guidance for prescribing exercise. *Med Sci Sport Exer*. 2011;43(7):1334-1359.

40. Wilmore JH, Green JS, Stanforth PR, et al. Relationship of changes in maximal and submaximal aerobic fitness to changes in cardiovascular disease and non-insulin-dependent diabetes mellitus risk factors with endurance training: the HERITAGE Family Study. *Metabolism*. 2001;50(11):1255-1263.

41. Cornelissen VA, Fagard RH. Effects of endurance training on blood pressure, blood pressure-regulating mechanisms, and cardiovascular risk factors. *Hypertension*. 2005;46(4):667-675.

42. Hambrecht R, Adams V, Erbs S, et al. Regular physical activity improves endothelial function in patients with coronary artery disease by increasing phosphorylation of endothelial nitric oxide synthase. *Circulation*. 2003;107(25):3152-3158.

43. Gordon DJ, Witztum JL, Hunninghake D, Gates S, Glueck CJ. Habitual physical activity and high-density lipoprotein cholesterol in men with primary hypercholesterolemia. The Lipid Research Clinics Coronary Primary Prevention Trial. *Circulation*. 1983;67(3):512-520.

44. MacDougall JD, Sale DG, Moroz JR, Elder GC, Sutton JR, Howald H. Mitochondrial volume density in human skeletal muscle following heavy resistance training. *Med Sci Sports Exer*. 1979;11(2):164-166.

45. Carroll TJ, Riek S, Carson RG. Neural adaptations to resistance training: implications for movement control. *Sports Med*. 2001;31(12):829-840.

46. Ploutz LL, Tesch PA, Biro RL, Dudley GA. Effect of resistance training on muscle use during exercise. *J Appl Physiol*. 1994;76(4):1675-1681.

47. Pollock ML, Franklin BA, Balady GJ, et al. AHA Science Advisory. Resistance exercise in individuals with and without cardiovascular disease: benefits, rationale, safety, and prescription: an advisory from the committee on exercise, rehabilitation, and prevention, council on clinical cardiology, american heart association; position paper endorsed by the american college of sports medicine. *Circulation*. 2000;101(7):828-833.

48. McCartney N, McKelvie RS, Martin J, Sale DG, MacDougall JD. Weight-training-induced attenuation of the circulatory response of older males to weight lifting. *J Appl Physiol*. 1993;74(3):1056-1060.

49. Ruiz JR, Sui X, Lobelo F, et al. Association between muscular strength and mortality in men: prospective cohort study. *BMJ*. 2008;337:a439.

50. Newman AB, Kupelian V, Visser M, et al. Strength, but not muscle mass, is associated with mortality in the health, aging and body composition study cohort. *J Gerontol A Biol Sci Med Sci*. 2006;61(1):72-77.

51. Colberg SR, Albright AL, Blissmer BJ, et al. Exercise and type 2 diabetes: American College of Sports Medicine and the American Diabetes Association: joint position statement. Exercise and type 2 diabetes. *Med Sci Sports Exer*. 2010;42(12):2282-2303.

52. Holten MK, Zacho M, Gaster M, Juel C, Wojtaszewski JF, Dela F. Strength training increases insulin-mediated glucose uptake, GLUT4 content, and insulin signaling in skeletal muscle in patients with type 2 diabetes. *Diabetes*. 2004;53(2):294-305.

53. Hu FB, Sigal RJ, Rich-Edwards JW, et al. Walking compared with vigorous physical activity and risk of type 2 diabetes in women: a prospective study. *JAMA*. 1999;282(15):1433-1439.

54. Lynch J, Helmrich SP, Lakka TA, et al. Moderately intense physical activities and high levels of cardiorespiratory fitness reduce the risk of non-insulin-dependent diabetes mellitus in middle-aged men. *Arch Intern Med*. 1996;156(12):1307-1314.

55. Kennedy JW, Hirshman MF, Gervino EV, et al. Acute exercise induces GLUT4 translocation in skeletal muscle of normal human subjects and subjects with type 2 diabetes. *Diabetes.* 1999;48(5):1192-1197.

56. Horton ES. Exercise in the treatment of NIDDM. Applications for GDM? *Diabetes.* 1991;40(suppl 2):175-178.

57. Rockhill B, Willett WC, Manson JE, et al. Physical activity and mortality: a prospective study among women. *Am J Public Health.* 2001;91(4):578-583.

58. Paffenbarger RS, Jr., Hyde RT, Wing AL, Hsieh CC. Physical activity, all-cause mortality, and longevity of college alumni. *N Engl J Med.* 1986;314(10):605-613.

59. Fried LP, Kronmal RA, Newman AB, et al. Risk factors for 5-year mortality in older adults: the Cardiovascular Health Study. *JAMA.* 1998;279(8):585-592.

60. Hsieh SD, Yoshinaga H, Muto T, Sakurai Y. Regular physical activity and coronary risk factors in Japanese men. *Circulation.* 1998;97(7):661-665.

61. Löllgen H, Böckenhoff A, Knapp G. Physical activity and all-cause mortality: an updated meta-analysis with different intensity categories. *Int J Sports Med.* 2009;30(3):213-224.

62. Lee DC, Sui X, Ortega FB, et al. Comparisons of leisure-time physical activity and cardiorespiratory fitness as predictors of all-cause mortality in men and women. *Br J Sports Med.* 2011;45(6):504-510.

63. Sesso HD, Paffenbarger RS, Jr., Lee IM. Physical activity and coronary heart disease in men: The Harvard Alumni Health Study. *Circulation.* 2000;102(9):975-980.

64. Swain DP, Franklin BA. Comparison of cardioprotective benefits of vigorous versus moderate intensity aerobic exercise. *Am J Cardiol.* 2006;97(1):141-147.

65. Manson JE, Hu FB, Rich-Edwards JW, et al. A prospective study of walking as compared with vigorous exercise in the prevention of coronary heart disease in women. *N Engl J Med.* 1999;341(9):650-658.

66. Weinstein AR, Sesso HD, Lee IM, et al. The joint effects of physical activity and body mass index on coronary heart disease risk in women. *Arch Intern Med.* 2008;168(8):884-890.

67. Leon AS, Myers MJ, Connett J. Leisure time physical activity and the 16-year risks of mortality from coronary heart disease and all-causes in the Multiple Risk Factor Intervention Trial (MRFIT). *Int J Sports Med.* 1997;18 Suppl 3:S208-215.

68. Sattelmair J, Pertman J, Ding EL, Kohl HW III, Haskell W, Lee IM. Dose response between physical activity and risk of coronary heart disease: a meta-analysis. *Circulation.* 2011;124(7):789-795.

69. Church TS, Earnest CP, Skinner JS, Blair SN. Effects of different doses of physical activity on cardiorespiratory fitness among sedentary, overweight or obese postmenopausal women with elevated blood pressure: a randomized controlled trial. *JAMA.* 2007;297(19):2081-2091.

70. Byers T, Nestle M, McTiernan A, et al. American Cancer Society guidelines on nutrition and physical activity for cancer prevention: reducing the risk of cancer with healthy food choices and physical activity. *CA Cancer J Clin.* 2002;52(2):92-119.

71. Ruiz JR, Sui X, Lobelo F, et al. Muscular strength and adiposity as predictors of adulthood cancer mortality in men. *Cancer Epidemiol. Biomarkers Prev.* 2009;18(5):1468-1476.

72. Holmes MD, Chen WY, Feskanich D, Kroenke CH, Colditz GA. Physical activity and survival after breast cancer diagnosis. *JAMA.* 2005;293(20):2479-2486.

73. Halle M, Schoenberg MH. Physical activity in the prevention and treatment of colorectal carcinoma. *Dtsch Arztebl Int.* 2009;106(44):722-727.

74. Pescatello LS, Franklin BA, Fagard R, et al. American College of Sports Medicine position stand. Exercise and hypertension. *Med Sci Sports Exer.* 2004;36(3):533-553.

75. Barlow CE, LaMonte MJ, Fitzgerald SJ, Kampert JB, Perrin JL, Blair SN. Cardiorespiratory fitness is an independent predictor of hypertension incidence among initially normotensive healthy women. *Am J Epidemiol.* 2006;163(2):142-150.

76. Manson JE, Rimm EB, Stampfer MJ, et al. Physical activity and incidence of non-insulin-dependent diabetes mellitus in women. *Lancet.* 1991;338(8770):774-778.

77. Meisinger C, Lowel H, Thorand B, Doring A. Leisure time physical activity and the risk of type 2 diabetes in men and women from the general population. The MONICA/KORA Augsburg Cohort Study. *Diabetologia.* 2005;48(1):27-34.

78. Weinstein AR, Sesso HD, Lee IM, et al. Relationship of physical activity vs body mass index with type 2 diabetes in women. *JAMA.* 2004;292(10):1188-1194.

79. Sieverdes JC, Sui X, Lee DC, et al. Physical activity, cardiorespiratory fitness and the incidence of type 2 diabetes in a prospective study of men. *Br J Sports Med.* 2010;44(4):238-244.

80. Gordon DJ, Probstfield JL, Garrison RJ, et al. High-density lipoprotein cholesterol and cardiovascular disease. Four prospective American studies. *Circulation.* 1989;79(1):8-15.

81. Williams PT, Haskell WL, Vranizan KM, Krauss RM. The associations of high-density lipoprotein subclasses with insulin and glucose levels, physical activity, resting heart rate, and regional adiposity in men with coronary artery disease: the Stanford Coronary Risk Intervention Project baseline survey. *Metabolism.* 1995;44(1):106-114.

82. Haskell WL, Lee IM, Pate RR, et al. Physical activity and public health: updated recommendation for adultsfrom the American College of Sports Medicine and the American Heart Association. *Med Sci Sport Exer.*2007;39(8):1423-1434.

83. Dishman RK, Rooks CR, Thom NJ, Motl RW, Nigg CR. Meeting U.S. Healthy People 2010 levels of physicalactivity: agreement of 2 measures across 2 years. *Ann Epidemiol.* 2010;20(7):511-523.

84. Sui X, LaMonte MJ, Laditka JN, et al. Cardiorespiratory fitness and adiposity as mortality predictors in old-eradults. *JAMA.* 2007;298(21):2507-2516.

85. Farrell SW, Finley CE, Radford NB, Haskell WL. Cardiorespiratory fitness, body mass index, and heart failure mortality in men: Cooper Center Longitudinal Study. *Circ Heart Fail.* 2013;6(5):898-905.

86. Manson JE, Greenland P, LaCroix AZ, et al. Walking compared with vigorous exercise for the prevention of cardiovascular events in women. *N Engl J Med.* 2002;347(10):716-725.

87. Lee IM, Shiroma EJ, Lobelo F, et al. Effect of physical inactivity on major non-communicable diseases world-wide: an analysis of burden of disease and life expectancy. *Lancet.* 2012;380(9838):219-229.

88. Loustalot F, Carlson SA, Fulton JE, Kruger J, Galuska DA, Lobelo F. Prevalence of self-reported aerobic physical activity among U.S. States and territories--Behavioral Risk Factor Surveillance System, 2007. *J Phys Act Health.* 2009;6(suppl 1):S9-S17.

89. Matthews CE, Chen KY, Freedson PS, et al. Amount of time spent in sedentary behaviors in the United States, 2003-2004. *Am J Epidemiol.* 2008;167(7):875-881.

90. Pratt M, Macera CA, Wang G. Higher direct medical costs associated with physical inactivity. *Phys Sportsmed.*2000;28(10):63-70.

91. Lobelo F, Duperly J, Frank E. Physical activity habits of doctors and medical students influence their counselling practices. *Br J Sports Med.* 2009;43(2):89-92.

92. Dunn AL, Trivedi MH, Kampert JB, Clark CG, Chambliss HO. The DOSE study: a clinical trial to examine efficacy and dose response of exercise as treatment for depression. *Control. Clin. Trials.* 2002;23(5):584-603.

93. Dunn AL, Trivedi MH, Kampert JB, Clark CG, Chambliss HO. Exercise treatment for depression: efficacy and dose response. *Am J Prev Med.* 2005;28(1):1-8.

94. McAuley E, Courneya KS, Lettunich J. Effects of acute and long-term exercise on self-efficacy responses in sed-entary, middle-aged males and females. *Gerontologist.* 1991;31(4):534-542.

95. McAuley E, Bane SM, Mihalko SL. Exercise in middle-aged adults: self-efficacy and self-presentational out-comes. *Prev Med.* 1995;24(4):319-328.

96. McAuley E, Lox C, Duncan TE. Long-term maintenance of exercise, self-efficacy, and physiological change in older adults. *J Gerontol.* 1993;48(4):P218-P224.

97. Allison MJ, Keller C. Self-efficacy intervention effect on physical activity in older adults. *West J Nurs Res.* 2004;26(1):31-46.

98. Ayotte BJ, Margrett JA, Hicks-Patrick J. Physical activity in middle-aged and young-old adults: the roles of self-efficacy, barriers, outcome expectancies, self-regulatory behaviors and social support. *J Health Psychol.* 2010;15(2):173-185.

3

Statistics for
Clinical Epidemiology

Ashley S. Long, PhD, LAT, ATC and Melanie Adams, PhD, CSCS, AT-Ret

CHAPTER OBJECTIVES

- Determine if a study is correlational or experimental from the abstract and relate the study design to the level of evidence the article provides.
- Understand basic statistical concepts, such as mean, median, confidence interval (CI), and significance.
- Interpret statistics that report incidence, risk, and effect of treatment.
- Describe common types of sample bias and identity the potential for error within a study.

INTRODUCTION

A single research study is not proof of a treatment's effect. To establish evidence for a particular treatment or intervention, several research studies must come to a similar conclusion. It takes more than 1 or 2 studies supporting a hypothesis. Instead, the majority of the literature (published studies on a single topic) need to agree for a hypothesis to become evidence-based practice. Not all research studies are equally weighted. Some types of studies are stronger than others and count more in terms of evidence for or against a specific treatment. When researchers begin work on a new topic, they start at the lower levels and build support for their hypothesis by testing it at each level until they have established a clear cause-and-effect relationship between the treatment and the outcome.

Adams M, Swiger W.
Epidemiology for Athletic Trainers: Integrating
Evidence-Based Practice (pp 41-63).
© 2016 Taylor & Francis Group.

Figure 3-1. Greater overlap implies greater association between two separate variables.

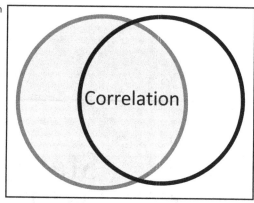

Relationships Between Variables

The goal of any research study is to examine the relationship between the independent and the dependent variable(s). The variable that causes or influences the change is called the *independent variable*, and the variable that is measured for change is the *dependent variable* or *outcome*. Independent variables are controlled by the researcher. A good way to learn the difference between the variables is that the dependent variable depends on the other, and the independent variable is independent of change.

The type of study used to examine this relationship determines how much one can learn about the relationship. To examine relationship, one must first examine descriptive data. With descriptive data, the researcher aims to determine whether a certain condition exists and, in terms of epidemiology, its prevalence. For example, a researcher reviews injury data and identifies how many cases of a particular injury occurred in a group of athletes.

After the researcher collects descriptive data, he or she may want to examine the possible relationship between variables. They may be correlated or associated. When 2 variables are correlated, they are occurring at the same time and are linked together. Figure 3-1 shows 2 overlapping circles. Each circle represents a variable. The amount of overlap can be measured; the greater the overlap, the more strongly the 2 variables are associated with each other. Association does not mean causation; it means that 2 things are related and could impact each other. Cross-sectional studies are an example of a study design that is made to examine the association between 2 or more variables. In this type of study, the researcher only measures variables once, instead of multiple measures over a period of time. Imagine taking height, weight, and girth measurements on different athletes and then asking them how many days a week they exercise. The mathematical relationship between weight and number of days a week they exercise can be assessed by examining the data. They may have no relationship at all or be strongly related based on the value of the correlation coefficient (from 0.00 to 1.00). Even if they are strongly related (values of .7 or greater), the researcher cannot say exercise causes lower or higher weight, but he or she can just that they are correlated.

The second relationship has the most influence on clinical decision making. It is called *cause and effect*, or *causal*. This relationship is harder to establish because the researcher has to control for all other possible reasons a specific outcome might occur. A cause-and-effect relationship is one in which one variable causes a change in the other variable (Figure 3-2). When an athletic trainer applies ice to an acute injury, he or she is trying to change something about the athlete's condition. The ice is the independent variable, and clinical measures, such as pain or range of motion (ROM), are the dependent variables.

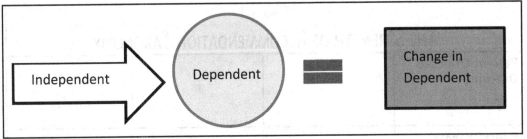

Figure 3-2. Cause-and-effect: Independent variable causes change in the dependent variable.

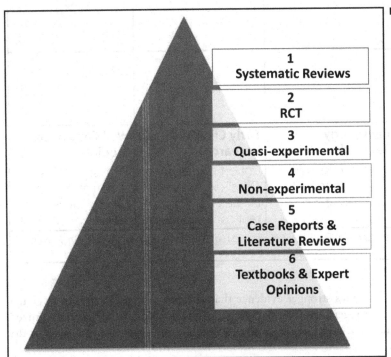

Figure 3-3. Evidence pyramid.

LEVELS OF EVIDENCE

The 6 levels of evidence form the shape of a pyramid (Figure 3-3). The base, level 6, provides the least amount of evidence. Included in this level are expert opinions and textbooks. One step up, level 5, are narrative reviews and case reports. Level 4 studies are those in which the researcher was not trying to change the dependent variable but, rather, examine its existence and look for possible correlations to other variables. Descriptive, cross-sectional, and longitudinal cohort studies are all nonexperimental and are level 4 evidence. Level 3 is quasiexperimental research. Here, the researcher is testing for a cause-and-effect relationship between an independent and a dependent variable but does not use a control group or did not randomly assign participants to treatment groups. Level 2 evidence consists of randomized, controlled trials (RCTs). These studies are stronger because participants are randomly put into treatment and control groups, which decreases the bias that participants have for a treatment. The strongest type of RCT is one in which neither the participants nor the researchers taking the measurements know to which group a participant is assigned. This is called a *double-blind RCT* and is used when testing prescription drug treatments. Within levels 3 to 5, there are strength differences, as well. For example, a narrative

TABLE 3-1 THE STRENGTH OF RECOMMENDATION TAXONOMY			
Patient-Oriented Outcomes Pain, RTP, cost, quality of life		B	A
Injury/Disease Markers Screening tests, bilateral deficit, ROM, strength		C	
Risk Factors Injury history, biomechanics, position, gender, level			
	Physiology Research Descriptive studies Case reports Clinical opinion	**Early Clinical Research** Cohort studies Quasi-experiments Limited or inconsistent controlled trials	**Well Controlled Studies** Consistent RCTs Systematic reviews Meta-analysis

Reprinted with permission from Slawson DC, Reed SW. Finding high-quality review articles. *Am Fam Physician.* 2009;15;79(10):875-877.

review or literature review provides stronger evidence than a case report in level 5. In level 4, a longitudinal cohort study is stronger than a cross-sectional study. A study with 2 nonrandomized groups provides better cause-and-effect evidence than a single group pre- to postdesign in the quasiexperimental studies.

The top level is for systematic reviews. Two types of studies are included here. The first is a meta-analysis, which combines the data of several RCTs to determine the effect size a particular independent variable has on a dependent variable. The second, called a *systematic review*, is a position paper. These are detailed literature reviews conducted by a group of experts that determines what the standard of care should be for clinicians in their field. The National Athletic Trainers' Association has produced several position papers in the past decade that set the standard of care for athletic trainers. Other medical organizations, such as the American Medical Association and American Physical Therapy Association, also develop practice guidelines with position papers. Often in position papers, the authors use another system besides the evidence pyramid to grade the support for practice standards. One such system is called the *Strength of Recommendations Taxonomy*. This system considers the strength of the study design and the type of dependent variables measured in the study. Measures that are closely tied to patient outcomes, such as changes in symptoms, level of function, cost, or quality of life, are given more weight than disease markers and risk factors. Using a grid (Table 3-1), the Strength of Recommendation Taxonomy grades the evidence as A, B, or C.

UNDERSTANDING THE DATA AND RESULTS

Information collected by researchers and clinicians about how well a patient is doing is called *data*. Quantitative data, which use numbers, can be gathered in several ways. Rating scales, such as a pain scale (0 to 10); graded performance, such as manual muscle testing (0 to 5); or number of errors (0 to 10) on a balance test are ways of measuring an aspect of someone's health or performance. Qualitative data are word based and not represented by a number. Qualitative research considers individual experiences and beliefs to increase understanding about a topic. This type of data is not analyzed statistically but is sometimes included in a study to help explain why patients did or did not do as expected.

Four types of data are used statistically. The first is nominal. These data categorize participants into groups. The groups are discrete, meaning that each participant can only belong to one group. Questions or tests that have yes or no answers produce nominal data. For example, the results of an x-ray are positive or negative. Ordinal data are the second type. This is a way of ranking a set of outcomes based on frequency, preference, or strength. Think of this as a team's seating in a tournament. Teams are ranked according to their record. The number one team may be way better than the number 2 team, but the team in third is just a little below second place. The key to ordinal data is that the distances between the numbers are not equal. For example, an athletic trainer might be asked to rank a list of modalities in order of most used to least used. The number assigned to the modality is the data. Although the numbers follow in successive order, they do not represent exactly how often they are used, and one cannot say that modality number 4 was used twice as much as modality number 2. The next type of data is called *interval*. Intervals are equally spaced numbers on a scale so that one is the same distance from 2 as 2 is from 3. Surveys that ask you to rate your level of agreement from 1 (strongly disagree) to 5 (strongly agree) are creating interval data. Ratio data are the last type and are similar to interval data. However, ratio data include zero, so that a score can be compared in multiples of another score. For example, one athlete could jump twice as high as another athlete—24 vs 12 inches. As with interval data, the distances between numbers are equal. Ratio and interval data are analyzed using parametric statistics. Nominal and ordinal data are used in nonparametric statistics.

Parametric statistics are based on the idea that data are normally distributed in a sample. This means that most people would score in the middle, and there will be roughly equal numbers of people above and below average. Figure 3-4 shows how a set of interval data would look if they were normally distributed. Because a normal distribution is assumed, parametric statistics examine the means and distances from the means (standard deviations [SDs]) of a particular measurement. Parametric statistics assess the probability of a piece of data being a certain distance from the mean and produce results that are used in comparisons.

Nonparametric data do not distribute normally because the choices were limited. If putting students in groups by grade in school, you would have a group of seventh graders, a group of eighth graders, and a group of ninth graders. There would be no one between the 3 distinct grades (Figure 3-5). Here, finding the average or mean grade does not tell you much about the students. Knowing how many were in each group (frequency) is more important. Nonparametric data use the frequency of answers to look for patterns and to find differences between groups.

Descriptive Statistics

Statistics that inform you about a set of participants or a measurement are descriptive. Statistics, such as the mean, median, and mode, tell you about the numbers in the middle of the distribution. The range and *SD* tell you how spread out the data are. The mean, or average, is an estimate of what was typical of the sample. If the mean score on a test is 82, that says that most people's results were near that 82; it does not mean that everyone scored an 82. The median is the number or score

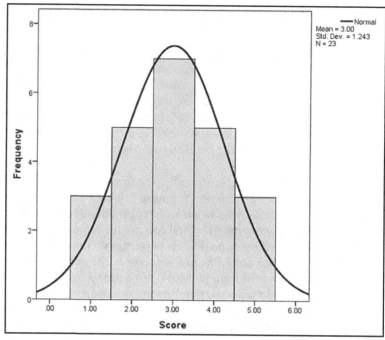

Figure 3-4. Normal distribution.

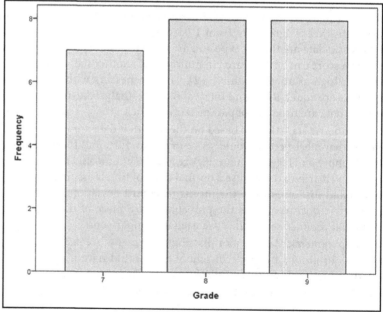

Figure 3-5. Non-parametric data do not distribute normally.

that is exactly middle of the range of the data, so that 50% of the data are below it and 50% are above it. This is why the median is sometimes referred to as the 50th percentile. The most common score in the sample is the mode. If 8 people took an examination and 5 people earned 85 points and 3 people earned an 80 points, then 85 points would be the mode. When data are normally distributed, the mean, median, and mode are all in the center of the normal curve (Figure 3-6).

Knowing how wide the numbers range in the data is as important as knowing the mean, median, or mode. The mean does not tell you how many people had high scores and how many people had low scores. Consider that the average of 60, 72, 86, 92, and 100 is 82. If you only looked at the

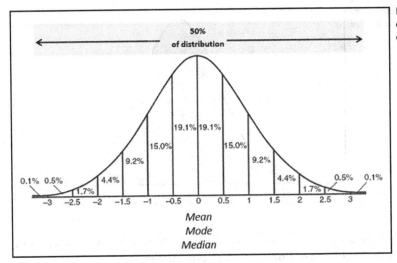

Figure 3-6. Percentages of data fall within each standard deviation.

mean, you would not know that one score was very low and one score was the highest possible. When there is a large range to the data, the mean is not a good representation of the sample. That is why the median is used when reporting data from a large population. Income, for example, is typically reported as the median of all incomes collected. *SD* is a commonly used statistic to describe the variation within a dataset. An *SD* represents a set distance from the mean. This distance could be to the right or left of the mean. *SDs* are reported as a ± after the mean. For example, the mean weight of a team is 165 lb with a *SD* of ± 1.5 looks like 165 ±1.5 lb. *SDs* are distances from the mean, not units, such as pounds. The numbers below the normal curve represent the *SDs* (see Figure 3-6). A specific percentage of the data will fall within each of the *SDs* based on a normal distribution. Data can be sectioned off into percentiles based on these percentages. Quartiles are a common way epidemiologists separate data and look for differences between people in the lowest quartile (bottom 25%) and the highest quartile (top 25%).

Inferential Statistics

Descriptive statistics provide general information about the study participants, but they do not test differences between groups or predict outcomes. Inferential statistics are tests that determine if there is a relationship between the independent and the dependent variables. Recall the difference between experimental and nonexperimental studies? Experiments show cause and effect, meaning that a change in the dependent variable was due to the independent variable. Cross-sectional and longitudinal cohort studies demonstrate how related the 2 variables are to each other. Each relationship has its own set of statistical tests. For example, the difference between pre- and post-treatment ROM in physical therapy patients can be evaluated by a *t*-test or analysis of variance (ANOVA). The relationship between patient pain and the number of treatments they have received can be tested by a Pearson correlation.

The term *statistically significant* is used when a relationship is unique or different from expected. In normally distributed data, you know that 68% of the data will fall within one *SD* of the mean. Ninety-six percent will be found between 2 *SDs* and 99% within 3 SDs. When the result of a statistical test is found at either end of the normal distribution, it is said to be significant because it is different than what would be found in the middle of the curve. Researchers set a threshold for significance prior to collecting data, called *alpha* (α). This is the probability that the result was not by chance. The lower the α, the farther away from the mean the result has to be to be significant. An $\alpha = 0.01$ means that there is a 99% probability that the results are not by chance. If the $\alpha = 0.05$, there is a 95% probability that the results are not a random accident. The α levels of some

Figure 3-7. Two-tailed test allows for chance of significance on each end of the curve.

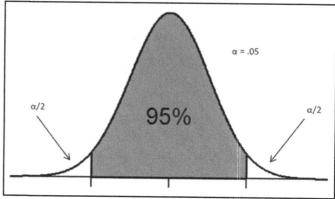

α = .05

α/2

95%

α/2

epidemiology studies can be very small (0.001 to 0.00001) because as the number of participants in the study increases, so does the likelihood of finding a significant relationship.

An inferential test can look for significance at one or both ends of the normal curve. These ends are called *tails*. A 2-tailed test means that half of the α value is placed on each end of the curve (Figure 3-7). A one-tail test takes all of the α and puts it on one side of the curve, giving it a better chance of finding a significant relationship on that particular side. One-tail tests are used when the researcher knows the direction of the relationship between the independent variable and the dependent variable. If you set up an experiment to examine the effect of a single ultrasound treatment on tendon extensibility, it seems obvious that any change in extensibility is going to be positive. You would use a one-tail test in this case. If you had no hypothesis about what would happen, a 2-tailed test would be appropriate.

Reading Statistics

Descriptive and inferential statistics are reported in the results section of a scientific article. This section is usually shorter than the other sections but is filled with Greek symbols, initials, tables, and graphs that can be confusing to the reader. Generally, the characteristics of the participants, such as age, weight, or activity level, are reported first using means (M) and SDs (s or SD). This is important information to have when considering to which type of patient (age, activity level, medical history, etc) the results can be applied. The M and SDs for the dependent variables are usually reported after the participant characteristics. Next, the researchers state the results of the inferential tests. Each test has been assigned a letter of the Greek alphabet (Table 3-2). If a test has a statistically significant result, the author will report the value for that test and the p-value (similar to α). For example, the ANOVA finds the value for f. A typical significant result would be written as $f(1,34) = 2.21, p = .03$. The numbers in parentheses are the degrees of freedom. The first is the number of groups minus 1. The second is the number of participants minus 1. The value of f was 2.21, which is significant because the p-value is less than .05. Prior to the study, the probability that a result is by chance is symbolized by α. After the study, an actual risk that the result is by chance is calculated, and p is its symbol. If the p-value is less than or equal to α, then the result is statistically significant. The term interaction is also used when discussing a study that has more than one treatment group. For example, if researchers were comparing the effect of static stretching to proprioceptive neuromuscular facilitation stretching, they would expect that ROM would increase in both groups and the posttreatment scores show some difference, but it is not clear if one treatment was really better. The interaction between the treatment group and the change in the dependent variable, in this case ROM from pre- to posttreatment, tells you if the treatment was the cause of the change. The ANOVA test is used to determine if there is a significant group × time interaction. When there is a significant change in the dependent variable and a significant

TABLE 3-2		
STATISTICAL SYMBOLS		
SYMBOL	**PRONUNCIATION**	**STATISTICAL TEST OR MEANING**
n	n	number of participants in the sample
M	mean	average of the data
s or SD	standard deviation	estimates the spread of the data
df	degrees of freedom	number of participants minus one
CI	confidence interval	range of 95% or 99% of the data
a	alpha	threshold for significance
r	rho	Pearson Product Moment Correlation
t	tee	T-test
f	f	Analysis of Variance (ANOVA)
x^2	chi-squared	Chi Goodness of Fit

TABLE 3-3					
MEANS, STANDARD DEVIATIONS, AND STATISTICAL SIGNIFICANCE					
	TREATMENT A **N = 40**			**CONTROL GROUP** **N = 24**		
	Baseline	Mid	Post	Baseline	Mid	Post
Pain rating	3.63±.69	3.36±.8$^{\#}$	3.61±.75$^{@}$	3.69±.75	3.39±.66$^{\#}$	3.27±.85*
Function score	3.78±.64	3.55±.67	3.59±.77	3.58±.87	3.35±.60	3.40±.80
Patient satisfaction	4.03±.93	3.54±.9$^{\#}$	3.88±.88$^{@}$	3.5±1.34	3.15±.97$^{\#}$	3.45±1.17$^{@}$
*baseline-post, p≤.05; #baseline to mid-point, p≤.05; @mid-point to post, p≤.05.					

group × time interaction, the author can conclude that the treatment was the cause of the change. Without a significant group × time interaction, the researcher cannot say that the treatment worked, even if there are significant improvements in the dependent variable.

Researchers also use tables and graphs to illustrate their data. Result tables contain the means and *SD*s for the outcome variables within the treatment groups. If the result has an asterisk (*) after it, that means the number is significantly different from another in the table. A key at the bottom of the table will provide the *p*-value and explain whether the difference was between the groups or a change from pre to post in a dependent variable (Table 3-3).

Graphs are another way to show relationships between the variables. They help illustrate differences between groups, changes in the dependent variable, and the direction of correlations between variables. Bar graphs are used for comparisons between groups and may contain multiple data points (pre, mid, and post) to show changes over time. The height of the bar represents the mean or the frequency of the measured variable. Some bar graphs include an estimate of the range of the data by adding a symbol that looks like a capital letter I to show the upper and lower limits of

Figure 3-8. Example of bar plot graph.

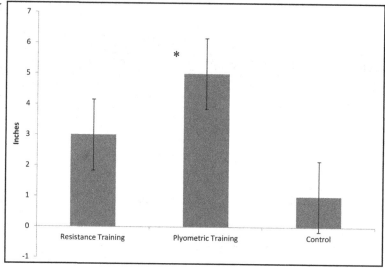

Figure 3-9. Dose-gradient graph.

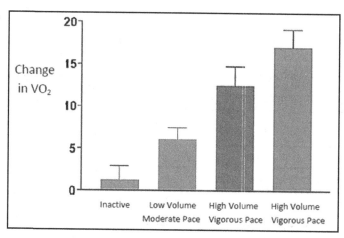

the data (Figure 3-8). When reading bar graphs, it is important to note the scale on the vertical (Y) axis. Differences between groups can be made to look larger than they are by decreasing the size of the scale. For example, if pain was the dependent variable and the scale was from 0 to 10, an author could exaggerate the difference between groups by narrowing the scale on the graph to 0 to 7. All statistically significant differences between groups are noted with an asterisk (*). Bar graphs that contain multiple levels of a treatment on the horizontal axis can illustrate dose-gradient and dose-response relationships. A dose-gradient graph shows increasing effects with greater exposures, or doses, of the treatment. For example, more intense exercise is related to greater improvements in oxygen uptake (Figure 3-9). The concept of dose-response is that there is a certain amount of a treatment that is needed to see a change in the dependent variable. This graph will show a step up or down at a particular level of the independent variable. Figure 3-10 illustrates the relationship between different volumes of physical activity and weight loss. While lower levels of physical activity are related to weight loss, there is a clear jump in the effect of physical activity on weight loss at 225 minutes/week.

The line graph is especially useful for showing relationships between 2 variables. These are common in nonexperimental research in which researchers are predicting the impact of risk factors on injury or disease. The direction and shape of the line defines the type of relationship. There

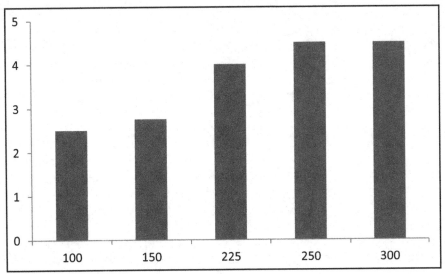

Figure 3-10. A jump in volume of weight loss occurs at exercising 225 minutes per week.

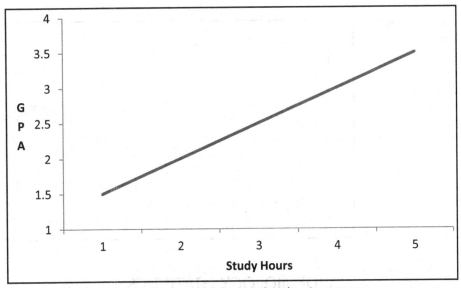

Figure 3-11. Positive correlation between study hours and grade point average.

are 3 general types of relationships between variables, including positive, negative, and curvilinear. Figure 3-11 shows a positive correlation between hours spent studying and grade point average; as study time increases, so does grade point average. This is also called a *linear relationship*. In a negative relationship, one variable increases as the other variable decreases. Another term for negative relationship is an *inverse relationship*, and the line slopes down to the right (Figure 3-12). The last type of relationship seen in line graphs is called *curvilinear*. Here, the relationship between the variables is more complex. At some points, the data are more strongly related than they are at other points (Figure 3-13). A curvilinear line is another way to illustrate a dose-response.

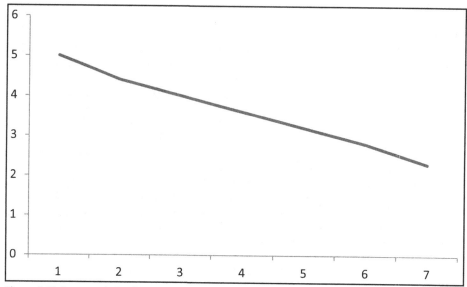

Figure 3-12. Inverse relationship.

Figure 3-13. Curvilinear relationship.

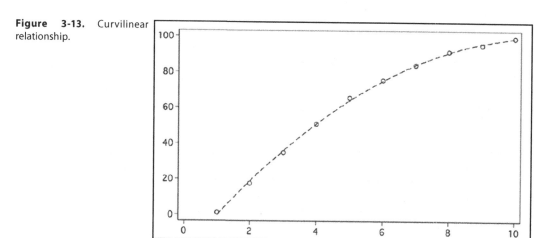

EPIDEMIOLOGY STATISTICS

Epidemiology is an important component of clinical practice. Gender, sport, time played, age, and other factors influence sport-related injuries. When athletes are exposed to their sport for a certain period of time, some conditions are more likely to arise; the risk depends on multiple factors. Physical characteristics, position played, surface type, etc, can contribute to the risk and rate of these injuries occurring. Athletic trainers should document injury occurrence, noting who is affected, identifying where and when injuries occur, and paying particular attention to what circumstances produce the best outcome.[1] Epidemiological data can inform special test selection, treatment parameters, prevention methods, etc. Clinicians must understand proper interpretation and usage of such information.

Incidence and Prevalence

Incidence and prevalence are commonly reported rates in injury literature. Incidence is a simple measure of the new cases occurring in a defined population over a specified period of time. It is a basic representation of risk. In athletics, the number of games and practices is typically multiplied by the number of players participating to quantify the population and exposure period.

These new cases contribute to the prevalence, a measure of the total number of cases in a population at risk during a specific period of time. There are 3 ways for the prevalence to change, including the following: there is an increase in onset of the condition (incidence), people are healed of the condition, or people with the condition die. The length of time to heal or die from the condition is described as duration. If the incidence rises, the prevalence rises, unless people are being healed or are dying at a higher rate than the new conditions are occurring. Because sports epidemiology is mainly focused on new cases, true prevalence statistics are not usually reported, and some authors use incidence and prevalence interchangeably.

Incidence and prevalence are often reported as rates of 100,000 people, but in athletic injury literature, there may be variations on reporting. Athlete exposure in games or training is multiplied by the number of players participating.[2] If one does not consider exposure when reporting incidence rates, one cannot reliably indicate the problem to compare injury incidence.

Another important factor of accurate reporting of incidence of injury involves the use of established definitions of injury. Objective, well-accepted measures should be used for coding and recording injuries. Best practices include having an individual record the information to increase intrarater reliability.[2]

For example, in a meta-analysis, Doherty et al[3] examined epidemiological studies about ankle injuries. They concluded that females experience a higher incidence of ankle sprains (13.6/1000 athlete-exposures [AEs]) than males (6.94/1000 AEs). They also reported that the highest incidence on ankle sprain was in indoor/court sports at 1.37/1000 AEs and 4.9/1000 hours of exposure. In this example, the authors are reporting incidence, or new cases, in a marked period of time. They are using exposure hours, which universally includes practices and competitions. They also report scores of the risk of ankle injury in a designated time frame (1000 hours). This example is a typical representation of epidemiological reporting on athletic injury.

Annual and Lifetime Prevalence

General medical and psychological concerns are reported in terms of annual or lifetime prevalence. Whereas a season of participation may define the time frame for athletes, the medical literature will use a longer period for reporting. Annual prevalence refers to an onset in the previous 12 months, and lifetime prevalence means any history of that illness or disease. Because lifetime prevalence covers a longer time period, it is significantly lower than annual prevalence data. For example, the lifetime prevalence of an eating disorder in adults in the United States is 4.7%, but the annual prevalence of eating disorders among the most at-risk group, teenagers, is 2.7%.

Validity of Clinical Tests

Clinical tests are an integral part of the injury evaluation. After a review of the patient's records, thorough history, and performance measures, the clinician will administer clinical diagnostic tests that may include the use of medical instruments or technology. Often, special tests and diagnostic tests have statistical information available to assist the clinician to properly implement and interpret the test. Through statistical analysis, one may discover that a test is not indicated or is best paired with others. A test's sensitivity and specificity must be taken into account when selecting a test and interpreting results. High sensitivity means the test correctly identifies those with the condition. High specificity means that the test rules out those without the condition. Both are important for an accurate diagnosis. Being an evidence-based clinician involves considering the

	+ Disorder	- Disorder
+ Test Result	True Positive (a)	False Positive (b)
- Test Result	False Negative (c)	True Negative (d)

Figure 3-14. 2×2 table test results.

available data about a clinical test and integrating it appropriately into the clinical examination. To be efficient, accurate, and effective, athletic trainers should research and use epidemiological evidence in their evaluations.

A 2×2 table is a useful tool to visualize clinical test results (Figure 3-14). Each box represents 2 pieces of information. First, it represents the test result being positive or negative. Second, it represents whether the patient has the condition. Therefore, box "a" represents a true positive, meaning the patient tested positive and truly has the disorder. Box "b" represents a false positive, meaning the patient tested positive when they did not have the condition. Box "c" represents a false negative, meaning the test result was negative, but the patient does have the condition. Therefore, the condition is undetected. Finally, box "d" represents a true negative, meaning the patient tested negative and does not have the condition. The information from the 2×2 table is used to calculate sensitivity and specificity. This statistical information is used to assist clinicians in knowing the strengths and weaknesses of diagnostic tests. Sensitivity and specificity are inversely proportional, meaning that if one goes up, the other goes down.[4] One cannot have a clinical test that has high specificity and sensitivity. Therefore, a combination of tests is often recommended.

Sensitivity: A test with high sensitivity is effective as correctly classifying the patient with the condition. Therefore, if a condition is suspected, and a special test with a high sensitivity is administered and yields a positive result, the clinician can feel confident that the patient has that condition. Sensitivity is expressed as a percentile and can be calculated using the following formula:

$$\text{Sensitivity} = \frac{\text{Patients without the condition who test positive}}{\text{All patients without the condition}}$$

Using the 2×2 table, the formula is Sensitivity = a / (a + c) × 100.

When a clinician obtains a negative result using a highly sensitive test, the clinician can have a high level of confidence that the condition can be ruled out. This concept is termed *SnNOut*. SnNOut is an acronym for sensitive (Sn), negative (N), condition ruled out (Out). Highly sensitive tests are good at identifying people with the condition.

An example of this from daily life could be drawn from going through security at the airport. Say there have been several threats of attack, and security is heightened. The metal detectors are turned on high and will beep, even with the smallest infraction. So, whereas a belt buckle may not have set it off in the past, even a small earring back will now trigger the alarm on the detector. Therefore, if someone passes through the detector and it does not beep (a negative test), one can be sure that they are not carrying a metal weapon. Because the detector has high sensitivity and there was a negative result, one can feel confident that the individual is not carrying a weapon. However, many people may receive a false positive, meaning that they receive a beep when they are not carrying a weapon.

Specificity: A test with high specificity is effective at correctly categorizing patients without the condition. Therefore, if a condition is suspected and a special test with a high specificity is

Term	Qualities	Questions Answered
Sensitivity	Good at detecting patients with the condition	"What is the probability that a test will indicate the condition among those with the condition?"
Specificity	Good at detecting patients without the condition	"What is the probability that the test will be negative in those without the condition?"

Figure 3-15. Descriptions of sensitivity and specificity.

administered and yields a positive result, the clinician can feel confident that the patient has that condition. Specificity is expressed as a percentile and can be calculated using the following formula:

$$\text{Specificity} = \frac{\text{Patients without the condition who test negative}}{\text{All patients without the condition}}$$

Using the 2×2 matrix, the formula for calculating specificity is Specificity = d / (d + b) × 100.

When a clinician obtains a positive result using a highly specific test, the clinician can have a high level of confidence that the condition can be ruled in. This concept is termed *SpPin* (Specific, Positive, In). Highly specific tests are good at correctly classifying people without the condition.

Here is an example using the Ottawa Ankle Rules. In 2013, Clifton et al[5] proposed a "Clinical Bottom Line" for the utilization of the Ottawa Ankle Rules. A meta-analysis revealed that the Ottawa Ankle Rules have a high sensitivity of 98.5%. Specificity ranges from the meta-analysis ranged from 26% to 50%. That is, if the clinician obtains a negative result using the Ottawa Ankle Rules, he or she can feel confident in ruling out an ankle fracture. The high sensitivity levels of this clinical prediction rule make it valuable in determining when to avoid referral. The authors noted that the poor specificity indicates that positive findings may not indicate a fracture and should not inform the clinician's decision-making process. This is a good display of the inverse relationship of sensitivity and specificity, as well as the proper and improper usage of a clinical test in decision making. Figure 3-15 provides the qualities and uses for sensitivity and specificity.

Predicting Risk

A large aspect of athletic training focuses on prevention. Knowledge of what increases risk of injury or illness is essential to preventing these events. Characteristics that contribute to predicting future outcomes are called *prognostic factors*. Predictors of adverse events are called *risk factors*. Risk can increase due to intrinsic factors, such as gender or body composition, or extrinsic factors, such as environment or equipment.

Relative Risk

In epidemiology, *relative risk* (RR) is the ratio of the probability of developing a disorder when exposed to a certain condition (risk factor), vs the risk of developing a disorder when not exposed to a risk factor. The RR of a condition can range from zero to infinity and is compared to a reference group, which has an RR of 1. Prospective longitudinal cohort studies collect data at baseline

	ACL injuries (3)	Athletic Exposures (5940) *(15 games + 120 practices) x 44 players*
Female	A (2)	B (2835)
Male	C (1)	D (3105)

Figure 3-16. 2×2 table showing the occurrence of ACL injuries and athletic exposures in male and female athletes.

and follow participants over months and years documenting which injuries occur. The RR of an injury is calculated by dividing the incidence of the exposed by the incidence of the unexposed. Sports epidemiologists consider exposed participants to be those who have the risk being examined for instance, a particular sport, position, or gender. The unexposed group is typically all other athletes in the study. Rather than just counting the number of players, one multiplies the number of players by the number of times they participate. This is called AE and can be defined as days or hours of participation.

The 2×2 table is the easiest way to calculate RR. Figure 3-16 shows the frequency of anterior cruciate ligament (ACL) injuries among one school's men's and women's soccer teams and their days of exposures (practices + games × # of players). The women's team had one more ACL injury than the men's team, but incidence does not describe the risk. RR compares groups or risk factors to each other to find the highest and lowest risk. In this case, males are the reference group (RR = 1), and females had a higher RR at 2.19. Although the incidence of an ACL injury was twice as high in the female soccer players, the actual risk of injury was more than 2 times that of the male players.

$$RR = \frac{A \div (A+B)}{C \div (C+D)}$$

$$RR = \frac{2 \div 2837}{1 \div 3106}$$

$$RR = \frac{0.0007049}{0.0003219}$$

$$RR = 2.19$$

Beynnon et al[6] reported a similar RR for females (2.10) and found a higher risk for ACL tears in college athletes (RR = 2.38) than high school athletes over 3 seasons. This study also examined the risk of ACL injury between 7 sports. Field hockey had the lowest RR at 0.47, and volleyball had the highest at 2.57. A RR less than 1 means a lower risk compared to the reference group. Compared to lacrosse athletes (RR = 1), field hockey athletes had half the risk of ACL injury.

Odds Ratio

The *odds ratio* (OR) expresses the odds that a patient with a risk factor had a condition/disorder as compared to the odds for a patient without that risk factor. OR can be expressed from the

	+ Ankle Injury (n=40)	- Ankle Injury (n= 360)
+ Air Cells in Shoe	A (26)	B (120)
- Air Cells in Shoe	C (12)	D(240)

Figure 3-17. Example of 2×2 table.

		Disease	
		Yes	No
Cohort	Exposed	a	b
	Unexposed	c	d

Figure 3-18. A 2×2 table can be used to calculate attributable risk.

numbers zero to infinity. Values less than 1 are classified as decreased odds. Values greater than 1 represent increased odds. An OR of 1 had no better chance of developing the condition than not. Retrospective longitudinal cohort studies, also known as case-control studies, use OR.

A 2×2 table can also be used to calculate OR. Let us create a 2×2 table representing the risk of ankle sprain related to the presence of air cells in the heel of the shoes (Figure 3-17). McKay et al[7] found that players wearing shoes with air cells in the heel were 4.3 times more likely to injure an ankle that those without. Hypothetically, 26 of the 40 injured athletes had air cells in their shoes and 12 did not. Also, 120 of the uninjured had air cells in their shoes, and 240 did not.

$$OR = \frac{AD}{BC}$$

$$OR = \frac{26x\ 240}{120\ x12}$$

$$OR = \frac{6240}{1440}$$

$$OR = 4.33$$

This means that athletes wearing shoes with air cells in the heel are 4.3 times more likely to injure an ankle than those wearing shoes without air cells. ORs can be helpful for the prediction and prevention of injury in athletes.

Attributable Risk

Attributable risk is defined as the difference in the rate of a disorder between an exposed population compared to an unexposed population. Using a cohort study design 2×2 table (Figure 3-18), the attributable risk can be calculated using the following formula:

Attributable Risk = Incidence in exposed individuals − Incidence in unexposed individuals or
Attributable Risk = a / (a + b) − c / (c + d)

Attributable risk is a valuable tool when measuring potential savings that would occur if the risk factor were removed in a population of patients.[8] By removing or attenuating risk factors, one can promote health and reduce injury.

Effect of Treatment

When treating patients, it is helpful to know the predictors of recovery. The clinician's understanding of effect size and numbers needed to treat (NNT) can assist him or her in knowing how likely a treatment is to be effective.

Prognosis Factors

A *prognosis* is the prior knowledge of the outcome of a condition, injury, or disease. A prognostic factor influences the chance of recovery from a condition or the chance of it recurring. These factors can be situational, conditional, or a patient characteristic. Often, many prognostic factors can assist the clinician in predicting the patient outcome. Some may be related to the injury or condition itself. For example, one can make return-to-play estimations based upon the severity of the injury, knowing that more severe injuries take longer to heal. However, other factors are related to the patient, such as age, gender, compliance to treatment, etc. Factors can be favorable, and lead to improved outcomes, or poor, and lead to decreased outcomes.

There is a difference between risk factors and prognostic factors. Risk factors are associated with causing the condition, whereas prognostic factors are those that influence the outcome. Therefore, risk factors are determined by examining the new cases, but prognostic factors are established by tracking and following up with those who have already suffered from the condition.[9]

Effect Size

Effect size is the amount of difference between 2 groups. Often, statistical significance is reported, and the authors make a conclusion on whether there is a statistical difference that exists between 2 groups. Less often, the size of the difference between groups is reported. Effect size can provide valuable information to the clinician because it provides commentary as to what degree a treatment, for example, is effective. It is a scale-free measure; therefore, it can interpret the size of the difference between groups no matter which units are being measured.

The problem with using statistical significance as a measure of effectiveness is that a *p*-value depends on the size of the effect and the size of the sample. If the effect was large but the sample was small, one would get a significant result. Or, if the effect was small, but the sample was large, one might calculate statistical significance. Therefore, differences between groups may be a function of the sample size, rather than the true effectiveness of the intervention. Often, the effect size is reported using a 95% CI, which is the equivalent of significance at $p \leq .05$. The benefit of effect size is that studies can be compared retrospectively using a meta-analysis, and the effect sizes can be compared and averaged.[10] Effect size provides a common comparison, even when studies have varying samples and designs.

Number Needed to Treat

The *NNT* provides the clinician with the number of patients he or she would need to treat with the intervention to prevent one event. More practically, it represents the proportion of patients likely to have treatment-specific effects. It is used as a measure of the effectiveness of an intervention and goes beyond statistical significance to assist the clinician in practice decisions. Similar to effect size, it is easy to compare between interventions. The NNT is a treatment-specific measure, comparing the treatment group to a control group in gaining a certain clinical outcome. To calculate and apply NNTs to clinical practice, clear clinical outcome measures must be used. NNTs established from systematic reviews of RCTs provide the highest level of evidence; therefore, an effort should be made to use NNTs that have been established by sound scientific techniques. Specific criteria of quality, validity, and size must be met before analyzing the NNT.

The best NNT is equal to 1. This would mean that everyone who experienced the treatment benefited as compared to the control group in which no one experienced an improved outcome. The worst NNT is -1, meaning that no one improved with the treatment and everyone improved on their clinical outcome in the control group. A well-defined NNT should include specifics about the comparator, the clinical outcome, the duration of treatment, and the 95% CI. The NNT can be calculated using the following formula:

$$NNT = \frac{1}{(proportion\ benefiting\ from\ treatment) - (proportion\ benefiting\ from\ control)}$$

An example of an NNT statistic that is valuable to athletic trainers can be found in report by Sugimoto et al.[11] The authors determined that when implementing primary ACL injury prevention programs, the NNT was 120 to prevent 1 ACL injury. This may present a dilemma when trying to gain support of implementation of such a program. Because so much time and effort is required to produce one positive outcome, this NNT does not support the value of such conditioning programs. More researchers need to corroborate this finding, and improvements to training programs may decrease the NNT.

Bias and Errors in Research

No one study is absolute proof of a hypothesis. It takes multiple studies with increasingly stronger designs to provide evidence of relationships. However, the study design is only one element in determining the quality of a particular study. In addition to the type of evidence the article provides—cross-sectional, longitudinal, or experimental—one must consider the overall validity of the study and reliability of the measurements used in the study. Despite researchers' best efforts, it is impossible to produce a perfect study. The results of a study are limited by who the participants were and how the data were collected. The following section highlights a few of the most common problems found in research. When reading articles, one should ask how well the author controlled for these biases and errors.

Validity and Reliability

To evaluate the quality of a study, one must understand the difference between *validity* and *reliability*. If a test or scale measures what it was intended to measure, it is a valid measurement tool. Data produced by valid tools or tests are considered accurate, or true. Clinical measures are considered valid if they are close matches to the gold standard way of measuring a variable. For example, the 12-minute run is a valid test of cardiorespiratory fitness because there is a strong correlation between athletes' measured maximal oxygen consumption and their performance on the run. This is called *criterion validity*. Measures that cannot be validated by comparing to a criterion may still be valid if they are logical and based on well-established evidence. These measures have what is known as face validity and construct validity.

Reliability is sometimes confused with validity. A test or measure is reliable if it produces similar results time after time on the same participants under the same conditions. Consider a clinical skill, such as consistently grading manual muscle tests. The ability to apply the 0-to-5 scale fairly over and over is the reliability. Practice will improve one's intertester reliability on clinical measures, meaning that one has more consistency when taking measures. Intratester reliability is how one compares to another evaluator. Research studies often need several people to take the same measures on a sample. Ensuring that the intratester reliability is high adds credibility to the data. The validity and reliability of a measure can be determined using statistics. These correlations test how well the data match a criterion (validity) or a repeated test using the same measure (reliability). Some examples include standard error of estimate, Cronbach's alpha, interclass correlations, and kappa coefficients.

Threats to Reliability

In studies that test the effect of a treatment on a dependent variable, it is critical that the dependent variable be measured reliably. If the measurement tool is not reliable, the researcher cannot say for sure that a change in the dependent variable was due to the treatment. It could be the result of the instability of the measurements. This is why studies should only be conducted with measures that have proven reliability in the specific population (age, gender, athletic/nonathletic) with which the researcher is working.

Even when a test or survey is reliable, a study's procedures could reduce that reliability. For example, if a list of words is given to participants for a memory test and the same words are used on multiple occasions, it is likely that the participants will have learned the words. The improvement of participants over time in this case was not due to a treatment but, rather, due to exposure to the test. This is called a *learning effect* and is common with physical skills or tests that require comprehension or math. Researchers can reduce learning effects by changing the order of tests in the assessment, increasing the time between data collections, or using different versions of validated tests. Poor inter- and intratester reliability is a threat to reliability. Authors should report statistics that measured the reliability of evaluators and describe what procedures were used by the evaluators to insure consistency. Another common issue for reliability is participant fatigue. Especially with survey measures or tests that require physical exertion, participants' attention, interest, or motivation may decrease if the testing is too long. Ways to minimize fatigue include breaking long data collection sessions into smaller sections, allowing rest breaks between tests, and scheduling data collection early in the day.

Internal Validity

A test or survey is valid if it measures what it was intended to measure (ie, it is accurate). An entire study is considered valid if it really tested what it claimed to be testing. This is called *internal validity*. A research study lacks internal validity if there are problems with participants, reliability, validity of measurements, or uncontrolled variables. Sample bias is one of the most difficult aspects of internal validity for a researcher to control. Recruiting and keeping participants in a study is time consuming, and who participants are and how they were recruited plays a large part in how useful the data will be. Health care studies tend to attract volunteers who have an interest in the topic. They may have prior knowledge or beliefs that could influence their compliance or the outcome. For example, if a doctor is seeking participants for a study on the effects of surgery on regaining function, the length and degree of disability someone has experienced may make them more or less willing to participate. It is likely that those with longer histories and more complications will consider the surgery vs a patient who may do well with the surgery but feels that he or she should explore other options first. Particularly for studies that involve physical therapy, participants will assume that the exercise should be improving their scores and will give better effort to prove it or will rate their perceptions of pain or benefit more positively. The Hawthorne Effect occurs if participants are influenced by the attention given to them rather than the actual effect of the intervention. Another problem comes from participants who do not finish the study. Potentially, something about the people who drop out is different than the ones that stay in. It could be that they have more or less severe injuries, they do not think there was any benefit to the treatment, or they were less motivated to comply with the procedures. And, when participants leave control groups at higher rate than they do the treatment group, it makes comparisons difficult because the groups are less similar than they were at the start. Social desirability is also a

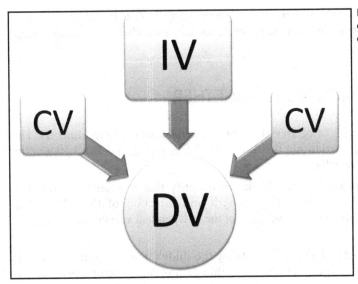

Figure 3-19. Independent and confounding variables influence dependent variables.

threat to internal validity. When participants provide self-reported data on health measures, such as exercise or diet or following medical orders, they tend to put themselves in the best light possible. They may not be consciously lying but have selective memory for how well they are doing with these behaviors. This is a key weakness of any study relying on survey data as the only measure of a dependent variable. A stronger method is to combine surveys with objective data (eg, measuring pain with a scale and counting the number of pain pills taken since the last visit).

An experiment or intervention with high internal validity has controlled for other factors that could change the dependent variable. These other factors are called *confounding variables*. A confounding variable is something besides the independent variable that could explain why a change occurred. If all confounding variables are not considered by the researcher beforehand, the conclusion is less reliable because there could be another cause-and-effect relationship besides the one between the independent and dependent variables. Figure 3-19 illustrates the relationship between the 3 variables. Imagine you are doing a study to see which treatment is better for delayed-onset muscle soreness pain—ice or heat. You measured the pain level of your participants before and after a 10-minute treatment. The treatment groups were randomized, and all participants had similarly high levels of pain 24 hours after the eccentric exercise. After treating one of the participants, he says to you that he does not think the ice or heat mattered as much as the ibuprofen he took this morning. You are panicked now because you realize that you did not control for any treatments the participants might have tried on their own. Without tight control over the confounding variables, you cannot say for certain that any decrease in pain was due to the treatment you provided.

There are 2 ways to control for confounding variables. But first, the researcher must identify as many factors that could impact the dependent variable as possible when planning the study. Then, they can use procedures that would minimize the effect. For example, in the delayed-onset muscle soreness study, you could have given participants clear instructions about what they could and could not do during the study. You could have double-checked this by asking participants prior to the treatment if they had taken anything for pain. The other option for controlling the influence of a third variable is to measure it during the study and use a special statistical analysis called *analysis of covariance*. This test allows you to see the effect of the independent variable on the dependent variable if the confounding variable is kept stable. This analysis is commonly used in epidemiology because there are many factors that could influence people's health. Age, gender, diet, education, occupation, level of physical activity, and medications are a few examples of confounding variables measured by researchers. If a confounding variable is found after the data has been collected, there is little that can be done about it, and the researcher has to acknowledge the error in their discussion.

BRINGING IT TOGETHER

- Research studies fall into 1 of 3 categories: descriptive, correlational, or experimental. The type of study is based on the relationship that the researcher is trying to define between the independent and dependent variable.

- The purpose of a descriptive study is to identify or quantify that a certain circumstance exists. A correlational study examines the strength and direction of the relationship between 2 variables. An experiment tests the effect of the independent variable on the dependent variable.

- The level of evidence provided is based on how strong the study's design is and how close it comes to showing a cause-and-effect relationship. Within each of the 6 levels there are stronger and weaker studies. Meta-analyses and position statements provide the best evidence for practice.

- Dose-gradient and dose-response are important concepts for clinicians. Each shows how the dependent variable reacts to changing levels of the independent variable. These are best shown with graphs. A dose-gradient is a linear relationship. The dose-response is a curvilinear relationship.

- Sports epidemiologists use RR and OR to show how much a risk factor increases the likelihood of injury. Attributable risk statistics show how much impact removing a risk factor has on the incidence of disease or injury. The NNT is another useful statistic that identifies how many patients must be given an intervention to prevent one occurrence.

- The term *statistical significance* means that the probability that the result was by chance is low. It is influenced by sample size so that larger numbers of study participants make it easier to find significant differences. For this reason, the effect size of a treatment is important to know. The larger the effect size, the more likely it is that an individual patient will notice an improvement.

- Reliability is the ability of a test or evaluator to produce consistent results when performed under the same conditions. Validity describes how well a test measures what it was intended to measure. Both are critical to the quality of a research study. Common problems for reliability and validity in research studies are sample bias, the Hawthorne Effect, social desirability, and confounding variables.

LEARNING ACTIVITIES

1. Calculate RR using data from your most recent athletic training clinical experience. Be sure to use the 2×2 table. Start with total injuries for the season and compare sports or genders.

2. How does NNT inform treatment selection and how has the use of modalities changed as research progresses? These two examples below illustrate both NNT and changes in modality use:

   - Olmsted LC, Vela LI, Denegar CR, Hertel J. Prophylactic ankle taping and bracing: a numbers-needed-to-treat and cost-benefit analysis. *J Athl Train.* 2004;39(1):95-100.

- Sugimoto D, Myer G, McKeon J, Hewett TE. Evaluation of the effectiveness of neuromuscular training to reduce anterior cruciate ligament injury in female athletes: a critical review of relative risk reduction and numbers-needed-to-treat analyses. *Br J Sports Med.* 2012;46(14):979-988.

REFERENCES

1. Caine DJ, Caine CG, Lindner KJ. *Epidemiology of Sports Injuries.* Champaign, IL: Human Kinetics; 1996:357-377.
2. Phillips LH. Sports injury incidence. *Br J Sports Med.* 2000;34(2):133-136.
3. Doherty C, Delahunt E, Caulfield B, Hertel J, Ryan J, Bleakley C. The incidence and prevalence of ankle sprain injury: a systematic review and meta-analysis of prospective epidemiological studies. *Sports Med.* 2014;44(1):123-140.
4. Parikh R, Mathai A, Changra Sekhar G, Thomas R. Understanding and using sensitivity, specificity and predictive values. *Indian J Opthalmol.* 2008;56(1):45-50.
5. Clifton D, Phan K, Zimmerman E. Utilizing Ottawa Ankle Rules to enhance clinical decision making. *NATA News.* 2013;24(3):42-43.
6. Beynnon BD, Vacek PM, Newell MK, et al. The effects of level of competition, sport, and sex on the incidence of first-time noncontact anterior cruciate ligament injury. *Am J Sports Med.* 2014;42(8):1806-1812.
7. McKay GD, Goldie PA, Payne WR, Oakes BW. Ankle injuries in basketball: injury rate and risk factors. *Br J Sports Med.* 2001;35(2):103-108.
8. Fleming ST. *Managerial Epidemiology: Concepts and Cases.* 2nd ed. Chicago, IL: Health Administration Press; 2008.
9. Phillps B. Risk vs. prognostic factors. *BMJ Blogs.* http://blogs.bmj.com/adc/2009/03/09/risk-vs-prognostic-factors/. Published March 9, 2009. Accessed May 28, 2014.
10. Coe R. It's the effect size, stupid: what effect size is and why it is important. http://www.leeds.ac.uk/educol/documents/00002182.htm. Published September 25, 2002. Accessed October 12, 2015.
11. Sugimoto D, Myer G, McKeon J, Hewett TE. Evaluation of the effectiveness of neuromuscular training to reduce anterior cruciate ligament injury in female athletes: a criticial review of relative risk reduction and numbers-needed-to-treat analyses. *Br J Sports Med.* 2012;46(14):979-988.

4

Injury Surveillance Systems

Wanda Swiger, EdD, ATC, CES

CHAPTER OBJECTIVES

- Identify and recall the basic concepts, terminology, and uses of injury and illness surveillance relevant to athletic training.
- Recognize the various Injury Surveillance Systems (ISSs) and describe the process for data collection in injury surveillance.
- Identify and describe measures used to monitor injury prevention strategies.
- Explain the importance of injury surveillance in identifying modifiable/nonmodifiable risk factors, mechanisms for injury, and injury prevention.
- Identify the issues surrounding surveillance that affect its validity.

INTRODUCTION

Participation in youth, interscholastic, and intercollegiate sports has increased over the past 3 decades and so has the incidence of sport-related injuries. In the United States (US), it is estimated that 20 to 30 million children (aged 5 to 17 years) participate in community youth sport programs.[3] Participation levels in National Collegiate Athletic Association (NCAA) athletics grew steadily for men (28%) and drastically for women (128%)[9] from 1981 to 2001. Sport-related injuries account for millions of visits to emergency departments by children and young adults. Injuries sustained by high-school athletes have resulted in more than 500,000 doctor visits, 30,000 hospitalizations, and a cost to the health care system of billions of dollars per year.[1,2] It is hypothesized that if one can understand the settings and mechanisms of these injuries, then sports medicine professionals can affect some control on these numbers.

Adams M, Swiger W.
Epidemiology for Athletic Trainers: Integrating Evidence-Based Practice (pp 65-81).
© 2016 Taylor & Francis Group.

As discussed in Chapter 1, epidemiology is the study of the distribution and determinants of disease. Epidemiological injury research involves the slow and thorough accumulation of precise data that can take years to obtain, and injury surveillance uses systematic methods for the rapid collection and dissemination of data. The most effective systems focus on an ongoing, embedded process that is easily used. Dependent on the methods, ISS can identify trends in sport injuries and evolve with new evidence to meet the changing needs of the sports medicine practitioners. Data collected on injury types, mechanisms of injury, IRs, body region, position, and predisposing risk factors are collected and analyzed to provide insight on sport safety. ISSs are important for several reasons.[2] They provide the following:

- Evidence for establishing prevention guidelines
- Rationale for rule or equipment changes
- Measures to define injury risk[2]

Exposure to risk is a critical component of ISS,[2] and consistency in data collection is critical to establishing rates of injury. Therefore, surveillance is thought to be the first step in preventing disease. Several surveillance systems request data to be collected by athletic trainers (high school, college, professional sport). Other systems use physicians and other health care professionals in hospitals and emergency departments,[2-4] and some community-based injury surveys have data reported by coaches.[2] Published sports injury articles are often difficult to interpret and compare because of different collection and/or analysis methods. Standard methods of data collection are needed for comparability and interpretation of data. Consensus on definitions would greatly improve the collection of comparable and reliable sports injury data. Specific issues regarding ISS data include the definition of a sports injury, how the population at risk is calculated (the denominator), and the method of data collection.[1] All sport ISSs should collect information about the rates of injuries, types of injuries, and mechanisms in a form that is relevant to a range of potential users (sport associations, sport governing agencies, physicians, athletic trainers, coaches, athletes, and parents) that allow for comparisons of trends, incidence, or risk.

BASIC COMPONENTS OF INJURY SURVEILLANCE

Over the past 40 years, injury data collection has increased the sports injury specialist's understanding of the nature and frequency of sport injuries. More recently, leaders in ISS data collection have identified the basic variables that are most valuable to enhancing this understanding. Consistent in surveillance systems are discrete variables, such as sport classification/type, activity type (practice/game), and mechanism of injury. Other components, such as defining an injury or determining the number of athlete-exposures (AEs), lack standardization. Although improved, ISS is not entirely uniform across collectors, agencies, or sports. Because of the lack of uniformity and standardization, surveillance systems can lack context.

Surveillance systems collect data that are used to identify risk factors associated with injury.[2] It answers the "who, what, where, when, and how" of a sports injury. The most common inquiries are which sport has the highest risk for injury, what are the most common injuries in sport, and what was the cause of the injury. However, deeper questions can be answered, such as the following:

- How do injuries vary based on playing position, gender, or from season to season?
- What types of injuries occur in which sports?
- Does the frequency of injury vary in practice vs game settings?
- Does the facility contribute to or limit injuries (ie, turf surface)?
- Do rules encourage or limit dangerous play?

- Is the use of certain equipment associated with more or fewer injuries?
- Is the physical condition of the athlete limiting or contributing to the frequency or severity of the injury?

Sport Classification

Nomenclature must be precise. Most classifications for surveillance systems are by sport name (ie, soccer, rugby, basketball, cheerleading).[2,7,8,12,14] Several classifications used in sport or epidemiology may not be consistently used in surveillance systems or may group sports based on similarities. Some terms include *noncontact, contact,* or *collision sport; team* or *individual;* or *equipment-intensive sport.* Some classifications come from the application of the surveillance data. For example, low risk, moderate risk, and high risk are used in determining the appropriate medical coverage.[28]

Type of Activity

Several surveillance systems request specific details about participation. Typically, this refers to variables, such as practice or game and position played.[2,7,8,12,14] This requires providing information regarding competition vs training injuries. Match or game exposure is defined as any activity that occurs between different teams or clubs. If a scrimmage is occurring within the same team, this would typically be defined as training or practice, unless specifically defined in the report. Training or practice exposure is team-based, noncompetition sessions. For most systems, a warmup pregame and cooldown postgame are also identified as training or practice. Individual training by the player who is unsupervised by the coach is not considered in surveillance. These injuries are not documented. Furthermore, any training exposure that is part of a player's rehabilitation is not considered training.[3,8,9]

When Did the Injury Occur?

Most surveillance systems require a time frame for the injury, based on when the activity occurred. This is typically the season (pre-, post-, or offseason). If the injury occurred during a tournament, the surveillance systems may request information regarding the round, heat, or group.[14] For example, a swimmer suffered a bicipital strain in the quarter final heat of a postseason competition. This information allows researchers to consider the role of fatigue in risk of injury. Designating time frames for injury has advanced the understanding of when injuries are more likely to occur.

Cause of Injury

The mechanism of injury is consistently reported.[2,7,8,12,14] Typically, one focuses on the extrinsic risk factors. The primary classifications are overuse, noncontact trauma, contact with opponent/teammate, contact with object (moving or stationary), and recurrent/previous injury.[14] Overuse is an injury that occurs due to repeated microtrauma with an insidious onset, meaning there was no single, identifiable event that caused the injury. Traumatic injuries are caused by a single, identifiable event, such as a collision with an opponent. Mechanisms can be further defined as noncontact, meaning there was no contact with another person or object, or contact, which are categorized as some degree of collision with another person, moving, or stationary object. The ISS may ask whether the action causing the injury was a violation of a sport rule.[8,14] These data allow people to track how well rules are implemented and followed and if they are effective in limiting injury. The type of surface played on or other environmental variables may be requested because they may have contributed to the mechanism. Playing surfaces can include types of grass, artificial grass or turf, or types of indoor playing surfaces or floor materials. Some surveillance systems may have a location for reporting hazards or worn surfaces (uneven surfaces) and weather if considered a factor (slippery surface).

Additional challenges arise when attempting to use surveillance data to research specific injuries, such as comparing noncontact and contact anterior cruciate ligament (ACL) injuries. These are additional terms, specific to an ACL injury, that appear to be inconsistent in the literature.[11] This focus in epidemiology is more on mechanism of injury or cause of injury. Most databases do not use these terms. Therefore, if epidemiologists want to investigate noncontact and contact anterior cruciate ligament injuries, this information would need to be added to the reporting information.

What Is a Definable Injury?

Clinically, definitions of injury often overlap with a diagnosis. An athletic trainer may evaluate and diagnose a basketball player with an injury based on the following:

- Location (ankle)
- Onset (acute [traumatic, macrotrauma] or chronic [insidious, overuse, microtrauma])
- Type of injury (sprain)
- Mechanism of injury (inversion)
- Severity (second degree)

This same clinician may determine severity of the injury by the following:

- Need for medical attention (evaluated and immediate treatment provided)
- Length of disability (restricted from practices and games for 3 days)
- Recurrence of injury (third ankle sprain in 8 months)

If the injury is a newly incurred injury, it should be reported. However, a recurrent or preexisting injury may be reported in some surveillance systems but not in others. The surveillance systems for international soccer records only new injuries.[14] There is much discrepancy regarding recurrent injury definitions and how they should be reported within ISS. Subsequent sport injuries may be coded[23] in ISS as the following:

- New injury = different location
- Local injury = same location but different type
- Recurrent injury = same location and same type

A clearer, standardized definition is needed for injury surveillance purposes. Within the international soccer ISS, an injury is defined as "any musculoskeletal complaint newly incurred due to competition or training that received medical attention."[8,14] This definition has several key variables that must be explored. First, it establishes all new injuries and excludes recurrent or preexisting injuries. Second, it excludes all nonmusculoskeletal injuries and illness. Third, it identifies all injuries requiring medical attention (not just injuries that resulted in time lost). However, medical attention is defined differently across surveillance systems (care provided by an athletic trainer vs referral to a physician). Fourth, it identifies when the injury occurred (training/practice or competition). Although competition is clearer and standard, training can be defined differently. Missing from this definition is a precise understanding of medical attention and training. One variable not included is time lost, meaning that an injury does not require missed participation to be counted.

As a result of surveillance systems, the term *reportable injury*[7-9,14] has been coined. Many systems define reportable differently and may link it to severity or time lost. There are several options for defining severity, including the following: by days of practice missed, games missed, or if a referral or hospitalization was required. Many ISSs arbitrarily base severity as days missed. Injuries resulting in restricted participation of 10+[9] days vs 30+[4] days have been reported as indicators of severity. The NCAA ISS requires time lost and needing medical attention in their definition of a reportable injury. The NCAA is more specific in its definition of an injury. Since 1995, a reportable injury has been defined as one that occurred as a result of participation in an organized intercollegiate event (practice or game, required medical attention (athletic trainer or physician), and restricted participation for more than 1 calendar day.[9]

A meaningful definition of injury should incorporate time lost from participation to reduce the bias associated with estimates of incidence.[1] However, systems that report all injuries are beneficial because studies of injury sequences support that minor injuries are often followed by moderate or major injuries, and acute complaints are a predictor of subsequent injuries.[23] The advantage of a broad definition of injury is that it allows for the assessment of the full spectrum of activities. A more narrow definition may assess musculoskeletal only, concussion only, or all dental injuries regardless of time lost but will likely exclude any chronic conditions, illnesses, or diseases. A clear definition within ISS decreases any misinterpretation by those collecting the data.

For best practice, a reportable injury should include the following multiple components:

- The injury occurred in a game or practice.
- The injury required medical attention.
- The injury resulted in a restriction or exclusion from participation for 1 or more days.[6-9,14]

Severity (Degree) of Injury

Some reporting systems may require additional severity information beyond the definition of reportable.[2,7,8,12-14] Additional classifications of injury severity are based on length of disability and are classified as mild (out of participation for <7 days)[2,7] or significant (out for ≥ 7 days).[2,7] More detailed ISS categorize severity as minor (1 to 7 days of absence), moderate (8 to 28 days of absence), and major (>28 days of absence).[13,29]

Severity is often defined by the number of days the athlete is withheld from participation. Some view time lost from sport as the main indicator of the severity of the injury,[8,14,20] and that time lost indirectly assesses severity.[3] Discrepancies often occur when coaches report injuries, which is typical of youth ISS. Seven days appears to be the most common time frame used in defining mild vs severe injury.[7] Usually, the day that an injury occurs is considered day zero and is not counted as time lost. For example, if a player is injured on Monday and returns to full participation the next day, Tuesday, the injury is reported as no time lost. An athlete who is unable to participate on Tuesday and Wednesday would be reported as 2 days of time lost. A career-ending injury is defined as an athlete who is unable to make a full return to sport.[8]

Location of Injury

Injuries can be classified by location (head), type (contusion), and body side.[2,7,8,12-14] Location of the injury refers to the area of the body that is affected.[2,7,8,12,14] There are main groupings by body region (head, upper limb, trunk, and lower limb) that are then divided into specific segments. For example, the main grouping for injury location may be the lower limb, with subcategories that include hip/groin, thigh, knee, lower leg/Achilles tendon, ankle, and foot/toe.[8] Body segments may also be combined into broader categories when the frequency of injury at a particular body area is low, such as with hand, wrist, and forearm injures. When using a coding system, such as the Orchard Sports Injury Classification System (OSICS), there are 24 injury locations and options for elaborating on the type of injury that the OSICS may identify, such as fracture, dislocation, etc.[17-19,24] Streamlined grouping is efficient for data collection. Issues may develop when users review longitudinal data to see trends for specific injuries because OSICS will denote knee sprain but will not denote knee medial collateral ligament sprain. Therefore, some systems add detail around the location and structure. For example, the 2003-2004 NCAA ISS for women's volleyball included a subcategory on knee injuries with knee structures identified (medial meniscus, lateral meniscus, ACL, posterior cruciate ligament, etc).[9]

Injury Classification

The tissue affected, rather than the location, is the main focus of injury diagnosis and care.[23] In surveillance systems, injury classification focuses on type of injury (contusion, sprain, strain). Injury type is summarized under a main heading (muscle, tendon, bone, ligament) and can be further defined into subcategories (concussion with or without loss of consciousness).[14] These subcategories identify the specific type of injury (dislocations/subluxations vs sprains/ligament injury).[8]

Clinically, when an injury occurs, a diagnosis is required by a clinician. These classifications can be turned into codes (numbers) for recordkeeping and billing. In general medicine, the International Statistical Classification of Diseases, Version 10 (ICD-10) is the preferred coding system used and is the gold standard. ICD-10 is used for tracking the general injuries and illness; however, the specificity of its codes limits its application for sport ISS.[21]

Surveillance systems may use a specific sport injury coding system. Examples of these systems include the OSICS,[17-19] the National Athletic Injury/Illness Reporting System (NAIRS),[20] and the Sports Medicine Diagnostic Coding System (SMDCS).[21] Injury classification systems are used in sports medicine for the following 2 main purposes[18]:

1. To accurately classify diagnoses for injury surveillance

2. To create a database from which cases can be extracted for research on particular injuries.

Orchard Sports Injury Classification System

OSICS is a 4-character, specific sport injury classification system that was developed to examine the incidence of injury in elite level Australian-rules football in 1992. At the time, there was no sports-specific injury classification system available. Provided it is appropriately acknowledged, OSICS is free for researchers and sports medicine professionals to use. It is similar to the ICD-10, and recent revisions have made it easier to use in a sports medicine setting. OSICS-10[1] was released in 2010 and is currently used by Union of European Football Associations and Fédération Internationale de Football Association.[8,15-17] For the most accurate version of OSICS, sports injury specialists should refer to the website: www.johnorchard.com/about-osics.html.

National Athletic Injury/Illness Reporting System

Kenneth Clarke and John Powell developed the National Athletic Injury/Illness Reporting System (NAIRS) at Pennsylvania State University in 1975.[12,18] NAIRS was originally developed to track football injuries and collected data from 1977 to 1981. All injuries were identified according to the American Medical Association's Standard Nomenclature of Athletic Injuries.[12] The initial system enhanced data collection and incorporated many important features, such as standardized definitions of injury/illness, standardized rates of AEs, and a larger longitudinal sample than previously attempted.[20] The NAIRS classifications are the basis of the NCAA ISS and are widely used in the United States. However, because the classifications are now embedded in data collection systems, it is difficult to find literature supporting its reliability.[18]

Sports Medicine Diagnostic Coding System

Developed in Canada in 1991, SMDCS is a numerical system that uses a 6-character structure denoting body region, structure, and diagnosis. It follows a systematic anatomical design, first listing the area (XX), then structure (.00), and then the type of injury (.00). For example, KN.53.06 is the code for complete tear of the ACL. The first pair of letters is assigned to the location (knee), the next pair of digits is assigned to structure (ACL), and the last pair of digits is assigned to the type of injury (sprain). This format permits data sorting on the basis of any pair of digits to allow analysis of the body region, structure, and diagnosis. The Canadian Intercollegiate Sport Injury Registry and international organizations associated with rugby currently use this system as part of their ISS.[19] For the most current version of SMDCS, sports injury specialists should refer to the University of Calgary's website (www.sportmed.ucalgary.ca/Sport_Medicine/smdcs).

EPIDEMIOLOGY DEFINITIONS AND CALCULATIONS

Current sport epidemiological research is limited by the lack of standard terminology across databases.[1,2,4,6-8] Many published studies define injury, selection criteria, and population sizes differently. This directly affects estimated rates of injury. Because the calculation of IRs used different variables, many early epidemiological studies must be viewed individually, and generalizing the results is difficult. In the United States, football has the dubious distinction of having the highest rate of reportable injuries and is the leader in the most catastrophic injuries and fatalities.[10] However, much of these data were not reported as a standard unit (AEs/1000) across studies. For example, when reviewing catastrophic and fatality data, football would be surpassed by ice hockey and gymnastics if AEs were calculated at the rate of participation per year instead of per season.[7] Therefore, any interstudy comparisons must be made critically and analyzed for discrepancies.

There are other confounding variables regarding what injuries are more prevalent in which sports. These include level of play (ie, elite vs novice), age, and gender.[7] This further limits the generalizability of data and requires additional analysis to determine risk based on level of performer, age, gender, or other variables.

How Do We Define a Population at Risk?

Overall athlete participation is a critical component of surveillance. For most, a population that is at risk is defined by identifying those injured and those not injured. Injury surveillance and epidemiology studies use different terms, variables, and calculations. For consumers of these data, it can be difficult to understand and apply the information provided. Some injury data do not report the number at risk in the population. As such, these types of databases are only reporting injury frequency. Sports epidemiologists and researchers express risk and incidence as ratios created from dividing a numerator by a denominator. Examples include rate ratios, risk ratios, incidence rates, and incidence proportion. These terms are often used interchangeably, which is incorrect. True IRs cannot be generated using the total population at risk as the denominator.[12]

Statistical Terminology

Prevalence is the proportion of individuals in a population who have an illness/injury at a particular time. This represents the number of athletes with a current injury (acute and chronic) relative to the population at risk.[6] True prevalence is not calculated in sport because conditions generally do not last longer than 1 year.

What was the prevalence of injury among the men's soccer team last season?

- Total number injured (N = 12) ÷ total number of players (N = 25)

  $12 \div 25 = .48$. Forty-eight percent of the men's soccer team was injured.

Incidence is the number of new occurrences of injury during a specified time. This quantifies the number of new cases relative to the population at risk.[6] It is also referred to as the IR.

What was the incidence of injury on the women's basketball team during last season?

- IR = total number of injuries (N = 13) ÷ total number of players (N = 16)

    13 ÷ 16 = .81. There were .8 injuries for each team member.

Incidence proportion (IP) is the average probability that any athlete will sustain at least one injury during the course of a single season. Here, the numerator is a subset of the denominator.[6] Instead of counting the number of injuries, one should count the number of injured athletes. Incidence proportion is a valid estimate of average risk. This is similar to prevalence as defined and calculated above.

What was the risk of injury in the women's basketball team last season?

- IP = total number of injured (N = 7) ÷ total number of players (N = 16)

    7 ÷ 16 = .44. There was a 44% chance of being injured on the women's basketball team.

Individuals may have other characteristics that would increase or decrease his or her risk for injury. These data can also be used to determine the risk of repeat injury. The numerator now becomes the denominator for 2 or more injuries.

- Repeat IP = number of athletes with more than 1 injury (N = 3) ÷ number of injured athletes (N = 7)

    3 ÷ 7 = .43. The probability of an athlete having a second injury during the season is 43%.

The IR is focused on the number of injuries that occurred, whereas the IP is based on the number of injured athletes.[6] Keep in mind that an athlete can have more than one injury in the same season.

The IR and IP use an absolute value in the denominator. The number of athletes on the team is not the best estimate of who is really at risk. Some athletes will play more than others, and some sports have longer seasons than others. A better way to compare the incidence of injury between sports, genders, levels of participation, and seasons is to standardize the amount of exposure to injury. Incidence rate is focused on the number of new cases divided by the total exposures. An exposure is any time an athlete participates in a practice or game and can be counted in number of events or by the hours of participation. By accounting for variations in the amount of time athletes are at risk, it directly measures injury incidence[6,9] and is the preferred estimator of occurrence.[6] The frequently asked questions about sport-related injury, including "What is the IR of sport X?" and "What is the incidence of injury in sport Y?", are not precise questions in understanding how often injury occurs. The more accurate question is, "What is the rate of injury per unit of exposure?"

The unit of exposure is termed *AE* and is a key concept to understand. It attempts to define the amount of time an athlete is exposed to potential injury.[2-4,6-9] Exposure time should be calculated as accurately as possible.[6] The NCAA ISS defines this as one athlete participating in one practice or one game, thus being exposed to potential injury.[4,6,9] The most commonly accepted definition in the United States is similar to the NCAA ISS and is "one athlete's participation in a practice or competition in which there is a possibility of sustaining an athletic injury."[4-7,9,11] For competition classification, "only those having played in the event" are counted as having game exposure. Unfortunately, AE can be calculated in several ways, including by total number of athletes, the number of exposing situations (practice, training, game), or the total time participating.[6-8,14] Several surveillance systems collect data based on number of hours[8] or minutes[6] of exposure. This exposure number is the denominator in the ratio that measures risk (IR). It is important to use the same type of AE denominator when comparing sports, teams, seasons, etc, so that calculations and similarities and differences are accurately identified across surveillance systems. Let us repeat the original IR calculation, this time using AE as the population at risk:

$$IR \text{ using } AE = \frac{total\ number\ of\ injuries}{[number\ of\ players\ x\ (number\ practices + games)}$$

$$= \frac{13}{16\ x\ (125+25)} = \frac{13}{2400} = 0.00542\ or\ 5.42\ per\ 1000AE\ (x\ by\ 1000)$$

Compared to the first IR of .81, the actual risk of injury is lower when the number of opportunities to be injured is considered.

To add to the confusion, IR has been calculated per 100, 1000, or 100,000 AEs. Others calculate by athlete-hours or athlete-minutes. For best practice, injury risk should be calculated using 1000 AEs. Some advocate for reporting all injury data as case rates per AEs, whereas others suggest reporting data in tables that allow the reader to calculate risk. The use of multiple denominators, athlete-hours of exposure and total athletes, provides the most precise information about IR and injury risk.[20]

A separate practice and game IR can be calculated by using only one type of participation in the AEs.

$$Game\ IR = \frac{total\ number\ of\ injuries\ in\ games}{number\ of\ players\ that\ completed\ x\ number\ of\ games}$$

$$= \frac{9}{16\ x\ 25} = \frac{9}{400} = .0225\ or\ 22.5\ per\ 1000AE$$

There were 22.5 injuries for every 1000 games this team played. To quantify how much higher the rate of one sport is compared to another, an additional calculation of rate ratio can be calculated. This is done by dividing one sport's (ice hockey) IR by the other (baseball) IR. This calculation is advantageous because it takes into account the number of games and practices and is helpful because it provides meaningful sport-to-sport comparisons. For this calculation to be accurate, the IR for each sport has to be calculated with the same denominator (AEs = 1000 vs AEs 100 or athlete-hours or athlete-minutes).[6,22]

INJURY SURVEILLANCE SYSTEMS RESEARCH DATABASES AND COLLECTION AGENCIES

Athletic trainers are typically the primary data collectors for ISS; therefore, it is important to be aware of the various sport databases and injury collection agencies. The accuracy of the data collected is critical to the quality control and validity of the system being used.

National Athletic Injury/Illness Reporting System

The NAIRS was the first attempt at a nationwide data collection process for IRs in sport. From 1977 to 1981, NAIRS focused on football injuries. During the original NAIRS work, more than 1 million AEs in a 3-year period were analyzed.[12] NAIRS stopped collecting high school and college data in 1983.[20] Issues with the NAIRS data collection were the length and complexity of the forms. NAIRS was the foundation of the current NCAA ISS.[12,17-20] Although NAIRS is no longer active, it was the first sport ISS in the United States.

National Collegiate Athletic Association Injury Surveillance System

The NCAA ISS data collection system has been in place since 1982. It is the largest continuous ISS in the United States. Its mission is to provide current and reliable data on injury trends in intercollegiate athletics to optimize student-athlete health and safety.[20] In 2003, the ISS transitioned from pen and paper to a Web-based system. The initial collection focused on 15 sports. Data are now collected on all NCAA championship sports. In conjunction with Datalys, a national nonprofit organization that conducts sport injury research, the NCAA has collected several decades of data.[2,4,5,9] These longitudinal data allow for trends and patterns of injury to emerge. The NCAA has set the standards for defining injury occurrence, severity, and exposure. A significant weakness of the system is the lack of data accessibility to researchers and clinicians. Annual summary reports are no longer available to the public.[2,4,5,9] However, publications and other information are available on the Datalys website (http://datalyscenter.org/programs/ncaa-injury-surveillance-program/).

National Center for Catastrophic Sport Injury Research

The National Center for Catastrophic Sport Injury Research (NCCSIR) is based out of Chapel Hill, North Carolina, and collects data on death and permanent disability injuries that occur in sport. The NCCSIR partners with the National Football League, NCAA, National Federation of High School Associations, and the American Football Coaches Association. Since its inception in 1965, NCCSIR monitors cases with a systematic data reporting system that allows for longitudinal investigation of athletes suffering from catastrophic injuries and illnesses. NCCSIR is not representative of all sport injuries; only catastrophic injuries are included in the center's database. Injury data are accessible on their website (http://nccsir.unc.edu/).

Center for Injury Research and Policy–Reporting Information Online

An Internet-based system developed in 2004, Reporting Information Online (RIO), is a surveillance system of time-loss injuries for high schools in the United States. It was designed using the footprint of the NCAA ISS. Based out of Children's Hospital in Columbus, Ohio, high schools across the country are invited to participate in the data collection process each year. Annual summary reports are provided to the public. Data can be pulled on injury patterns and trends, specific sporting activities, participant demographics, and specific body parts that were injured.[2,4,5] Injury data are available on their website (www.nationwidechildrens.org/cirp-rio).

United States Consumer Product Commission National Electronic Injury Surveillance System

For more than 30 years, the United States Consumer Product Commission National Electronic Injury Surveillance System (NEISS) has collected demographic data, injury type, severity, mechanism of injury, injury location, and products involved. Patient information is collected from each NEISS hospital for every emergency visit involving an injury associated with consumer products. This system allows for tracking of injuries associated with sports protective equipment, such as helmets and shoulder pads. Analysis can identify faulty equipment and can lead to the recalls of the equipment. Information is available on their website (www.cpsc.gov/en/Research--Statistics/NEISS-Injury-Data/).

ISSUES WITH DATA COLLECTION

The quality of any injury statistic is dependent upon the standardization of definitions, statistical terms, and the population at risk. The struggle with comparing data collection systems/ISS is that there is not full consensus on the definition of a reportable injury, injury severity, and risk exposure.[1,2,4] In addition, the quality of the data may be confounded by personnel collecting the data, the frequency of the recording of data, the system's ease of use, and the process for submitting the data.

Who Is Collecting the Data?

Data entry and quality control may vary based on the professional entering the information.[2,5,24] For example, data collected by a medical professional may be more reliable than that of a coach, and that of a coach may be more reliable than that of a parent. Because of the need for a working knowledge of the terms being used, individuals who are trained in ISS data entry tend to report findings more thoroughly.[24] Data entered by medical professionals is of higher quality than that entered by a coach or reported by a parent.[4,13,24] A confounding factor for physicians or the athletic trainers may be whether the data are entered as part of the professional's job description vs considering the data entry as extra work.[2] Athletic trainers or other sports injury specialists are not the ones entering the data in many cases. Sport epidemiology could be enhanced if there was a focus on increasing the number of athletic trainers in each public and private high school who were responsible for injury surveillance. The Fairfax County (Virginia) Public School System Injury Surveillance Database is an example of this type of model. As part of their job description, certified athletic trainers, at each of the public high schools in the county, are required to enter data on all injuries through a computerized data collection system called Sport Injury Management System. Athletes are followed throughout their 4-year careers. As a result, Fairfax County has more than 12 years of cumulative data with more than 15 million AEs.[2]

How Are the Data Being Collected?

The goal is to collect the widest range of injuries possible while also collecting the data to calculate AEs accurately. The method of data collection varies depending on geographical location and the organization of sport in that area.[1] Many ISSs have moved from paper to computer for convenience. One example of paper reporting decreasing over time is with the improvement of the RIO.[2] As previously discussed, adding to one's workload can result in poor data collection. Easier data entry would ensure that an athletic trainer is able to perform the task. Further improving data collection, a single system for ISS, and clinical recordkeeping is needed. There are several athletic injury management software systems that have several fields that parallel ISS databases. Furthermore, several of these systems have the ability to export to the Datalys managed by the NCAA ISS.[2,5] This allows data in regular daily recordkeeping to be automatically exported to the NCAA ISS, which significantly decreases the workload. The more electronic medical records systems that can be interfaced with many of these national surveillance systems, the more likely the records collected will have higher-quality controls.[2,5] Datalys currently has 3 certified vendors, including ATS, NExTT solutions, and Sport Injury Management System. This approach reduces, if not eliminates, the need for double data entry.[5]

How Often Are the Data Being Collected?

Frequency of reporting is another variable that may affect the quality of the data. It appears that data entered daily or on a real-time basis are more accurate than when reported weekly or monthly.[2,5] In 1998, when the NCAA ISS began its data collection, pen and paper forms were mailed from the participating athletic trainer/college to the NCAA and were then entered by hand into the database. In the 1990s, they began to electronically scan the forms but still had to enter the information into the database by hand. Since the 2004-2005 season, the NCAA ISS has converted to a completely online system. This has decreased the time from injury to data submission. Historically, data were submitted by season, month, or week to the NCAA. Now, with electronic, Web-based systems, the accuracy of the data has increased because of the real-time submission of data.[5] Early sport epidemiological studies reported injuries for a specific group for a specific period of time (ie, one soccer team for one season).[2,7] ISS reporting in real-time or daily tends to be more reliable than weekly or monthly.[5] Most sport ISS systems require weekly data entry.[3-5,9]

The NCAA is not the only Internet-based ISS. The Center for Injury Research developed RIO. These types of systems are increasing the ability of athletic trainers, coaches, and parents[5] to provide real-time reporting.[2] These Web-based systems have led to the ability to evaluate the reliability of these ISSs. The Centers for Disease Control and Prevention has established criteria to evaluate these systems.[4]

Who Is Using Injury Surveillance System Data?

ISS data have been referenced in journal articles and medical textbooks and have been applied to modification of sports rules, policies, and issues by a variety of administrative and sports medicine groups.[1] These data have been used in studies of IRs by sport, gender, position, concussion rates, and on the effectiveness of prophylactic knee braces and football helmets. Surveillance data collection has led to collaboration between the American Medical Society for Sports Medicine, American College of Sports Medicine, American Orthopedic Society for Sports Medicine, Centers for Disease Control and Prevention, and the National Athletic Trainers' Association (NATA).[20] Collaboration efforts have benefited collegiate athletics, as well as the entire sports medicine community. The NATA, NCAA, and high school athletic associations continue to use ISS to improve the health and safety of all athletes.

OUTCOMES OF INJURY SURVEILLANCE

Surveillance databases are important resources that can affect sport rules, safety equipment, and sports medicine administration and policy.[20] Due to the potential to use incidence rates and risk factors associated with athletic injury to alter sport rules or modify equipment, much of the ISS has been driven by government agencies or sports associations.[2,4,22] Others may use the data to identify injury causes in an attempt to develop better equipment or injury prevention protocols. Although all types of information are critical for athletic trainers,[2,4] athletic trainers may also use these data to assess needs for staffing and coverage.[20] For example, the primary audience for the ISS system was originally the NCAA Committee on Competitive Safeguards and Medical Aspects of Sports and relevant NCAA sport rules committees, who used the information as a resource upon which to base recommendations, rules, and policies impacting student-athlete health and welfare.[20] Other reliable ISS databases are also used by sport rules committees at the Olympic,[14] professional,[8] high school,[5] or youth level.[3,13] However, the audiences interested in this information have expanded to include individual colleges and universities, sports medicine researchers, other administrative and sports medicine organizations, the media, and the general public.[20]

Rule and Equipment Changes

Sport injury surveillance and epidemiological data have had a significant impact on rules and equipment changes. After reviewing longitudinal data from several sport injury database systems, rules committees have implemented rule changes. The most noticeable measure to decrease rates of severe injury in sport is to decrease AE. Of late, the NCAA has attempted to implement this concept with new rules limiting the number of contact days allowed for spring football.[7] Although some rule changes have been instituted to decrease IRs of specific injuries within that sport, other rule changes are specific to readiness, age, and physical maturity.[7] Youth sport competition is organized by age group. However, some sports also allow movement between age groups. Each organization requires additional information based on readiness or maturity. An example of a multifactorial determination of participation occurs within the rules for USA Gymnastics competition. A participant can petition to participate in a higher level of competition with submission of age verification and proof of skill level development with participation at the preceding competition level. However, to compete at the highest levels, gymnasts must have documentation of minimum scores at those preceding levels to be eligible for competition at the platinum and diamond division.[25] Rule and equipment changes have been most evident in football. Cervical spine injuries have decreased with the banning of spear tackling, and knee injuries have decreased with the banning of chop blocking. Moreover, there have been changes to the type of helmet used (leather to plastic), the strength of the helmet (polycarbonate material), and the requirement of the face mask.[7] Requirements for additional safety equipment have increased across types of sport and levels of participation. Chapter 11 describes changes in rules and equipment as a way of preventing injury. These types of changes are an attempt to make sport safer; although physical activity has an inherent risk of injury, these modifications can significantly reduce risk.[1,22] Governing organizations will continue to use ISS data to implement changes in rules, policies, and equipment.

Acceptable Level of Injury Risk

Risk of athletic injury is problematic at all levels, from youth to professional sport. Sport sociologists frequently discuss why people select sports in which to participate. Is it based on likes and dislikes or skill level? For many parents, allowing their child to participate or not may be based on risk. The relative safety of one sport over another may deter parents from allowing their sons or daughters to participate in any given sport. Perhaps the rationale for sport selection varies as a child ages and matures. Parents may allow some sports at a certain age and allow different sports at a more mature age. USA Football, a national governing body for youth football (partially funded by the National Football League), recently reported that participation among players ages 6 to 14 years fell from 3 to 2.8 million in 2011, a 6.7% decline.[26] The nation's largest youth football program, Pop Warner, saw participation drop 5.7% from 2010 to 2011 and another 4% drop between 2011 and 2012.[26] Concussion risk and awareness may play a part in parents' reluctance to allow their children to participate in football. Although concussion has occurred in other sports, the IR is significantly higher in American football than other sports. However, when looking at injuries beyond concussion, female cross country running has the highest IR/1000 AEs (15.9).[7]

Prevention

Prevention programs can be developed once injury mechanisms and risk factors are well understood. Many times, ISS provides necessary data to identify injury clusters and trends with sport. Moreover, it can ascertain if longstanding assumptions are facts or misconceptions. A 5-year study of NCAA ISS data published in 1995[27] revealed a significant increased risk of ACL injury in female collegiate soccer and basketball athletes when compared to male soccer and basketball athletes. This large sample over a 5-year period supported the anecdotal evidence that women were at higher risk of ACL tears, at least in basketball and soccer. This information then led to a surge in research trying to explain the root cause of the gender difference and determine how to reduce the risk for female athletes. A critical component in determining the effectiveness of prevention interventions is for data to be collected pre- and postintervention. Early prevention interventions only had the postintervention incidence data and, thus, do not have the ability to confirm positive findings.[1,2] In order for ISS to truly impact prevention intervention procedures, ongoing prevention studies will need to use several epidemiology and surveillance techniques to assess the effectiveness of these programs.

Staffing and Coverage

For athletic trainers working at a middle school, high school, or a college, staffing and proper coverage are always areas of concern. Athletic trainers can use ISS data to identify sports that are of higher risk for injury and adjust coverage plans accordingly. Also, by tracking injury occurrence over several years, athletic trainers can identify the time of year or type of events that are associated with higher rates of injury. For example, do multiday events, such as a wrestling tournament, warrant more staff than a single match?

The NATA Recommendations and Guidelines for Appropriate Medical Coverage of Intercollegiate Athletics (AMCIA) were established in 2000 to create a more justifiable and objective system for determining the health care needs of each institution. The most up-to-date injury information provided by the NCAA ISS further supported AMCIA Recommendation and Guidelines amendments in 2003, 2006, and 2010. These empirical data informed changes in calculating health care units and were dictated by increased participation opportunities and IR changes as reported by NCAA ISS.[28]

Appropriate medical coverage, as determined by the NATA Committee of College and University Athletic Trainers involves basic emergency care during sports participation and other health care services for student-athletes. This includes[27] but is not limited to the following:

- Determination of athletes' readiness to participate

- Injury prevention

- Evaluation of athletic injuries/illnesses

- Immediate treatment of athletic injuries/illnesses

- Rehabilitation and reconditioning of athletic injuries.

These recommendations are for collegiate level athletics and are not requirements. Sports that are considered lower risk include baseball, softball, cross country, swimming, outdoor track, and tennis, must have an individual physically present who possesses the minimum qualifications as stated in the NCAA Sports Medicine Handbook (cardiopulmonary resuscitation, first aid, automated external defibrillator, and bloodborne pathogen training). Sports considered moderate risk, including women's basketball, field hockey, lacrosse (men's and women's), soccer (men's and women's), indoor track, and volleyball, should have a certified athletic trainer or a designated staff member with minimal qualifications. If the athletic trainer is not present, he or she must be able to respond in less than 5 minutes. Sports with increased risk include football, ice hockey (men's and women's), wrestling, men's basketball, and gymnastics should have a certified athletic trainer physically present for all practices.[27] Some institutions may determine from their own ISS data that sports considered lower risk outside may be at a higher risk during their indoor season (ie, baseball in a gymnasium) and, therefore, justify having a certified athletic trainer at these practice events. Overall, AMCIA recommendations can be critical to determining if staffing is limited and provide factual information to justify additional staffing.

BRINGING IT TOGETHER

Sports injury surveillance has formed the backbone of injury epidemiology research, serving to highlight the types and patterns of injury that warrant additional investigation. Injury surveillance has been integral in guiding rule changes, improving equipment, and developing training regimens that decrease modifiable risk factors. Limited by definitions and methodology, ISS is not entirely uniform across collectors, agencies, or sports. With this broad scope, ISS can, at times, lack context. Specific issues revolve around a lack of standardized nomenclature (definition of a reportable injury, selection criteria [new injury, recurrent injury], severity [time lost]), lack of standardized exposure rates (definition for exposures [events, hours]; varying denominator variables [100 or 1000 AEs]), and data collection procedures (reporting time [monthly, weekly], personnel [trained, medical background]). Overall athlete participation is a critical component of surveillance because the actual number of players that participated in any given sport or event is used to calculate AE. Although attempts have been made to create consistency across databases, the most critical factor for all injury data is hindered by the exposure denominator. Although it is recommended to use AE 1000, it is not universally reported this way. Therefore, sport injury specialists will continue to review each study as separate case reports, limiting their abilities to make interstudy comparisons or to generalize across types of populations.

REVIEW QUESTIONS

1. What should be included in the definition of an injury?
2. Describe the purpose of injury classification systems, such as the OSICS or NAIRS.
3. Explain the difference between IR and IP.
4. Calculate the IR/1000 AEs from the following data: athletes = 35, practices = 250, games = 17, and reportable injuries = 47. IR = 5.03/1000 AEs.
5. What situations produce the most accurate and reliable injury information for ISS?
6. How are data from injury surveillance used?

LEARNING ACTIVITIES

1. Identify similarities and differences in reporting data.
   a. Students will break into groups to review the primary ISSs and inform classmates on the data the athletic trainer will need to identify and report.
      i. www.nationwidechildrens.org/cirp-rio
      ii. www.cpsc.gov/en/Research--Statistics/NEISS-Injury-Data
      iii. http://datalyscenter.org/programs/ncaa-injury-surveillance-program
      iv. http://nccsir.unc.edu
2. Electronic Medical Records
   a. Design an injury reporting system that would interface with an ISS.
   b. Investigate various types of electronic medical records and determine pros and cons for interfacing with ISS. (Students can also analyze the medical records system in their current clinical course.)

3. A certified athletic trainer is newly hired and given the responsibility for care of all 8 college teams. What are all of the considerations that he or she must make when addressing coverage? (Teams include men's/women's soccer, men's/women's ice hockey, men's/women's lacrosse, and baseball/softball.)

4. Use published articles to show the variations in reporting IR, particularly for the same injury in the same population. Ask students to convert AEs into the same metric, if possible. Suggested articles include the following:

   a. Ruhe A, Gänsslen A, Klein W. The incidence of concussion in professional and collegiate ice hockey: are we making progress? A systematic review of the literature. *Br J Sports Med.* 2014;48(2):102-106. (Athlete-hours and AE are used in the same study comparing rates of concussion between college and professional hockey.)

   b. Marar M, McIlvain NM, Fields SK, Comstock RD. Epidemiology of concussions among United States high school athletes in 20 sports. *Am J Sports Med.* 2012;40(4):747-755. (Uses 10,000 AEs.)

   c. Lincoln AE, Caswell SV, Almquist JL, Dunn RE, Norris JB, Hinton RY. Trends in concussion incidence in high school sports: a prospective 11-year study. *Am J Sports Med.* 2011;39(5):958-963. (Uses 1000 AEs.)

REFERENCES

1. Goldberg AS, Moroz L, Smith A, Ganley T. Injury surveillance in young athletes: a clinician's guide to sport injury literature. *Sports Med.* 2007;37(3):265-278.
2. Hinton RY. Sports injury surveillance systems. *Sports Medicine Update.* 2012;January/February:2-7.
3. Radelet MA, Lephart SM, Rubinstein EN, Myers JB. Survey of injury rate for children in community sports. *Pediatrics.* 2002;110(3):e28.
4. Kucera KL, Marshall SW, Bell DR, DiStefano MJ, Goerger CP, Oyama S. Validity of soccer injury data from the National Collegiate Athletic Association's Injury Surveillance System. *J Athl Train.* 2011;46(5):489-499.
5. Schiff MA, Mack CD, Pollissar NL, Levy MR, Dow SP, O'Kane JW. Soccer injuries in female youth players: comparison of injury surveillance by certified athletic trainers and Internet. *J Athl Train.* 2010;45(3):238-242.
6. Knowles SB, Marshall SW, Guskiewicz KM. Issues in estimating risks and rates in sports injury research. *J Athl Train.* 2006;41(2):207-215.
7. Armsey TD, Hosey RG. Medical aspects of sports: epidemiology of injuries, preparticipation physical examination, and drugs in sports. *Clin Sports Med.* 2004;23(2):255-279.
8. Fuller CW, Ekstrand J, Junge A, et al. Consensus statement on injury definitions and data collection procedures in studies of football (soccer) injuries. *Br J Sports Med.* 2006;40(3):193-201.
9. Dick R, Agel J, Marshall SW. National collegiate athletic association injury surveillance system commentaries: introduction and methods. *J Athl Train.* 2007;42(2):173-182.
10. Garrick JG, Requa RK. Injuries in high school sports. *Pediatrics.* 1978;61(3):465-469.
11. Marshall SW. Recommendations for defining and classifying anterior cruciate ligament injuries in epidemiologic studies. *J Athl Train.* 2010;45(5):516-518.
12. Milner EM. The epidemiology of sports injuries or caveat emptor! http://www.isss-sportsurfacescience.org/downloads/documents/6EGQHIOVRC_Milner.pdf. Accessed June 1, 2014.
13. Beachy G, Rauh M. Middle school injuries: a 20-year (1988-2008) multisport evaluation. *J Athl Train.* 2014;49(4):493-506.
14. Junge A, Engebretsen L, Alonso JM, et al. Injury surveillance in multi-sport events: the international olympic committee approach. *Br J Sports Med.* 2008;42(6):413-421.
15. Ekstrand J, Gillquist J. Soccer injuries and their mechanisms: a prospective study. *Med Sci Sports Exerc.* 1983;15(3):267-270.
16. Dvorak J, Junge A, Chomiak J, et al. Risk factor analysis for injuries in football players. Possibilities for a prevention program. *Am J Sports Med.* 2000;28(5 suppl):S69-S74.
17. Orchard J. Orchard sports injury classification system (OCISCS). *Sport Health.* 1995;11:39-41.
18. Rae K, Britt H, Orchard J, Finch C. Classifying sports medicine diagnoses: a comparison of the International classification of diseases 10-Australian modification (ICD-10-AM) and the Orchard Sports Injury Classification System (OSICS-8). *Br J Sports Med.* 2005;39(12):907-911.

19. Rae K, Orchard J. The orchard sports injury classification system (OCISCS) version 10. *Clin J Sport Med.* 2007;17(3):201-204.

20. Zemper ED, Dick RW. Epidemiology of athletic injuries. In: McKeag DB, Moeller J, eds. *ACSM Primary Care Sports Medicine.* Philadelphia, PA: Wolters Kluwer Health: Lippencott, Williams and Wilkins; 2007:11-28.

21. Meeuwisse WH, Wiley JP. The sport medicine diagnostic coding system. *Clin J Sport Med.* 2007;17(3):205-207.

22. van Mechelen W, Hlobil H, Kemper HC. Incidence, severity, aetiology and prevention of sports injuries. A review of concepts. *Sports Med.* 1992;14(2):82-99.

23. Finch CF, Cook J. Categorising sports injuries in epidemiological studies: the subsequent injury categorisation (SIC) model to address multiple, recurrent and exacerbation of injuries. *Br J Sports Med.* 2014;48(17):1276-1280.

24. Finch CF, Orchard JW, Twomey DM, et al. Coding OSICS sports injury diagnoses in epidemiological studies: does the background of the coder matter? *Br J Sports Med.* 2014;48(7):552-556.

25. National Women's Program Committee. 2014 - 2015 women's program rules and policies. Published August 1, 2014. https://usagym.org/PDFs/Women/Rules/Rules%20and%20Policies/2014_2015_w_rulespolicies.pdf. Accessed October 13, 2015.

26. Fainaru S, Fainaru-Wada M. Youth football participation drops. ESPN Outside the Lines. November 13, 2014. http://espn.go.com/espn/otl/story/_/page/popwarner/pop-warner-youth-football-participation-drops-nfl-concussion-crisis-seen-causal-factor. Accessed October 13, 2015.

27. Arendt EA, Dick R. Knee injury patterns among men and women in collegiate basketball and soccer. NCAA data and review of literature. *Am J Sports Med.* 1995;23(6):694-701.

28. National Athletic Trainers' Association. Recommendations and Guidelines for Appropriate Medical Coverage of Intercollegiate Athletics. http://www.nata.org/appropriate-medical-coverage-intercollegiate-athletics. Revised January 2010. Accessed January 12, 2015.

29. Hägglund M, Waldén M, Bahr R, Ekstrand J. Methods for epidemiological study of injuries to professional football players: developing the UEFA model. *Br J Sports Med.* 2005;39(6):340-346.

5

Evidence-Based Practice

Thomas Cappaert, PhD, ATC, CSCS

CHAPTER OBJECTIVES

- Define evidence-based practice (EBP) and explain the 5 steps for finding and applying research.
- Describe importance of EBP in clinical decision making.
- Identify and construct different types of clinical questions using the patient, intervention, comparison, and outcome (PICO) format.
- Perform critical appraisal of research to answer clinical question using a 5-step process.

INTRODUCTION

Effective clinical practice requires that health professionals make a series of choices. What is the most effective way to diagnose a condition? What is the best treatment option? Should the clinical practice change based upon new research? These decisions are based on a clinician's experience, knowledge, skills, attitudes, and available resources. The patients' concerns, expectations, abilities, and willingness to change must also be considered.

The term *evidence-based medicine* (EBM) was first used by Sackett et al[1] in the early 1990s and was intended to integrate the best available research evidence with clinical expertise and patient considerations to achieve the best possible patient outcomes. A critical characteristic of EBM is clinical expertise (professional expertise is based on learned knowledge, experiences, and specialization). Patient considerations may include patient values, culture, and expectations. Another characteristic of EBM is the use of high-quality information to avoid making decisions without valid evidence to support them. The evidence is empirical research from studies of clinical outcomes. Following the steps of EBM helps health professionals sort through volumes of information and find the best evidence.

Adams M, Swiger W.
Epidemiology for Athletic Trainers: Integrating Evidence-Based Practice (pp 83-102).
© 2016 Taylor & Francis Group.

There is a large gap between research results and clinical practice.[2] So much research is published in so many formats today that clinicians are often unaware of it, do not have time to access it, or do not have the skills to understand and apply the results. In many cases, clinical decisions are made without the support of valid research but are based upon expert opinion, anecdotal evidence, common practice, or trial and error. Insurance reimbursement and resource allocation is often based on the effectiveness of the treatment, usually measured in terms of patient outcomes and cost. It is imperative for clinicians to seek and use the best evidence for clinical practice to reduce the information gap and provide the best care possible. Consider the analogy of purchasing a new appliance, such as a washing machine. Before deciding which model to buy, one would compare the load size, consumer ratings, and costs of all the available washers. In the same way one would shop for an appliance, clinicians should review studies of patient outcomes and select treatments that are appropriate and effective for a particular patient. Following the 5 steps of EBP allows clinicians to locate and synthesize information on a topic in a timely manner.

Most clinicians receive information from a variety of sources on many topics that interest them and then take away what they think may be useful one day (just in case learning). EBP principles ask clinicians to deliberately seek information in a focused way and to apply it to an immediate situation (just in time learning).

How to Perform Evidence-Based Practice?

EBP relies on a series of systematic steps to find and apply the required information.[3]

1. Construct an answerable clinical question.
2. Find the best evidence of clinical outcomes available.
3. Critically evaluate the evidence.
4. Apply the evidence to the desired clinical situation.
5. Evaluate the efficacy and efficiency of the practice.

Step 1: Construct an Answerable Clinical Question

One of the most difficult aspects of EBP is that the clinician must admit that he or she may not know the answer to a clinical question. As research expands, standards of care can change. What was once considered an effective treatment may be less so as new approaches are developed. It is impossible to know a definitive answer to every clinical question, so EBP provides clinicians with a method for finding answers to questions of which they are unsure.

When constructing a clinical question, use the PICO format. This takes the key components of a clinical question and structures it in a way that makes it easier to find the evidence. The majority of clinical questions can be separated into the following elements[3]:

P   The patients or population
     Who are the participations in the studies? Are they similar to my patient?

I   The intervention or indicator
     What is the treatment, diagnostic procedure, or risk factor in which you are interested?

C   The comparison or control group
     What is the control, alternate treatment, procedure, or factor to which you will be comparing to your treatment, procedure, or risk factor?

O   The outcome
     What are the consequences or results relative to the patient? How was effectiveness measured?

The most common clinical question is how best to treat a patient with a particular disease or condition. This is known as an intervention question. The clinician or researcher is attempting to change or intervene in the patient's condition. Not all clinical questions will be about interventions.

Other types of questions include the following:

- Frequency/occurrence: How often does the problem occur?
- Etiology/risk factors: What causes the problem?
- Diagnosis/testing: Does this patient have the problem?
- Prediction: Who will get the problem?
- Phenomena: What types of problems may be occurring in a population?

Each type of clinical question can be answered using the PICO format, except phenomena that likely consist of only the P and O. The following examples show how to match key parts of a clinical situation with the PICO letters.

Intervention PICO

A 16-year-old high school basketball player presents with recurrent lateral ankle sprains (4 over the past 2 years). He has been treated and rehabilitated to full activity after each injury. He asks if there is a way to prevent this injury, such as taping or bracing. To convert this to an answerable clinical question, first select the relevant PICO information:

P   Population/patient = athletes with recurring lateral ankle sprains
I   Intervention = prophylactic taping or bracing
C   Control = no treatment
O   Outcome = reduction in reoccurrence of lateral ankle sprains

Then, combine the elements into a question, such as the following:

In athletes with recurring lateral ankle sprains, does prophylactic taping or bracing reduce the recurrence rate compared to no treatment?

Etiology/Risk Factors PICO

Questions about etiology or risk factors are used to determine what causes a disease or injury as opposed to questions about how best to treat them. Consider the following situation: a college football player says that he recently began taking an herbal supplement containing St. John's Wort to lose weight. He heard that St. John's Wort can increase the risk of heart arrhythmias or heart attacks. The clinician does not know much about the supplement and wants to give him good advice.

P   Population/patient = adult males
I   Intervention = herbal supplement containing St. John's Wort
C   Control = no supplement
O   Outcome = cardiac arrhythmia or myocardial infarction

Possible Question: In men, does taking a supplement containing St. John's Wort increase the risk of cardiac arrhythmia or myocardial infarction compared to not taking it?

Frequency/Occurrence PICO

Questions of frequency deal with how many people in the population have a particular condition (number of ankle injuries in soccer athletes) or compare the timing of an injury (winter vs summer).

Say a clinician is talking with the parents of a preadolescent female (10 years old) who are asking about the risk of injury in youth volleyball and soccer. Their daughter is interested in both, and the parents want to know which sport tends to have the highest injury rate for children her age.

P   Population/patient = preadolescent females
I   Intervention = volleyball athletes
C   Control/comparison = soccer athletes
O   Outcome = injury occurrence

Possible Question: Which sport has the highest risk of injury for preadolescent girls, volleyball or soccer?

Diagnosis/Testing PICO

Diagnosis questions are concerned with how accurate a diagnostic procedure or test is in determining whether someone has a particular condition. These are often compared to a criterion or gold standard measurement.

For example, a clinician is observing a knee evaluation at an orthopedic clinic. After conducting a thorough history, visual examination, and palpation of the area, the physician's assistant performs one special test (Lachman's) to determine the diagnosis of an anterior cruciate ligament (ACL) injury. The clinician is curious as to how the physician's assistant can be so certain after only one diagnostic test. The clinician decides to investigate by searching the literature for the validity of the Lachman's test compared to arthroscopy, which would have the least number of false-positive results.

P   Population/patient = patients with suspected ACL injuries
I   Intervention = Lachman's test
C   Control/comparison = knee arthroscopy (criterion measure)
O   Outcome = accurate diagnosis of ACL injury

Possible Question: For suspected ACL injuries, can Lachman's test accurately diagnose the presence or absence of an ACL injury compared to knee arthroscopy?

Prediction PICO

Prediction questions examine how likely an outcome is in a particular population with certain characteristics or risk factors. For example, heat illness can be frightening for athletes, and they often want to know how likely they are to have another episode of heat illness. To help athletes understand their risks, clinicians need data showing how likely a second episode of heat illness is for someone with a previous history.

P   Population/patient = athlete
I   Intervention = previous episode of heat illness
C   Control/comparison = no previous episode of heat illness
O   Outcome = subsequent episodes of heat illness

Possible Question: In athletes with a previous history of heat illness, what is the risk of subsequent episodes compared with athletes with no history of heat illness?

Phenomena PICO

A phenomenon is an event or occurrence that is not well understood. These questions can relate to any aspect of clinical practice, such as poorly understood treatments, barriers to exercise adherence, health behaviors, or professional burnout. A common phenomenon in rehabilitation is poor adherence to the prescribed exercise program. If one wants to understand possible reasons for poor adherence, he or she should start with reviewing reports of other similar patients. In this case, only the P and the O need to be used.

P   Population/patient = patients with orthopedic injuries and poor exercise adherence
O   Outcome = reasons for poor adherence

Possible Question: What reasons are given by patients for poor exercise/rehabilitation adherence?

Eventually, one will want to see how other clinicians have improved adherence by adding the I and the C. Some phenomena are so new to research that one will only find descriptions of them rather than ways to change them.

TABLE 5-1 COMMONLY USED DATABASES FOR SPORTS MEDICINE		
NAME	**DESCRIPTION**	**URL**
The Cochrane Library	A collection of systematic reviews, registered clinical trials, and abstracts of systematic reviews; generally allows free access.	www.cochranelibrary.com
PubMed	The National Library of Medicine provides free access to article abstracts on the MEDLINE database. Clinical Queries is a search tool within PubMed for systematic reviews and controlled trials. Add /clinical to URL.	www.ncbi.nlm.nih.gov/pubmed
PEDro	Stands for the Physiotherapy Evidence Database and contains access to randomized trials, systematic reviews, and clinical practice guidelines related to physical therapy and rehabilitation.	www.pedro.org.au
CINAHL	The Cumulative Index to Nursing and Allied Health Literature contains all types of published literature on medicine and health care. It can be searched for clinical trials and systematic reviews. Access is limited to subscription.	www.ebscohost.com/cinahl
SPORTDiscus	This collection emphasizes sports medicine and related fields. Content areas range from exercise physiology and sports psychology to physical education and recreation. It is accessed by subscription.	www.ebscohost.com/academic/sportdiscus

Step 2: Find the Best Evidence of Clinical Outcomes Available

To find the best evidence to answer clinical questions, one should use several databases that contain articles from medical and research journals or reviews written by research centers, called *white papers*. Depending on the clinical question, one may have to search several databases to find relevant articles. Descriptions of several databases used for sports medicine searches and their URLs are provided in Table 5-1. One can search topics that span all aspects of health care. The volume of information available is overwhelming, and it is critical to limit the search by using the PICO components as keywords. The best evidence comes from studies that are near the top of the evidence pyramid (Figure 5-1; meta-analysis and position statements, also known as systematic reviews). If a systematic review is not available on the clinical question, one can search for any published randomized, controlled trials. If there are a few randomized, controlled trials, one will have to consider the evidence provided by quasiexperiments, longitudinal cohort studies, cross-sectional studies, and expert reviews. EBP asks for the best available evidence, which may not always be Level I or II. The next step shows how to critically appraise the quality of a study to determine the value of nonsystematic reviews.

Basics of Computerized Searching

Databases use keywords to find relevant articles and filter out unrelated ones. The PICO components used to develop the question now become the search terms. One should keep in mind that researchers may use other terms than that were searched. Think of possible synonyms for the

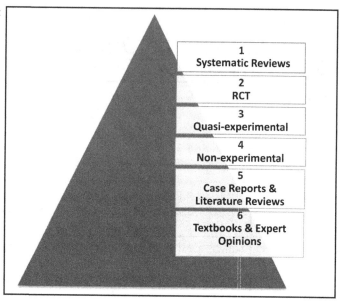

Figure 5-1. Levels of evidence with most useful evidence at top of the pyramid.

| 1 |
| Systematic Reviews |
| 2 |
| RCT |
| 3 |
| Quasi-experimental |
| 4 |
| Non-experimental |
| 5 |
| Case Reports & Literature Reviews |
| 6 |
| Textbooks & Expert Opinions |

TABLE 5-2
SEARCH TERMS FROM PICO

QUESTION COMPONENT	SEARCH TERM	SYNONYMS
Population/patient	Athletes	Player, physical activity
Intervention	Prophylactic taping, bracing	Prevention, neoprene sleeve, wrapping
Control/comparison	None	-
Outcome	Ankle sprain	Lateral ankle sprain, ankle injury, anterior talofibular ligament

search terms. Table 5-2 provides an example of correct search terms and synonyms for the first PICO question on prophetic ankle taping/bracing. Using multiple search terms focuses the search to only the articles that include those terms. Combining keywords produces fewer results that are more targeted to the question. For example, if one just used the term *taping*, one would see all articles in which taping is mentioned for any joint. Adding the term *ankle sprain* narrows that the result to taping for that specific injury. Adding *prophylactic* to the search will reduce the number of relevant articles further. This overlap of the search terms can be represented in a Venn diagram (Figure 5-2).[4] The overlap between each pair of terms is larger than the convergence of all 3 key terms under the star.

Once the study question has been broken into search terms, different combinations can be constructed by using the Boolean operators AND and OR. The operators improve the specificity of the search. If one wishes to capture articles that have taping or bracing, then OR is used (eg, bracing OR taping AND ankle sprain). The OR includes articles with bracing or taping. The AND limits the articles to just those that include ankle sprains. The overlap of all 3 terms will provide articles that are the most relevant to the clinical question. There are situations in which an overlap between all terms does not exist, so an overlap of just 2 terms may be the only information available.

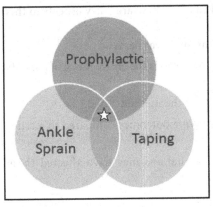

Figure 5-2. Venn diagram showing overlap of search terms.

Incorporating synonyms or variations of search terms can be a useful way to expand the number of articles found. For example, adding prevention to taping or injury to ankle sprain can increase the number of articles available (eg, taping OR prevention AND ankle sprain OR ankle injury). NOT is the Boolean operator that stops a term from being included in a search. This can be helpful for limiting the population of the studies. If one only wants articles for adults (ages 18 years or older), use NOT to filter out adolescents and children (eg, bracing AND taping AND adults NOT adolescents).

Like any clinical skill, using a computer database to search for articles takes practice. The following are tips and tricks to help get started:

- Tip 1: Boolean operators AND, OR, and NOT can be selected from the pull-down selection boxes or entered directly within the search text boxes. Use parentheses to separate components when entering a complex search directly in text box with mixed Boolean operators. Example: (ligament injury OR sprain) AND (ankle AND foot).

- Tip 2: The AND operator is used by default between search terms. The string ice application will match records where both words are included in any order or proximity. Search for exact phrases by enclosing a string in quotation marks. Example: "therapeutic ultrasound" matches the exact term.

- Tip 3: Use an asterisk (*) as a wildcard character. Realize that autopluralization and autosingularization are active. Example: athlete matches athlete, athletes, athletic, and athletics.

- Tip 4: Use the wildcard character (*) at the end of a term to search for diseases that could appear in the text with different endings, such as Alzheimer or Alzheimer's disease. Example: alzheimer* disease.

- Tip 5: Articles retrieved can be restricted in several ways, including by date of publication, language, whether an abstract is present, etc. Check the advance search tab of the database.

- Tip 6: Use so or [so] at the end of a term to search for studies from a specific source. Example: concussions AND JAMA [so].

- Tip 7: Use the Medical Subject Heading list to find synonyms and other terms and subtopics related to the search terms (www.nlm.nih.gov/mesh/MBrowser.html).

Step 3: Critically Evaluate the Evidence

The previous steps describe how to formulate an answerable clinical question and how to search for evidence using computer databases. This section outlines how to evaluate the quality of the articles that were found. Not all studies are equally strong in terms of determining cause and effect. Unless one has been fortunate enough to find a systematic review or position statement about his or her question, one will have to form an opinion about the best clinical practice. To do that, one will need to weigh the strength of the evidence available. There are 5 key aspects to this evaluation, including the following:

1. Identify the research study design and know its strengths and weaknesses.

2. Consider the similarities of the study participants to the patient. (Is the entire range of patients included? Is the patient included in the range?)

3. How were treatments conducted? (Determine the quality of the methods used.)

4. What was the accuracy of the outcome measurements? (Were outcomes compared to a criterion? Were clinically useful statistics used?)

5. What other explanations exist for the results? (What limitations may have affected these results?)

Research Study Design and Clinical Questions

The hierarchy of study designs was introduced in Chapter 3 (see Figure 5-1). Recall that Level I evidence comes from meta-analyses and position statements from medical organizations. As the levels progress downward, the impact of the research decreases, as does the value of the evidence. In the absence of systematic reviews, a thorough critical appraisal of the studies is needed. Table 5-3 summarizes the type of study and which clinical question can be answered by that design. It is important to understand the basic types of research designs that can be undertaken. They generally fall into 3 categories (descriptive, correlational, and experimental [cause and effect]). Each has its benefits and limitations. The 3 types can be viewed as a continuum from simple to complex. Descriptive questions are considered the simplest, and experimental studies are the most complex. A correlation study assumes that one can first describe (by measuring or observing) each variable. An experimental study assumes that the variables are related to each other. Experimental designs are the best design to determine causal relationships. A summary of the purpose, characteristics, limitations, and statistical analysis of each type are summarized in Table 5-4. Once a database search has been completed, one may have several articles to choose from to an attempt to answer a clinical question. There will be several types of studies, so it is important to choose article(s) that use a research design that is best suited to the clinical question one wants to answer and also ones that provide the best evidence. If one has several articles to choose from in answering a clinical question, choose the articles that are as close to the top of the pyramid as possible. The Oxford Centre for Evidence-Based Medicine (CEBM)[4] created a table matching the levels with the type of clinical question one may be asking. It can be downloaded from www.cebm.net/ocebm-levels-of-evidence/. A simplified version is found in Table 5-4.

Critical Appraisal Questions

More than the level of evidence is needed to determine if a study provides solid evidence for a clinical question. Not all studies are as carefully planned out or executed as others and may be limited by the type of participants or reason a variable was measured. This section describes what to look for in individual studies to decide if the results are valid and clinically useful. The following list of questions asks about characteristics that are present in studies that provide the best evidence. When a study falls short of one of the guidelines, it is said to have a limitation and that the reader should take that limitation into account before applying the results. These are basic appraisal questions for intervention studies and can be slightly modified with other types of research articles and clinical questions. By consistently asking these questions when reading an article, one will learn how to pick out key information that is likely to help answer the clinical question. The Critical Appraisal Worksheet at the end of the chapter provides a format to follow when evaluating articles. The CEBM[5] has also created Critical Appraisal Worksheets that depend on the type of article one may be evaluating (www.cebm.net/critical-appraisal).

1. Were the treatment groups representative and comparable?

	TABLE 5-3 SUMMARY OF RESEARCH ARTICLE TYPE	
BEST STUDY DESIGN	**DESCRIPTION**	**CLINICAL QUESTION TYPE**
Meta-analysis	Technique that combines and analyzes the results of similar published, high-quality research studies and bases a conclusion upon statistical data	All
Systematic review	A review of literature that critically examines and summarizes high-quality research relating to a specific, focused research purpose	All
Randomized, controlled trial	Experimental research technique that randomly assigns participants to a treatment group or control group; one group receives the treatment, but the other does not. Differences between the groups in their response (or nonresponse) to the treatment are analyzed statistically to draw conclusions about the treatments effects.	Intervention, etiology
Cohort	Two groups of participants are studied forward (prospectively) over time to determine the effects of a treatment. One group receives the treatment, whereas the other group does not.	Etiology, frequency, prediction
Case control	The effects of a condition are studied back through time (retrospectively) by comparing differences between a group of people who had the condition (case group) and a group of people who did not have the condition (control group).	Etiology
Cross-sectional with random sample	An independent, blind comparison with a "gold standard" test	Diagnosis
Case series/ case report	Descriptive report on the characteristics of patients with a particular condition or who followed a particular course of treatment; no comparison group is used; designed to assess the range and presence of issues.	Phenomena

- Participants should be similar to the population they represent. If not, the study results may not be applicable to other members of that population. For example, were the older adults in a resistance training study healthier and more physically active to start with than typical older adults? Are the study participants similar in most ways to the current patient? Age, gender, socioeconomic and education level, comorbidities, and health behaviors are some of the many characteristics to consider.

- In experimental studies, participants are put into control or treatment group(s). If participants of one group are not similar to the other group, one of the dissimilar characteristics (confounding variable), rather than the treatment, may explain differences between the groups. Consider the older adults again. If the resistance training group was more physically active from the start than a group that is given tai chi classes, maybe the better balance

TABLE 5-4
THREE BASIC RESEARCH DESIGNS

PURPOSE/QUESTION	CHARACTERISTICS	TYPE OF DESIGN AND LEVEL (HIGH TO LOW)	LIMITATIONS	STATISTICAL ANALYSIS
Describe what is going on or what exists. Example: What percentage of athletes exhibit signs of disordered eating?	Observation/measures existing groups Variables measured as they naturally occur Data usually gathered by survey, interview, or available records Attempts to determine the frequency or typical amount of a behavior, characteristic, trait, or opinion	Descriptive Level IV: cross-sectional Level V: case series, case report	Ability to generalize results limited by sample size and characteristics Cannot explain why a condition is happening	Descriptive statistics, frequency, mean/median, ratios
Examine the relationship(s) between 2 or more variables Example: What is the relationship between hamstring flexibility and vertical jump height?	Interested in the associations, trends, or interactions among 2 or more variables Observation/measures existing groups Variables measured as they naturally occur	Correlational Level IV: cohort studies, cross-sectional	Ability to generalize the results limited by sample size and characteristics Explaining why is difficult Presence of a relationship does not imply causation	Correlation coefficient

(continued)

Table 5-4 (continued)
Three Basic Research Designs

PURPOSE/QUESTION	CHARACTERISTICS	TYPE OF DESIGN AND LEVEL (HIGH TO LOW)	LIMITATIONS	STATISTICAL ANALYSIS
Determine whether one or more variables causes a change in one or more outcome variables. Example: Does spinal mobilization reduce chronic low back pain?	Groups that receive an intervention are compared to groups that receive no intervention or a placebo Ideally, participants are randomly assigned to the groups Environment of the experiment is highly controlled Cause and effect is implied Population-based inferences can be made	Experimental Level I: meta-analysis Level II: double-blind randomized, clinical trial; randomized, clinical trial Level III: nonrandom groups, single group	Confounding variables and bias may interfere with the ability to detect true causation Time and resource intensive Cannot assign injury, making study of sport-related injuries a challenge	Inferential statistics, t-tests, analysis of variance

of the resistance training group at the end of study was due to their higher activity level and not because of the exercise treatment. Characteristics that are used to match participants in addition to those previously mentioned are socioeconomic and education levels, smoking status, medical conditions, and fitness level.

- The best technique for creating equal groups is through random assignment. There are several ways researchers will randomize their samples. Picking colored marbles from a bag, using a computerized number generator, or doing a coin toss could be used to assign a participant to a treatment or control group. Participants must have an equal chance of being assigned to either group. Using order of appointments or having participants make groups by counting off 1 or 2 is not random.

- Participants who leave the study early should be accounted for in the analysis. It is common for participants, especially those in the control group, to drop out of studies. Researchers should show whether the lost participants made the groups less similar.

2. Was participant or researcher bias controlled for?

- Sample bias is when the participants, because of who they are or what they know, can shift the results. Participants who know they are receiving the study treatment are more likely to report that they had improvements or will subconsciously work harder to show that the treatment is effective. The term *blinded* refers to hiding the group assignment from the participants so they cannot influence the outcome variables. In exercise and physical modality studies, it is difficult to blind participants to their treatments.

- Researchers and those collecting the study data also have knowledge about how the treatment may or may not work. They may unintentionally tip off or cue participants as to the desired outcomes of an experiment, known as demand characteristics. To prevent this bias from impacting the results, some studies are double-blinded. This means that the participants and the person taking the measurements do not know to which treatment the participants are assigned. This strong study design is what is used in drug studies.

3. Were the groups given comparable treatments or placebos?

- The only difference between the 2 groups should be the treatment being tested. All other aspects of the procedures should be identical for each participant. When giving a placebo or sham treatment, the procedure must be identical to the actual treatment. For example, if one is studying the effects of ultrasound on an injury, the sham ultrasound treatment should include all of the prep and clean-up steps of the real ultrasound treatment.

4. Were the outcomes measured accurately?

- Researchers used a valid technique to measure the dependent variable. Validity is the ability of the technique to measure what it is intended to measure. Researchers may choose a gold standard measurement (known to have the highest level of validity) or may attempt to show how closely related their measurement was to a criterion measurement. For example, the gold standard for measuring percentage of body fat is dual energy x-ray absorptiometry scanning. Due to cost and availability, a researcher will discuss the level of agreement between dual energy x-ray absorptiometry and skinfolds taken by trained personnel.

- The way in which the measurements were taken must also be consistent. Reliability is the ability to accurately repeat the measurement over and over so that any changes in the data are due to the intervention. There are several potential threats to reliability in a study. There could be changes to the instrument or how the instrument is being used. For instance, the evaluator making the pretest measurement may not follow the same protocol at the posttest, which shows low intratester reliability. If multiple evaluators are being used to measure range of motion, there may be differences in how each performs, causing poor intertester reliability. Researchers should analyze and report the reliabilities of their measurements. There are several statistics for reliability, but, generally, a coefficient of .70 is needed.

- The way in which the tests were set up could also influence their reliability. Participants may get fatigued or bored and not perform their best on physical or mental tasks. When a variable is measured multiple times, the participants may experience a learning effect. For example, while performing an agility task, participants may become more proficient from practice with the test. Also, the fact that the patients are being observed and monitored closely may result in different responses to treatment. Lastly, measurements taken in experimental settings can produce different results from ones taken in a natural setting. For example, if a balance test is administered individually to soccer athletes in a quiet laboratory, their levels of focus and their scores may be different from that of on-field tests. In this way, highly controlled laboratory studies may not translate to real-world situations.

- Other common threats to reliability include the following:
  - Hawthorne effect: Subjects respond to the attention given by the researchers rather than to the actual treatments.
  - John Henry effect: The control group becomes aware of its secondary status and tries to outperform the experimental group.
  - Placebo effect: Participants improve based on the belief that the treatment will work, even if given a sham treatment.

5. Could the results have been due to chance, error, or a confounding variable?

- In the methods and results sections, the researcher should explain how a positive outcome was determined. The P-value that most commonly determines statistical significance is .05. Higher P-values mean a greater possibility that the results are due to chance. However, statistical significance does not mean clinically significant. The author should also report measures such as confidence intervals and effect size to estimate how useful the treatment is likely to be.

- Did the researcher consider all the possible explanations for the result besides the treatment? Possibly, some error or a confounding variable influenced the outcome. These limitations should be addressed in the discussion section. One should consider possible problems that the researcher did not by thinking about the sample, type of study, measurements, and treatment protocol. There is a wide range in the quality of research available, and it is important to be critical of anything that seems too good to be true.

- An example of a confounding variable is found in the following scenario. A researcher gave the experimental group a specific weight loss diet to follow and simultaneously asked the control group to eat as they normally would. The amount of physical activity performed by the participants was not controlled or monitored in either group. The experimental group, as expected, lost more weight, but because there was no way to sort out the influence of physical activity, it was difficult to trust that the difference in outcomes was due solely to the diet.

Hill's Criteria for Causation

A complementary approach to the aforementioned questions is a set of considerations proposed by Hill.[6] The criteria evaluate the likelihood that a cause-and-effect relationship exists between 2 variables and is helpful when there are few experimental studies to use as evidence. Hill[6] proposed this systematic approach for making inferences of causation from statistical associations observed in epidemiological data. He outlined 9 criteria, or in his words, viewpoints, to consider when judging whether an observed association is a causal relationship. He did not intend for his viewpoints to be used as a formal checklist and he did not believe any concrete rules of evidence could be adhered to. He emphasized that his 9 viewpoints were neither necessary nor always sufficient for causation. They provide a useful framework for systematically examining observed associations for causation.

1. Strength of Association: The magnitude of the correlation between the variables impacts the likelihood of causation. A small association does not preclude a causal effect; however, the larger the association, the more likely that it is causal. High relative risk and odds ratio are examples of strong associations between risk factors and disease occurrence that border on cause and effect.

2. Consistency: Consistent findings observed by different researchers using different settings, populations, and time frames strengthens the likelihood of an effect. Strong associations should be reproduced over and over to ensure consistency.

3. Specificity: Causation is likely if a specific causal factor produces a specific effect/disease/ injury at a specific site with no other likely explanation. This can be difficult to establish because a single risk factor may be associated with multiple outcomes. The more specific an association between a factor and an effect is, the bigger the probability of a causal relationship. The effect of cigarette smoking on mortality is a commonly cited example.

4. Temporal Sequence: The potential cause has to precede the effect. If there is a delay between the cause and expected effect, the effect must occur after that delay. If there is a cause-and-effect relationship between general knee laxity and ACL injury, the laxity must exist prior to the ACL injury.

5. Biological Gradient (Dose-Gradient Relationship): Greater exposure should generally lead to greater incidence of the effect. However, in some cases, the mere presence of the factor can trigger the effect. In other cases, an inverse proportion is observed. Greater exposure leads to lower incidence. If the causative factor is removed, the effect will disappear or be reduced. An example is a causative relationship between use of an orthotic insole and the presence of foot pain. If there is causation, consistent use of the insole would result in consistent reduction in pain. If the insole is removed, the pain returns.

6. Plausibility: There needs to be a theoretical basis for proposing a cause-and-effect association between 2 variables. It must make physiological sense. For example, a relationship may exist between the price of bananas and the prevalence of low back pain, but there is not likely to be any logical connection between the 2 events. Conversely, the discovery of a correlation between social media use and the incidence of eating disorders has a foundation in societal and peer pressure being a trigger for those behaviors. Research that conflicts with established theory is not necessarily faulty. It may call for a reexamination of accepted principles.

7. Coherence: Agreement between epidemiological and laboratory findings increases the likelihood of an effect. For example, studies of blows to mannequin heads in biomechanics laboratories point to angled and side blows as being more injurious than frontal blows, which has been noted in injury surveillance studies.

8. Experiment: Evidence shows that the effect can be prevented or limited when exposed to appropriate experimental designs. For example, the incidence of a second heart attack is reduced if the patient completes a cardiac rehabilitation program.

9. Analogy: When one causal factor is known, other similar factors are likely to produce similar outcomes, and the standards for causation can be lower for this new factor.

A final step in the evaluation of the evidence is to organize the findings into a format that allows one to analyze and assess relevance. If one feels that he or she has collected sufficient information on which to act, he or she will need to determine the clinical bottom line, which provides guidance about how the evidence relates to the care one will provide.

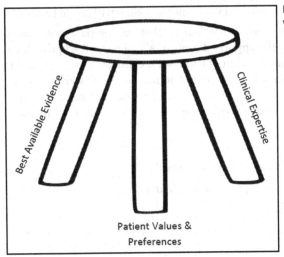

Figure 5-3. Three pillars of evidence-based practice work together to support best clinical practice.

Step 4: Apply the Evidence to the Desired Clinical Situation

If you have located quality evidence to use in clinical decision making, you must determine if the evidence is generalizable to your patient, feasible in your situation, and matches your patient's expectations. Establishing the generalizability of a study centers around how similar your patient is to the participants in the study. Your patient is more likely to respond according to the study if he or she is a member of that population. Consider age, gender, level of competition/experience, length of injury/recovery, and prior injuries. Next, is the treatment feasible in your facility and with your level of experience? Be sure that your interest in trying a new technique is not overshadowing some practical issues. Do you have the same equipment? Can you provide the same frequency and duration of treatments? Are you knowledgeable enough to perform the treatment or test? If not, are there ways for you to learn more or practice in advance? Finally, do the potential benefits outweigh the potential harms for the patient?

EBP provides a 3-pronged approach to patient-centered care. Such as with the legs of stool, all prongs are equally weighted (Figure 5-3). The first leg is using the best available evidence in decision making. Leg 2 takes advantage of the clinician's expertise and experience to provide the highest quality care. The third leg supports the patient's needs and preferences about his or her care. Ask yourself if this treatment is suitable for this patient. Consult with your patient and involve him or her in the final decision before implementing the treatment.

If the patient's preferences and values are not taken into consideration, patient compliance, persistence, and follow-through may be lacking, and the treatment will lose a measure of effectiveness. For example, if the patient finds that the core strengthening program you prescribed for his or her back injury is too difficult, time consuming, or complicated, his or her compliance will suffer, and the potential for a positive outcome is reduced. There are many issues to discuss with patients, such as the following:

- Their outcome goals and expectations
- What support they have from family and friends and whether their family and friends have to help with the treatment (eg, transportation, self-care, or encouragement)
- Whether the proposed treatment is in line with their religious, moral, cultural, or ethical beliefs
- How rigorous, complicated, or time demanding the treatment be will
- The potential side effects or less-than-ideal outcomes

- Whether the financial costs of the treatment (missed work, medical bills) will create hardship.

One commonly used method for creating a usable document that summarizes and stores evidence and the clinical bottom line is a critically appraised topic (CAT). The CEBM[4] provides a method for writing CATs (www.cebm.net/catmaker-ebm-calculators/). Clinicians can also locate CATs in various professional journals (ie, Journal of Sports Rehabilitation). CATs are typically limited to 2-page document that include a summary of the search process and results. It also includes a summary table of the articles that were appraised.[4] The components of the CAT include, but are not limited to, the following:

- Focused clinical question (PICO)

- Search strategy (terms used, databases; inclusion/exclusion criteria)

- Summary of the findings (number of articles, types of research articles)

- Best evidence (summary of level of evidence)

- Best evidence/key findings (summary of key points, similarities, or differences in articles)

- Clinical bottom line (based on key findings; what you will apply).

Step 5: Evaluate the Efficacy and Efficiency of the Practice

Well-defined, objective measures should be used to determine the clinical benefit of the treatment and the patient's experience. Clinically oriented outcomes include measures of pain, range of motion, strength, and scores on functional tests. Patient-oriented outcome measures relate to meeting patient goals and expectations and may include return to work or play, ratings of satisfaction with the treatment, and perceived benefits. Clinical measures should be taken prior to treatment, every few sessions thereafter, and at the end of the treatment plan. Patient-oriented measures typically occur after the last session and may be done less formally through conversation. Review the data and assess how well the treatment worked. This is also the time to determine if there are any factors that helped or hurt the outcome. These factors become new evidence to be used in the future.

When beginning to perform regular searches on clinical questions, it is also important to catalog and periodically update the searches as more evidence becomes available. At first, this step appears to be very time consuming, but establishing a regular day and time allotment helps. The goal is not to answer every question you have, but to seek new ideas and stay involved in the literature. You can engage colleagues by sharing your questions and results. The following questions will help guide you:

- Are you consistently asking and following through on your clinical questions?

  ○ What questions or interesting ideas have presented themselves recently in your practice?

  ○ How could you use the EBP principles to improve your clinical practice?

  ○ What colleagues might be resources for new questions or help you critically appraise evidence?

- What is your success rate in answering your clinical questions?

  ○ Are you finding the evidence you need to answer questions? If not, how will you adjust your process?

  ○ If you do not feel successful, you may need to refine your search strategies or your writing of clinical questions.

  ○ How many sources of evidence are you using? Are you constantly relying on 1 or 2?

  ○ How long is it taking to find and appraise evidence?

  ○ Might there be a more efficient way to conduct searches and review articles?

- How have you applied new evidence in your clinical practice?
  - What new questions or factors did you consider during this process?
  - Check for more recent articles. Possibly, the questions or factors you noticed have been investigated.

BRINGING IT TOGETHER

- The 3 components of EBM are clinical expertise, scientific research, and patient values and characteristics.
- EBP helps to improve clinical decision making and provides answers to clinical questions that are based on the best available evidence.
- The 5 steps of EBP include developing a clinical question, conducting a search, critically appraising the research, applying the evidence by integrating the clinical bottom line with clinical expertise and patient values, and evaluating the effectiveness and efficacy of the clinical bottom line.
- The PICO method allows clinicians to frame a clinical question based on clinical characteristics so that the best available evidence will be located.
- The type of database used may depend on the type of PICO question being asked.
- Critical appraisal of the best evidence provides the information that assists in answering the clinical question and develops the framework for applying the answers to clinical practice.
- Depending on the type of article being reviewed, the critical appraisal will use different metrics to evaluate the quality.
- Based on the available evidence, clinician expertise, and the patient's needs, the best treatment option is determined. A plan of care with specific patient outcomes will evaluate the effectiveness of the clinical intervention.

LEARNING ACTIVITIES

1. Construct a clinical question using PICO from the scenarios below. What type of clinical question is it (eg, intervention, etiology/risk factor, frequency/occurrence, diagnosis/testing, prediction, or phenomena)?

   A: An athlete asks you about using creatine supplements. He has heard it can make a big difference in improving muscle strength and power. He is a cross-country runner and has had little improvement in his performance lately. He is hoping to improve his aerobic capacity. Should he try it?

   B: A football coach is considering purchasing a new artificial turf practice field to replace the grass field but is concerned about the effect this may have on athlete injury rates (especially ACL injury). You know there is some relationship between the 2 but want to give him a more precise answer. Develop a clinical question to answer the coach's concern.

2. Conduct a search using one of the PICO questions. Develop a list of keywords or search terms and a list of synonyms for searching. Then select 2 databases/search engines to locate articles. Finally, record the findings in a research log; include information on search history, terms, combining terms, number of articles retrieved, and how you limited your search.

Critical Appraisal Worksheet

Clinical Question: _____

Article Citation:_____

A. INTERNAL VALIDITY

1. Were the groups of subjects representative and comparable?	
(a) Was the selection and assignment of subjects to groups randomized?	
What is best practice?	Where do I find this information?
Subjects should be randomly selected from the population of interest, but if the subjects are volunteers then an inclusion/exclusion should be specific and clearly outlined. The number of subjects should be large enough to be representative (>12 subjects per group is a minimal rule of thumb). Group assignment should be random and concealed.	The METHODS section should tell you how subjects were selected and allocated.
Answer: YES Comment:	NO UNCLEAR
(b) Were the groups similar at the start of the trial?	
What is best practice?	Where do I find this information?
If the randomization process was appropriate, the groups should be similar. The paper should indicate if that was checked and if the groups were different it should be mentioned if the differences were statistically significant	The RESULTS section should have a table of subject characteristics comparing groups on a number of variables relevant to the research question. If not, these should be described in the narrative of the RESULTS section
Answer: YES Comment:	NO UNCLEAR
(c) Were the groups treated equally (aside from the treatment or placebo)?	
What is best practice?	Where do I find this information?
Apart from the intervention, the subjects should be exposed to the same exact procedures. If a placebo was used it should be made to resemble the treatment as closely as possible.	The METHODS section should detail how the procedures were designed and executed.
Answer: YES	NO UNCLEAR

Comment:

(d) Were all the subjects that entered the study accounted for at the end?	
What is best practice?	Where do I find this information?
Losses of subjects should be minimal (less than 20%) but these losses should be reported and subjects should be analyzed in the groups to which they were randomized.	The RESULTS section should show how many subjects were randomized and analyzed and reasons for the losses (if any).

Answer: YES	NO	UNCLEAR

Comment:

2. Was the outcome measurement accurate?

(a) Were the subjects and investigators kept blind to which group each subject was assigned?	
What is best practice?	Where do I find this information?
It is ideal if both subjects and investigators are unaware of group assignments (double-blinding). Blinding is less critical if the outcome is objective (e.g. sustained injury) than if it is subjective (e.g. pain or function).	The METHODS section will indicate if subjects were blinded, how the outcome was measured and whether the investigators were blinded.

Answer: YES	NO	UNCLEAR

Comment:

(b) Were the outcomes measured the same way for all groups?	
What is best practice?	Where do I find this information?
It is important that outcomes are measured exactly the same way for all subjects regardless of group membership.	The METHODS section should describe how the outcomes were measured. The RESULTS section should show actual measures obtained.

Answer: YES	NO	UNCLEAR

Comment:

B. RESULTS

1. What measure was used and how large was the treatment effect?

2. Could the effect be random or due to chance?	
p-value	
Confidence Interval	

CONCLUSION
Internal validity:

Results:

Other Critical Appraisal Tools

Randomized Clinical Trials
- **Physiotherapy Evidence Database (PEDro)**
  Scores articles based upon a 1-10 score
  http://www.pedro.org.au/english/downloads/pedro-scale/
- **Jadad Scale**
  Scores articles based upon a 1-5 score
  http://www.anzjsurg.com/view/0/JadadScore.html

- **Quality of Reports of Meta-Analyses of Randomized Controlled Trials** (QUORUM)
  Checklist to use while reading evidence
  www.oxfordjournals.org/our_journals/humrep/for_authors/quoromcheck.doc

- **Preferred Reporting Items for Systematic Reviews and Meta-Analyses (PRISMA)**
  Modified QUOROM checklist
  http://www.prisma-statement.org/index.htm

REFERENCES

1. Sackett DL, Rosenberg WM, Gray JA, Haynes RB, Richardson WS. Evidence based medicine: what it is and what it isn't. *BMJ.* 1996;312(7023):71-72.
2. Sackett DL, Rosenberg WM. On the need for evidence-based medicine. *J Public Health Med.* 1995;17(3):330-334.
3. Straus SE. *Evidence-Based Medicine: How to Practice and Teach It.* 4th ed. Edinburgh, Scotland: Elsevier Churchill Livingstone; 2011.
4. Colorado State University Libraries. How to Do Library Research: Venn diagrams. http://lib.colostate.edu/howto/others/venn.html. Accessed March 1, 2015.
5. Oxford Centre for Evidence Based Medicine. http://www.cebm.net/index.aspx?o=5653. Accessed March 1, 2015.
6. Hill AB. The environment and disease: association or causation? *Proc R Soc Med.* 1965;58:295-300.

SUGGESTED READINGS

Glazebrook M. Symposium: evidence-based medicine: what is it and how should it be used? Introduction. *Foot Ankle Int.* 2010;31(11):1033-1037.

Greenhalgh T. *How to Read a Paper: The Basics of Evidence-Based Medicine.* 4th ed. Hoboken, NJ: Wiley-Blackwell; 2010.

Guyatt G, Drummond R, Meade M. *Users' Guides to the Medical Literature: A Manual for Evidence-Based Clinical Practice.* 2nd ed. New York, NY: McGraw-Hill Medical; 2008.

Journal of the American Medical Association Evidence. http://www.jamaevidence.com/. Accessed March 1, 2015.

Mayer D. *Essential Evidence-Based Medicine.* 2nd ed. Cambridge, UK: Cambridge University Press; 2010.

Steves R, Hootman JM. Evidence-based medicine: what is it and how does it apply to athletic training? *J Athl Train.* 2004;39(1):83-87.

II

Sport-Related Epidemiology

6

Sport-Related Concussion

Johna K. Register-Mihalik, PhD, LAT, ATC

CHAPTER OBJECTIVES

- List sports at most risk for concussive injuries.
- Identify important risk factors for concussion.
- Discuss barriers and limitations to epidemiological studies of concussion.
- Understand the need for a multimodal assessment (clinical examination, symptom assessment, cognitive assessment, and balance assessment) when evaluating concussions.

INTRODUCTION

No other injury has received the scrutiny and media attention that concussion has over the past 5 years. Careful attention should be paid to understanding the epidemiological, risk, and management factors surrounding concussions. These factors provide important evidence that will drive clinical practice. The current attention has allowed for an increased knowledge base and a general increase in awareness of concussion inside and outside of the sport. However, despite this attention and a growing body of knowledge concerning the acute and long-term effects of concussion, many of these injuries continue to go unidentified and mismanaged.[1,2] Concussion is one of the most difficult injuries to assess and manage. Currently, no gold standard of diagnosis exists. Diagnosis is largely based on self-reported symptoms with the incorporation of balance and memory tests.[3,4] Because much of this diagnosis relies on self-disclosure, many injuries are never identified. These factors further complicate how concussions are assessed and managed. Because of the complexity of concussive injury, a management model, including a team of sports medicine team professionals, is ideal. Athletic trainers, because of their unique skill set and position in sport, play a key role in identifying and properly managing these injuries.

Adams M, Swiger W.
*Epidemiology for Athletic Trainers: Integrating
Evidence-Based Practice (pp 105-118).*
© 2016 Taylor & Francis Group.

One specific issue concerning concussion is the continued evolution of the injury definition. The definition of concussion has evolved to be more clinically applicable and straightforward over the past decade. However, there are many variations on the definition, leading to potential problems for identification of the injury. One of the most commonly accepted definitions comes from the International Consensus Conference on concussion in sport, which states that, "concussion is a brain injury and is defined as a complex pathophysiological process affecting the brain, induced by biomechanical forces."[4]

This definition goes on to highlight many of the complexities and common misnomers about concussion that lead to issues in identification and management of the injury, such as a lack of a gold standard for diagnosis and that, in some cases, symptom presence may be prolonged. In addition, it illustrates that signs and symptoms may last beyond the acute phase. The recently updated National Athletic Trainers' Association (NATA) Position Statement[3] defines concussion using the broader definition from the American Academy of Neurology, which states that concussion is a "trauma-induced alteration in mental status that may or may not involve a loss of consciousness."

A leading issue for researchers and clinicians is the potential for long-lasting effects from concussions. These range from cognitive issues and motor issues in the days following injury[5,6] to the development of psychological or neurological conditions later in life.[7-10] These negative effects raise significant concerns in the medical community and among athletes, schools, sporting organizations, and parents. The science behind these effects continues to advance, and better epidemiological and clinical studies are needed to further understand the potential outcomes. The key studies reviewed in this chapter and position statements may be used to inform clinical practice and decision making for concussed athletes.

INCIDENCE OF CONCUSSION IN YOUTH, COLLEGE, AND PROFESSIONAL SPORTS

Traumatic brain injury (TBI) results in more than 1,224,000 emergency department visits, 290,000 hospitalizations, and 51,000 deaths each year.[11] Disabilities following TBI, even from mild injuries, lead to many problems that may decrease an individual's quality of life, including emotional, physical, academic, cognitive, and social dysfunction.[12-14] The Centers for Disease Control and Prevention estimates that between 1.6 and 3.8 million sport-related traumatic brain injuries occur each year. Concussions account for approximately 10% of all sport-related injuries.[15,16] A high incidence of concussion, specifically among contact sports, no matter the level, is well documented in the literature.[17-21]

Youth Sports

Among youth athletes (14 years and younger), there are few comprehensive epidemiological studies of concussion. This age group was previously difficult to study due to the lack of sports medicine professionals present at events and the transient nature of athletes across seasons and teams. One of the few studies to examine the incidence of concussion (combined practices and games) in American youth football found the incidence rate (IR) of concussion to be 1.76 concussions/1000 athlete-exposures (AEs; 95% confidence interval [CI], 0.99, 2.54), with the IR in games being 6.16/1000 AEs (95% CI, 3.76, 9.54) and in practices being 0.24/1000 AEs (95% CI, 0.04, 0.79).[22] These numbers are comparable to known rates for the high school and collegiate populations participating in American football, with the game IR being higher than reported for the older age groups.

Among youth and middle school female soccer players, the IR has been reported to be 1.2/1000 AE hours (95% CI, 0.9, 1.6) overall, with a cumulative incidence of 13%.[23] There are currently no national, regional, or state-wide surveillance systems in place to comprehensively evaluate the epidemiology of concussion at the youth sports level. The Institute on Medicine's report on sport-related concussions in youth specifically outlined the need for this type of surveillance to be implemented.[24] Furthermore, there are typically no sports medicine professionals, particularly athletic trainers, staffing youth sport events, making surveillance more difficult because many of the epidemiological studies of concussion include settings in which athletic trainers are staffed.

High School Sports

Epidemiological data among high school athletes are more widely available, but varying definitions and greater awareness of concussion are likely factors in the differences in the numbers seen today compared to 10 years ago. Recent studies indicate that concussion rates have increased across most high school sports in recent years.[25] Prominent studies of high school concussion include studies by Lincoln et al[25] and Gessel et al,[26] which report similar overall concussion rates.

However, Lincoln et al[25] had a longer data collection period (1997 to 2008) and discussed increases in concussion incidence over time. Lincoln et al[25] reported the following incidence rates for common high school sports per 1000 AEs: football, 0.60; boys' lacrosse, 0.30; boys' soccer, 0.17; girls' soccer, 0.35; boys' basketball, 0.10; girls' basketball, 0.16; wrestling, 0.17; baseball, 0.06; softball, 0.11; field hockey, 0.10; and cheerleading, 0.06. The overall incidence of concussion in this study was reported to be 0.24.

Gessel et al[26] used data collected during the 2005-2006 school year and suggested the overall incidence of concussion to be 0.23/1000 AEs. These data were some of the first to highlight potential gender differences, with females' concussion incidence being greater than that of boys in specific sports. Gessel et al[26] reported the following incidence rates/1000 AEs for high school sports: football, 0.47; boys' soccer, 0.22; girls' soccer, 0.36; girls' volleyball, 0.05; boys' basketball, 0.07; girls' basketball, 0.21; wrestling, 0.18; baseball, 0.05; and softball, 0.07. These sports are those with the greatest risk of concussion because participants often receive direct blows to the head and face. An additional study estimated the incidence of concussion in boys' lacrosse to be 0.28/1000 AEs and the incidence in girls' lacrosse to be 0.21/1000 AEs.[27] The incidence of concussion among cheerleaders has been estimated to be as high as 0.09 (0.02 to 0.17) per 1000 AEs.[28] The incidence of concussion in ice hockey is thought to be one of the highest across all sports. Despite this high incidence, few studies address concussions at the high school level. In 1987, Gerberich et al[20] reported that concussion may account for more than 10% of injuries in hockey, which is higher than other sports.

College Sports

Studies suggest that in collegiate sports, concussion accounts for approximately 6% of all injuries, with incidence rates being higher in the collegiate age group than in the high school age group. In addition, many of the gender differences observed in the high school age group are not as prevalent in the collegiate age group.[26] Two of the most recent studies, both published in 2007, highlight the following incidence rates for college sports per 1000 athlete-hours[26,29]: football, 0.37 to 0.61; men's lacrosse, 0.26; men's soccer, 0.28 to 0.49; wrestling, 0.25 to 0.42; men's basketball, 0.07 to 0.09; women's soccer, 0.41 to 0.63, women's lacrosse, 0.25; women's basketball, 0.22 to 0.43; softball, 0.14 to 0.19; and field hockey, 0.18. Few other recent profiles outline the incidence of concussion in collegiate athletics.

Professional Sports

Although professional sports is the most publicized arena of sports, there are few epidemiological studies of concussion in the professional setting. One of the comprehensive studies of overall concussion epidemiology in the National Hockey League found the incidence rate of concussion to be 1.8/1000 player-hours. Another interesting finding of this same study found that time loss increased on average 2.5 days for every subsequent (recurrent) concussion during the study period (1997 to 2004).[30] One of the most recent studies of concussion in the National Football League found the incidence rate to be 64.3/10,000 AEs (6.43/1000 AEs).[31]

Neurodegenerative conditions potentially from head trauma have been studied in professional athletes, although it is predominately cross-sectional evidence. These studies have observed associations among former professional American football players between previous history of concussion and depression, mild cognitive impairment, and other psychological and memory-related issues.[8,32,33] Studies among professional ice hockey players have observed similar findings.[34] Varying results for the effects of professional soccer on some of these same measures, particularly heading, have been reported.[35] A recent study found that once retired, former elite soccer athletes risk of neurodegenerative issues fell in line with the general population.[36] However, others have suggested that exposure to head impacts, even purposeful heading, may be a precursor to neurodegenerative issues as an individual ages.[37,38] Boxing has often been the sport of reference when discussing potential long-term and cumulative effects of head trauma because some of the first research positing potential links centered on boxers.[39,40]

Another issue that is of increasing concern is chronic traumatic encephalopathy (CTE). CTE is often characterized by mental deterioration (including psychological deterioration), confusion, slowing of speech, and Parkinson-like symptoms. Pathologically, there is typically more a diffuse accumulation of Tau protein in the brain with other specific changes.[41] Athletic trainers are often the first health care providers approached if an individual or his or her family has concerns about CTE. Currently, CTE can only be diagnosed postmortem through an autopsy despite many providers claiming that individuals may have CTE. Recent studies suggest that various forms of imaging may be able to pick up the Tau protein deposits characteristic of CTE; however, these are yet to be fully clinically validated.[42] The current studies of CTE are laboratory and pathology based. To date, no prospective or causal study has been conducted to fully uncover the factors that place an individual at risk for the disease. It is estimated that approximately 10% of individuals who receive multiple impacts as a result of sport will develop the disease.[33,43,44] More research is needed to fully understand the pathology of CTE and what risk factors exist around the disease.

Future research in this area is essential to understanding the true epidemiology of the condition and its relationship to sport participation. Overall, there are few prospective epidemiological studies of concussion among professional sports presented in the literature. This group is often hard to study because data are not widely available for analysis and review. More detailed epidemiological profiles and prospective studies of concussion in this population are needed.

Recovery Patterns Across All Sport Levels

Clinicians want to see postconcussive athletes make a safe and progressive return back to activity. As such, one of the primary indicators of recovery is time to return to play (RTP). A recent study examining high school athletes during the 2007-2009 school years found that following a concussion incident, the probability of RTP within 1 to 2 days of injury was 2.5% (95% CI, 0.3, 6.9), 71.3% (95% CI, 59.0, 82.9) for 7 to 9 days postinjury, and 88.8% (95% CI, 72.0, 97.2) for 10 to 21 days postinjury.[45] However, previous studies have illustrated more premature returns, or at least return to participation not in compliance with existing RTP guidelines. The most recent NATA position statement recommends no athlete return to participation while symptomatic. Academic accommodations may be necessary during the recovery period, and, prior to return to activity,

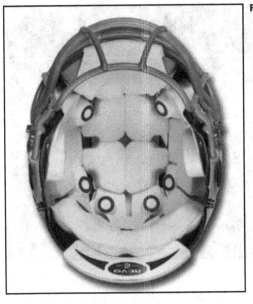

Figure 6-1. Head impact telemetry system.

a gradual and progressive approach should be used.[3] A study during the 2005-2008 school years observed that 15% percent of concussed football athletes who sustained a loss of consciousness returned to play in less than 1 day. In addition, approximately 40% of concussed athletes returned to play prematurely under American Academy of Neurology guidelines and 15% according to International Consensus RTP guidelines. Males were more likely than females to return 1 to 2 days after sustaining more severe injuries (12% vs 5.9%, respectively).[46] Few studies have addressed return to learn or school activities.

PROBLEMS IN EPIDEMIOLOGICAL PROFILES OF CONCUSSION

Although the number of studies examining the epidemiology of concussion has increased rapidly over the past 10 years, there are barriers and issues related to the collection of these data. One of the most notable is the definition of concussion. Ten to 15 years ago, the definition of concussion involved a loss of consciousness[47]; therefore, these studies grossly underestimated the incidence of concussion across all levels of sport and activity. Because concussion has no gold-standard measure for diagnosis, many clinicians and researchers use varying definitions. Many model a multimodal approach that encompasses the clinical evaluation, symptom assessment, cognitive assessment, and balance assessment.[3,4] Furthermore, many concussions are identified through self-report or disclosure, and studies have indicated that more than 50% of concussive injuries may go unreported and unidentified.[1,2] Despite the recent advances in head impact biomechanics, including measurement of head impact acceleration magnitudes, location, and direction (Figure 6-1), there is currently no threshold for concussive injury, also making it difficult to identify all concussions.

Various settings in which concussions may be managed, such as the emergency department, clinic, or school, also make interpretation of findings difficult. However, an epidemiologic profile and knowledge of patients in various settings is essential to better understanding the injury.

Adding further issue to the full understanding of the epidemiology of concussion are the definitions concerning recovery. Varying definitions are used in studies to define recovery, ranging from asymptomatic to full return to sport.[45,48,49] These definitions can make it difficult to determine the course of recovery because times for these variables may be affected by

Figure 6-2. Impact forces.

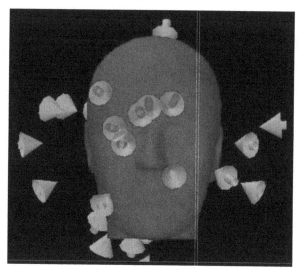

self-reporting and clinician bias and decision making. In addition, there are issues of studying recurrent and multiple concussions. Studies show that once an athlete sustains a concussion, he or she is more likely to sustain another.[50] Recent studies attempt to address recurrent injuries, at least within the context of a single season. However, over longer study periods, this becomes more difficult. Understanding recurrent concussion is important from epidemiological and clinical standpoints, given the growing body of evidence linking multiple concussions to issues later in life. Sports medicine professionals should be aware of these potential limitations when reading the literature and attempting to apply them to clinical practice.

CONCUSSION ETIOLOGY AND ASSESSMENT

The complex pathophysiology of concussions makes it difficult to clearly diagnose and define. Signs and symptoms and the duration of disability vary greatly among athletes. This section describes the known mechanism, neurophysiology, and risk factors, as well as the current assessment protocols, including symptom scales, computerized assessment, and balance measures.

Mechanism and Pathophysiology

A concussive injury results from acceleration-deceleration forces transmitted through the brain. Coup (same side) and/or contrecoup (opposite side) injury may also result from these forces. The coup-contrecoup pressure phenomenon states that contrecoup injury may produce the majority of deficits in a closed head injury.[51] However, some studies concerning concussion have theorized that rotational forces result in more severe brain injury and produce increased dysfunction as rotational forces (Figure 6-2) cause shearing of the tissue within the brain.[52,53] Although the majority of what is known regarding the neurophysiology of concussion comes from animal studies, new functional imaging techniques are giving insight and paralleling these findings in humans.[54-56] Recent preliminary in vivo (in living person) head impact research has found no relationships between concussive injury and impact magnitude or location.[57-59]

The forces causing concussion produce what is known as a complex neurometabolic cascade of events leading to the variety of signs and symptoms following a concussion. Acutely following injury, there is an abrupt ionic shift, resulting in changes in cellular physiology. During this complex cascade, the sodium potassium pump goes into overdrive, leading to increased energy needs (need for adenosine triphosphate). As a result, there is a significant increase in glucose metabolism, which occurs while there is also decreased cerebral blood flow. This disparity between glucose supply and demand triggers an ongoing energy crisis, which is thought to be the cause of postconcussive vulnerability.[60] During this period of vulnerability is when individuals often present with the initial symptoms of concussion, such as headache and difficulty concentrating. Next, the brain then goes into a phase of depressed metabolism. Increases in calcium may further impair cell function and fuel the ongoing energy crisis. The increased and unchecked calcium accumulation may also lead to cell death. The diffuse nature of the injury and the level at which it occurs leads to poor identification, which is a problem in understanding the epidemiology of concussion across all levels of sport.[60]

Risk Factors

Due to the complex individualized nature of concussive injuries, there are few prospective risk factor studies in the literature. A primary risk factor among athletes is participation in a collision sport, such as football, boys' ice hockey, and boys' lacrosse.[26,61-63] One of the most cited studies concerning risk highlights previous concussion as a risk factor for subsequent injury. This study suggested the risk of sustaining a concussion is 5.8 times greater for individuals with a history of previous concussion (95% CI, 4.8, 6.9).[50] An additional study identified concussion history, participation in contact sports, and being in the bottom quintile for body mass index to be some of the strongest predictors of concussion rates.[28]

More recent studies also suggest that females may be more at risk for concussion than male athletes, specifically among female soccer and basketball athletes.[26,64] The growing body of literature suggests that in comparable female sports, the risk may be 2 times greater.[25,62] However, when all males and females are grouped together, few gender differences have been observed. Schulz et al[28] reported that the high school concussion injury rate per 100,000 athlete practices was 4.01 (95% CI, 1.25, 6.77) for females and 5.81 (95% CI, 3.30, 8.31) for males overall. The only gender difference observed in this study was between male (2.67/100,000 AEs) and female (7.94/100,000 AEs) soccer athletes.

Gender differences concerning reporting of concussions are not well understood or studied. Covassin et al[64] reported that female athletes sustain a higher percentage of concussions during games than males. Many theories exist around why these differences are observed. Concussion disclosure behaviors may contribute to the increased relative incidence among females reported in the literature. Health behavior literature reports that females are more likely to seek medical care and report symptoms of many medical conditions than males.[65,66] These studies are largely focused on more severe health problems and chronic pain, which may not directly translate to athletic injury. A study related to TBI in individuals of all ages found no difference in gender on seeking care for concussion. However, many of these individuals were older, and some had more severe brain injuries.[67] There continues to be speculation concerning other potential risk factors for concussion, including neck strength, physical characteristics, location, and cumulative magnitude of impacts; however, limited data exist concerning these factors. Other factors, such as fair play, equipment, and play through pain cultural standards may be risk factors. These are discussed in the rules and equipment sections in Chapter 11.

Concussion Assessment

Current literature and experts suggest a comprehensive approach using a clinical evaluation, symptom assessment, balance assessment, and neurocognitive assessment. Broglio et al[68] reported that using a combination of a symptom checklist, balance assessment, and neuropsychological testing yields sensitivity of greater than 90%, whereas neurocognitive testing alone is about 79%, symptom

TABLE 6-1 SYMPTOM SCALE						
SYMPTOM	NONE	MILD		MODERATE		SEVERE	
Headache	0	1	2	3	4	5	6
Nausea	0	1	2	3	4	5	6
Vomiting	0	1	2	3	4	5	6
Dizziness	0	1	2	3	4	5	6
Poor balance	0	1	2	3	4	5	6
Sensitivity to noise	0	1	2	3	4	5	6
Ringing in the ear	0	1	2	3	4	5	6
Sensitivity to light	0	1	2	3	4	5	6
Blurred vision	0	1	2	3	4	5	6
Difficulty concentrating	0	1	2	3	4	5	6
Feeling mentally "foggy"	0	1	2	3	4	5	6
Difficulty remembering	0	1	2	3	4	5	6
Trouble falling asleep	0	1	2	3	4	5	6
Drowsiness	0	1	2	3	4	5	6
Fatigue	0	1	2	3	4	5	6
Sadness	0	1	2	3	4	5	6
Irritability	0	1	2	3	4	5	6
Neck pain	0	1	2	3	4	5	6

assessment is 68%, and balance assessment is 62%. In addition, Register-Mihalik et al[69] identified this multimodal approach as significantly more sensitive than any measure used in isolation.

A symptom checklist is one of the most commonly used clinical measures in the assessment of concussion. Symptom checklists (Table 6-1) have been used in various studies and have been shown to be valid and reliable.[70-72] Studies suggest that variations of the tool are reliable and valid when administered by clinicians and across age groups, from children to adults.[70,72] However, these tools are all based on self-reports, which can be subjective; thus, there is need for a comprehensive approach inclusive of more objective measures.

Computerized neurocognitive assessments provide an objective assessment of cognitive function and, thus, have risen to the forefront of concussion evaluation over the past 15 years.[73-76] Recent literature questions the utility of many of these tests and batteries due to low reliability and limited psychometric research.[77,78] In addition, these tests were developed from the framework of more traditional paper and pencil neuropsychological tests, which have more clinician interaction. Research on the reliability of these computerized tasks is limited by the testing environment and the time elapsed between test sessions. The environment, such as a noisy room or the presence of many other athletes, also often limits many studies related to neuropsychological performance. Various products are available for computerized assessment, including the ImPACT (ImPACT Applications, Inc), Concussion Vital Signs (CNS Vital Signs), and Cogstate CCAT (Axon Sports). Each of these measures some form of cognition, and all have the limitations previously mentioned.

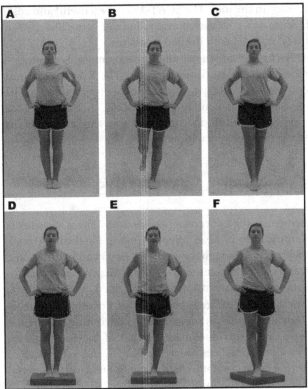

Figure 6-3. Balance Error Scoring System. (Reprinted with permission from Stiffler M, Mihalik JP, Register-Mihalik JK, Ingriselli JM. Cognition and balance performance following a single-task training intervention in healthy collegiate recreational students: A preliminary study. *Athletic Training & Sports Health Care.* 2013;5(2):63-68.)

Nonetheless, these tests can provide valuable information following possible injury. Many consensus statements have recommended the use of some form of neurocognitive assessment in the evaluation of concussion.[79-81] Measurement of basic cognitive function involves use of a mental status examination, such as the Standardized Assessment of Concussion (SAC). The SAC has been shown to be sensitive to concussion and is often used in research studies assessing the acute effects of concussive injury. It is most useful and sensitive within the first 48 hours following a concussion.[82]

Balance assessment has also been recommended as a component in a concussion assessment program. Like neurocognitive testing, there are many ways to assess balance, from a simple Romberg test to computerized force-plate measures.[76] The clinical field test, the Balance Error Scoring System, offers a cheap, objective way to assess balance on the field following a possible concussive injury (Figure 6-3). The athlete performs 6 trials consisting of 3 different stances done on firm and foam surfaces. The stances include double leg, single leg (on the stance leg), and tandem (with the stance leg in the back). Errors are recorded if individuals lift their hands off of their iliac crest; abduct or flex their hip to greater than 30 degrees; step, stumble or fall; open eyes; lift their toes; or remain out of the testing position for greater than 5 seconds. A higher score indicates a greater deficit in postural stability. Due to individual variability, baseline measures are important to determine the severity of deficit following injury.[83]

The Sport Concussion Assessment Tool–3 (SCAT-3) encompasses some form of all of the aforementioned pieces in the concussion assessment.[4] Recently revised, it now includes sectioned scoring instead of a composite score and asks more questions about the athlete's injury. The SCAT-3 is free to the public, and all athletic trainers have access to the tool. The tool encompasses a Sideline Checklist, a Background section, the Glasgow Coma Scale, Maddux questions, Symptom Evaluation (with checklist), the SAC, a neck examination, the modified Balance Error Scoring System, and a tandem gait task. The tool also provides general RTP information and interpretation of the information for each of the tasks included in the tool. The SCAT-3 may be a useful and cost-effective way to ensure that the essential pieces of a concussion evaluation are being included in the process in an objective fashion for athletic trainers with limited resources.

Additional measures, such as the King-Devick test[84] and the Vestibular Oculomotor Screening,[85] may provide even more objective information to the assessment process. The King-Devick test incorporates visual scanning and assesses a patient's ability to scan quickly and accurately. The Vestibular Oculomotor Screening assesses visual and oculomotor function and may provide indications of vestibular-ocular dysfunction. These additional tests are supplemental tools for clinicians to use in the assessment and management of concussion.

POSITION AND CONSENSUS STATEMENTS

Numerous position and consensus statements exist concerning concussion. These statements likely lead to increased awareness and identification of head injuries among medical personal, contributing to the increased concussion incidence. Although they vary in content and are directed at different audiences, these position statements all recommend a comprehensive approach to concussion assessment, including the multimodal assessment approach presented in the literature.

The position statements are guidelines for what is considered best practice. For athletic trainers specifically, knowledge of the NATA's recently updated position statement concerning concussion is essential.[3] The most widely cited of these consensus documents is that of the International Concussion in Sport Group.[4] A summary of best practices from the NATA and International Concussion in Sport Group includes gathering baseline data when feasible and possible, serial evaluation of the injury, appropriate home care instructions, symptom free prior to return to physical activity, management of academic conditions as needed, and a gradual increase in volume and intensity in physical activity prior to full return to sport. These position statements often drive clinical practice and research metrics, which can lead to changes in the epidemiological profile of the injury. These position statements, in addition to a recent Institute of Medicine report on youth concussion,[24] highlight the need for better concussion surveillance across all levels of sport.

BRINGING IT TOGETHER

Recent increases in concussion rates, mostly at the high school level, are likely due to increased awareness and better detection of these injuries. Studies now include a more comprehensive definition of concussion, which allows for more broad identification of the injuries. Recent literature highlights that females, compared to matched-sport male counterparts, may be more than twice as likely to suffer a concussion. There are now more links than ever illustrating association with potential long-term effects after concussion that leave many clinicians and athletes questioning just how mild an injury may truly be when recovery is considered. A combination of assessments provides the best evaluation procedure for concussion and should be undertaken prior to participation and multiple times during recovery.

REVIEW QUESTIONS

1. What are the key components recommended in the literature as part of the multimodal assessment of concussion?

2. List 2 barriers to epidemiological studies of concussion discussed in this chapter and explain why these may be problematic in understanding the epidemiology of concussion.

3. List at least one risk factor for concussion and describe why this may be a risk factor.

Learning Activities

1. Administer the SCAT-3 to friends and classmates. Repeat the test after a dizzy bat race.

2. List 3 things sports medicine professionals can do to decrease the incidence of concussion, both new and recurring.

3. Do an Internet search on the construction of sports helmets and the organizations that certify helmets.

    a. Identify materials used for youth vs adult helmets as well as repeated-blow and single-impact type helmets.

    b. Select a sport (hockey, lacrosse, football, Nordic skiing, equestrian, or mountain biking), determine which agency sets the standard for the helmet used, and identify the industry standard for testing energy attenuation.

    c. For repeated-blow helmets, identify the recommendations for the reconditioning of helmets.

References

1. Register-Mihalik JK, Guskiewicz KM, McLeod TC, Linnan LA, Mueller FO, Marshall SW. Knowledge, attitude, and concussion-reporting behaviors among high school athletes: a preliminary study. *J Athl Train.* 2013;48(5):645-653.

2. McCrea M, Hammeke T, Olsen G, Leo P, Guskiewicz K. Unreported concussion in high school football players: implications for prevention. *Clin J Sport Med.* 2004;14(1):13-17.

3. Broglio SP, Cantu RC, Gioia GA, et al. National Athletic Trainers' Association position statement: management of sport concussion. *J Athl Train.* 2014;49(2):245-265.

4. McCrory P, Meeuwisse WH, Aubry M, et al. Consensus statement on concussion in sport: the 4th International Conference on Concussion in Sport held in Zurich, November 2012. *Br J Sports Med.* 2013;47(5):250-258.

5. De Beaumont L, Théoret H, Mongeon D, et al. Brain function decline in healthy retired athletes who sustained their last sports concussion in early adulthood. *Brain.* 2009;132(pt 3):695-708.

6. Parker TM, Osternig LR, van Donkelaar P, Chou LS. Recovery of cognitive and dynamic motor function following concussion. *Br J Sports Med.* 2007;41(12):868-873.

7. Guskiewicz KM, McCrea M, Marshall SW, et al. Cumulative effects associated with recurrent concussion in collegiate football players: the NCAA Concussion Study. *JAMA.* 2003;290(19):2549-2555.

8. Guskiewicz KM, Marshall SW, Bailes J, et al. Recurrent concussion and risk of depression in retired professional football players. *Med Sci Sports Exerc.* 2007;39(6):903-909.

9. Chen JK, Johnston KM, Petrides M, Ptito A. Neural substrates of symptoms of depression following concussion in male athletes with persisting postconcussion symptoms. *Arch Gen Psychiatry.* 2008;65(1):81-89.

10. Ahman S, Saveman BI, Styrke J, Björnstig U, Stålnacke BM. Long-term follow-up of patients with mild traumatic brain injury: a mixed-method study. *J Rehabil Med.* 2013;45(8):758-764.

11. Rutland-Brown W, Langlois JA, Thomas KE, Xi YL. Incidence of traumatic brain injury in the United States, 2003. *J Head Trauma Rehabil.* 2006;21(6):544-548.

12. Mainwaring LM, Hutchison M, Bisschop SM, Comper P, Richards DW. Emotional response to sport concussion compared to ACL injury. *Brain Inj.* 2010;24(4):589-597.

13. Kontos AP, Covassin T, Elbin RJ, Parker T. Depression and neurocognitive performance after concussion among male and female high school and collegiate athletes. *Arch Phys Med Rehabil.* 2012;93(10):1751-1756.

14. Soberg HL, Røe C, Anke A, et al. Health-related quality of life 12 months after severe traumatic brain injury: a prospective nationwide cohort study. *J Rehabil Med.* 2013;45(8):785-791.

15. Guskiewicz KM, Weaver NL, Padua DA, Garrett WE Jr. Epidemiology of concussion in collegiate and high school football players. *Am J Sports Med.* 2000;28(5):643-650.

16. Powell JW, Barber-Foss KD. Traumatic brain injury in high school athletes. *JAMA.* 1999;282(10):958-963.

17. Buckley WE. Concussions in college football. A multivariate analysis. *Am J Sports Med.* 1988;16(1):51-56.

18. Bruce DA, Schut L, Sutton LN. Brain and cervical spine injuries occurring during organized sports activities in children and adolescents. Clin *Sports Med.* 1982;1(3):495-514.

19. Cantu RC. Minor head injuries in sports. *Adolesc Med.* 1991;2(1):141-154.

20. Gerberich SG, Finke R, Madden M, Priest JD, Aamoth G, Murray K. An epidemiological study of high school ice hockey injuries. *Childs Nerv Syst.* 1987;3(2):59-64.

21. Gerberich SG, Priest JD, Boen JR, traub CP, Maxwell RE. Concussion incidences and severity in secondary school varsity football players. *Am J Public Health.* 1983;73(12):1370-1375.

22. Kontos AP, Elbin RJ, Fazio-Sumrock VC, et al. Incidence of sports-related concussion among youth football players aged 8-12 years. *J Pediatr.* 2013;163(3):717-720.

23. O'Kane JW, Spieker A, Levy MR, Neradilek M, Polissar NL, Schiff MA. Concussion among female middle-school soccer players. *JAMA Pediatr.* 2014;168(3):258-264.

24. Graham R, Rivara FP, Ford MA, Spicer CM. *Sport-Related Concussions in Youth: Improving the Science, Changing the Culture.* Washington, CD: The National Academies Press; 2014.

25. Lincoln AE, Caswell SV, Almquist JL, Dunn RE, Norris JB, Hinton RY. Trends in concussion incidence in high school sports: a prospective 11-year study. *Am J Sports Med.* 2011;39(5):958-963.

26. Gessel LM, Fields SK, Collins CL, Dick RW, Comstock RD. Concussions among United States high school and collegiate athletes. *J Athl Train.* 2007;42(4):495-503.

27. Lincoln AE, Hinton RY, Almquist JL, Lager SL, Dick RW. Head, face, and eye injuries in scholastic and collegiate lacrosse: a 4-year prospective study. *Am J Sports Med.* 2007;35(2):207-215.

28. Schulz MR, Marshall SW, Yang J, Mueller FO, Weaver NL, Bowling JM. A prospective cohort study of injury incidence and risk factors in North Carolina high school competitive cheerleaders. *Am J Sports Med.* 2004;32(2):396-405.

29. Hootman JM, Dick R, Agel J. Epidemiology of collegiate injuries for 15 sports: summary and recommendations for injury prevention initiatives. *J Athl Train.* 2007;42(2):311-319.

30. Benson BW, Meeuwisse WH, Rizos J, Kang J, Burke CJ. A prospective study of concussions among National Hockey League players during regular season games: the NHL-NHLPA Concussion Program. *CMAJ.* 2011;183(8):905-911.

31. Myer GD, Smith D, Barber Foss KD, et al. Rates of concussion are lower in National Football League games played at higher altitudes. *J Orthop Sports Phys Ther.* 2014;44(3):164-172.

32. Guskiewicz KM, Marshall SW, Bailes J, et al. Association between recurrent concussion and late-life cognitive impairment in retired professional football players. *Neurosurgery.* 2005;57(4):719-726.

33. Gavett BE, Stern RA, McKee AC. Chronic traumatic encephalopathy: a potential late effect of sport-related concussive and subconcussive head trauma. *Clin Sports Med.* 2011;30(1):179-188.

34. Caron JG, Bloom GA, Johnston KM, Sabiston CM. Effects of multiple concussions on retired national hockey league players. *J Sport Exerc Psychol.* 2013;35(2):168-179.

35. Matser JT, Kessels AG, Lezak MD, Troost J. A dose-response relation of headers and concussions with cognitive impairment in professional soccer players. *J Clin Exp Neuropsychol.* 2001;23(6):770-774.

36. Vann Jones SA, Breakey RW, Evans PJ. Heading in football, long-term cognitive decline and dementia: evidence from screening retired professional footballers. *Br J Sports Med.* 2014;48(2):159-161.

37. Webbe FM, Ochs SR. Recency and frequency of soccer heading interact to decrease neurocognitive performance. *Appl Neuropsychol.* 2003;10(1):31-41.

38. Stålnacke BM, Tegner Y, Sojka P. Playing soccer increases serum concentrations of the biochemical markers of brain damage S-100B and neuron-specific enolase in elite players: a pilot study. *Brain Inj.* 2004;18(9):899-909.

39. Jordan BD, Jahre C, Hauser WA, et al. CT of 338 active professional boxers. *Radiology.* 1992;185(2):509-512.

40. Jordan BD, Relkin NR, Ravdin LD, Jacobs AR, Bennett A, Gandy S. Apolipoprotein E epsilon4 associated with chronic traumatic brain injury in boxing. *JAMA.* 1997;278(2):136-140.

41. Brandenburg W, Hallervorden J. Dementia pugilistica with anatomical findings [in German]. *Virchows Arch.* 1954;325(6):680-709.

42. Small GW, Kepe V, Siddarth P, et al. PET scanning of brain tau in retired national football league players: preliminary findings. *Am J Geriatr Psychiatry.* 2013;21(2):138-144.

43. McKee AC, Cantu RC, Nowinski CJ, et al. Chronic traumatic encephalopathy in athletes: progressive tauopathy after repetitive head injury. *J Neuropathol Exp Neurol.* 2009;68(7):709-735.

44. Gavett BE, Stern RA, Cantu RC, Nowinski CJ, McKee AC. Mild traumatic brain injury: a risk factor for neuro-degeneration. *Alzheimers Res Ther.* 2010;2(3):18.

45. McKeon JM, Livingston SC, Reed A, Hosey RG, Black WS, Bush HM. Trends in concussion return-to-play time-lines among high school athletes from 2007 through 2009. *J Athl Train.* 2013;48(6):836-843.

46. Yard EE, Comstock RD. Compliance with return to play guidelines following concussion in US high school athletes, 2005-2008. *Brain Inj.* 2009;23(11):888-898.

47. Powell JW, Barber-Foss KD. Injury patterns in selected high school sports: a review of the 1995-1997 seasons. *J Athl Train.* 1999;34(3):277-284.

48. McCrea M, Guskiewicz K, Randolph C, et al. Incidence, clinical course, and predictors of prolonged recovery time following sport-related concussion in high school and college athletes. *J Int Neuropsychol Soc.* 2013;19(1):22-33.

49. Lau BC, Kontos AP, Collins MW, Mucha A, Lovell MR. Which on-field signs/symptoms predict protracted recovery from sport-related concussion among high school football players? *Am J Sports Med.* 2011;39(11):2311-2318.

50. Zemper ED. Two-year prospective study of relative risk of a second cerebral concussion. *Am J Phys Med Rehabil.* 2003;82(9):653-659.

51. Drew LB, Drew WE. The contrecoup-coup phenomenon: a new understanding of the mechanism of closed head injury. *Neurocrit Care.* 2004;1(3):385-390.

52. May PR, Fuster JM, Haber J, Hirschman A. Woodpecker drilling behavior. An endorsement of the rotational theory of impact brain injury. *Arch Neurol.* 1979;36(6):370-373.

53. Greenwald RM, Gwin JT, Chu JJ, Crisco JJ. Head impact severity measures for evaluating mild traumatic brain injury risk exposure. *Neurosurgery.* 2008;62(4):789-798.

54. Chen JK, Johnston KM, Collie A, McCrory P, Ptito A. A validation of the post concussion symptom scale in the assessment of complex concussion using cognitive testing and functional MRI. *J Neurol Neurosurg Psychiatry.* 2007;78(11):1231-1238.

55. Lovell MR, Pardini JE, Welling J, et al. Functional brain abnormalities are related to clinical recovery and time to return-to-play in athletes. *Neurosurgery.* 2007;61(2):352-359.

56. Ptito A, Chen JK, Johnston KM. Contributions of functional magnetic resonance imaging (fMRI) to sport concussion evaluation. *NeuroRehabilitation.* 2007;22(3):217-227.

57. Guskiewicz KM, Mihalik JP, Shankar V, et al. Measurement of head impacts in collegiate football players: relationship between head impact biomechanics and acute clinical outcome after concussion. *Neurosurgery.* 2007;61(6):1244-1252.

58. McCaffrey MA, Mihalik JP, Crowell DH, Shields EW, Guskiewicz KM. Measurement of head impacts in collegiate football players: clinical measures of concussion after high- and low-magnitude impacts. *Neurosurgery.* 2007;61(6):1236-1243.

59. Mihalik JP, Bell DR, Marshall SW, Guskiewicz KM. Measurement of head impacts in collegiate football players: an investigation of positional and event-type differences. *Neurosurgery.* 2007;61(6):1229-1235.

60. Giza CC, Hovda DA. The neurometabolic cascade of concussion. *J Athl Train.* 2001;36(3):228-235

61. Meehan WP III, d'Hemecourt P, Comstock RD. High school concussions in the 2008-2009 academic year: mechanism, symptoms, and management. *Am J Sports Med.* 2010;38(12):2405-2409.

62. Marar M, McIlvain NM, Fields SK, Comstock RD. Epidemiology of concussions among United States high school athletes in 20 sports. *Am J Sports Med.* 2012;40(4):747-755.

63. Castile L, Collins CL, McIlvain NM, Comstock RD. The epidemiology of new versus recurrent sports concussions among high school athletes, 2005-2010. *Br J Sports Med.* 2012;46(8):603-610.

64. Covassin T, Swanik CB, Sachs ML. Sex differences and the incidence of concussions among collegiate athletes. *J Athl Train.* 2003;38(3):238-244.

65. Verbrugge LM, Wingard DL. Sex differentials in health and mortality. *Women Health.* 1987;12(2):103-145.

66. Dick RW. Is there a gender difference in concussion incidence and outcomes? *Br J Sports Med.* 2009;43(suppl 1):i46-i50.

67. Setnik L, Bazarian JJ. The characteristics of patients who do not seek medical treatment for traumatic brain injury. *Brain Inj.* 2007;21(1):1-9.

68. Broglio SP, Macciocchi SN, Ferrara MS. Sensitivity of the concussion assessment battery. *Neurosurgery.* 2007;60(6):1050-1057.

69. Register-Mihalik JK, Guskiewicz KM, Mihalik JP, Schmidt JD, Kerr ZY, McCrea MA. Reliable change, sensitivity, and specificity of a multidimensional concussion assessment battery: implications for caution in clinical practice. *J Head Trauma Rehabil.* 2013;28(4):274-283.

70. Mailer BJ, Valovich-McLeod TC, Bay RC. Healthy youth are reliable in reporting symptoms on a graded symptom scale. *J Sport Rehabil.* 2008;17(1):11-20.

71. Piland SG, Motl RW, Guskiewicz KM, McCrea M, Ferrara MS. Structural validity of a self-report concussion-related symptom scale. *Med Sci Sports Exerc.* 2006;38(1):27-32.

72. Lovell MR, Iverson GL, Collins MW, et al. Measurement of symptoms following sports-related concussion: reliability and normative data for the post-concussion scale. *Appl Neuropsychol.* 2006;13(3):166-174.

73. Broglio SP, Macciocchi SN, Ferrara MS. Neurocognitive performance of concussed athletes when symptom free. *J Athl Train.* 2007;42(4):504-508.

74. Collins MW, Field M, Lovell MR, et al. Relationship between postconcussion headache and neuropsychological test performance in high school athletes. *Am J Sports Med.* 2003;31(2):168-173.

75. Collins MW, Grindel SH, Lovell MR, et al. Relationship between concussion and neuropsychological performance in college football players. *JAMA.* 1999;282(10):964-970.

76. Guskiewicz KM, Ross SE, Marshall SW. Postural stability and neuropsychological deficits after concussion in collegiate athletes. *J Athl Train.* 2001;36(3):263-273.

77. Randolph C. Neuropsychological testing: evolution and emerging trends. *CNS Spectr.* 2002;7(4):307-312.

78. Randolph C, McCrea M, Barr WB. Is neuropsychological testing useful in the management of sport-related concussion? *J Athl Train.* 2005;40(3):139-152.

79. Aubry M, Cantu R, Dvorak J, et al. Summary and agreement statement of the First International Conference on Concussion in Sport, Vienna 2001. Recommendations for the improvement of safety and health of athletes who may suffer concussive injuries. *Br J Sports Med.* 2002;36(1):6-10.

80. Guskiewicz KM, Bruce SL, Cantu RC, et al. National Athletic Trainers' Association position statement: management of sport-related concussion. *J Athl Train.* 2004;39(3):280-297.

81. McCrory P, Johnston K, Meeuwisse W, et al. Summary and agreement statement of the 2nd International Conference on Concussion in Sport, Prague 2004. *Br J Sports Med.* 2005;39(4):196-204.

82. McCrea M, Kelly JP, Randolph C, et al. Standardized assessment of concussion (SAC): on-site mental status evaluation of the athlete. *J Head Trauma Rehabil.* 1998;13(2):27-35.

83. Riemann BL, Guskiewicz KM. Effects of mild head injury on postural stability as measured through clinical balance testing. *J Athl Train.* 2000;35(1):19-25.

84. Galetta KM, Brandes LE, Maki K, et al. The King-Devick test and sports-related concussion: study of a rapid visual screening tool in a collegiate cohort. *J Neurol Sci.* 2011;309(1-2):34-39.

85. Collins MW, Kontos AP, Reynolds E, Murawski CD, Fu FH. A comprehensive, targeted approach to the clinical care of athletes following sport-related concussion. *Knee Surg Sports Traumatol Arthrosc.* 2014;22(2):235-246

7

Sudden Death in Sport

Brendon P. McDermott, PhD, ATC and
William M. Adams, MS, ATC

CHAPTER OBJECTIVES

- Identify the risks associated with the most common conditions or accidents that lead to sudden death in sport, including sudden cardiac arrest, cervical spine trauma, exertional heat stroke (EHS), and exertional sickling associated with sickle cell trait.
- Explain the prevention guidelines associated with the leading causes of sudden death during physical activity, including, but not limited to, sudden cardiac arrest, EHS, exertional sickling, cervical spine injury, and lightning strike.
- Describe elements of an evidence-based plan to screen for potentially fatal conditions for athletes and assess the effectiveness of current assessments for pathologies that predispose athletes to sudden death in sport.
- Recognize and discuss the need for an appropriate emergency action plan (EAP) focused on recognition and treatment of potentially fatal conditions for athletes.

INTRODUCTION

Physical activity can stress the human body and increases the risk of fatality. The term *sudden death* is used in sport to denote that death is a direct result of physical activity. Physiologically, activity increases exposure to harsh environments, stresses the cardiovascular system, and can serve as the trigger for potentially fatal conditions. Furthermore, sport activity can increase the risk of trauma, which can result in death. The National Center for Catastrophic Sport Injury Research recorded 857 sport-related deaths during a 30-year period (1982 to 2012). More than three-quarters of catastrophic injuries occurred at the high school level (81%).[1] Not all sudden death related to physical activity results from organized sporting activities. Case reports have

Adams M, Swiger W.
Epidemiology for Athletic Trainers: Integrating
Evidence-Based Practice (pp 119-135).
© 2016 Taylor & Francis Group.

been published on sudden death following recreational hiking,[2] snow shoveling,[3] and distance running.[4] The American College of Sports Medicine recommends a minimum of 150 minutes/week of physical activity to protect against chronic disease. The long-term cardiovascular and respiratory adaptations from physical activity can prevent myocardial infarction and stroke and lead to healthier body composition.[5] Although physical activity can stress the body, the risks do not outweigh the benefits of regular physical activity.

The majority of National Collegiate Athletic Association (NCAA) student-athlete fatalities result from off-field activities or accidents.[4] However, traumatic and nontraumatic injury as a direct result of playing sports is a potential that warrants attention. Beyond injuries resulting from trauma in sports, a few potentially fatal conditions have been highlighted as preventable in recent years (cardiac conditions, exertional sickling, EHS, and lightning strikes). This chapter focuses on a few of the most common reasons that sudden death occurs in athletes. Athletic trainers bear the clinical responsibility to maximize survival at the following 2 critical time points in the sudden death scenario: screening/prevention and acute care.[8]

SUDDEN CARDIAC DEATH

Sudden cardiac death (SCD) is the term used for any fatality resulting from an infarction or stoppage of the heart due to structural or electrical disturbance. SCD is the leading cause of sudden death in high school and collegiate athletes.[8] Structural abnormalities are often found postmortem and are signs of underlying pathology. Hypertrophic cardiomyopathy (HCM), in which the ventricular wall and/or septum is abnormally enlarged, is the most common cause of SCD.[9,10]

Commotio cordis and coronary artery abnormalities, defects in the location or structure of the arteries supplying blood to the myocardium, are the second and third most prevalent causes of SCD.[1,10] Commotio cordis is a traumatic hit to the chest or thorax that causes ventricular arrhythmia upon absorbing impact. Structural defects represent the most common form of sudden cardiac pathology. However, commotio cordis remains a potential in sports with fast-moving projectiles (hockey, baseball, softball, lacrosse, etc) and collisions between players.[10]

Other developing or congenital pathologies may affect cardiac function, including mitral valve prolapse, Wolff-Parkinson-White syndrome, etc. The most common underlying conditions that predispose one to SCD are myocarditis, Marfan syndrome, ventricular dysplasia, and valvular heart disease.[7] Marfan syndrome, for example, leads to aortic enlargement secondary to excessive production of connective tissue. When the aorta enlarges, it can occlude blood flow or cause excessive ventricular contractility, either of which can lead to fatality. Because accurate diagnosis is so critical and the possibility of multiple conditions exists, any athlete who presents with signs or symptoms should be referred for testing to accurately diagnose the cause.[8]

Incidence of Sudden Cardiac Death

Over a 5-year span, 16% of deaths in college athletes were the result of cardiac pathology. The annual incidence of SCD is 1/43,770.[6] Basketball players have the greatest risk among all NCAA athletes for SCD. Male Division I athletes had an incidence of 1/3126 from 2004 to 2008.[6] Given that there are 350 NCAA Division I institutions with more than 10 players per team, this represents more than 1 cardiac death per year in Division I men's basketball. Other divisions of basketball presented decreased risk.[6]

In high school and collegiate football, the incidence of SCD has been 0.41/100,000 participants since 1990.[10] The risk is much higher in college football players (86%) compared to high school football players (14%). This equates to a relative risk that is 100% greater in college compared to high school football players with SCD. Unfortunately, the specific cause of SCD is unknown in about 63% of fatalities due to differences in how data were recorded.[10]

Athletes from all sports need appropriate medical care because all are at risk. For example, there were 4 SCDs in a 19-year span in male cross country, basketball, and wrestling.[11] SCD is not isolated to basketball and football athletes.

Risk Factors of Sudden Cardiac Death

Potential risk factors for SCD that have been analyzed include a family history of SCD, race, gender, or a lack of screening. Although physical exertion increases risk, death rates from athletes are similar to the general population for sudden death, and some student-athlete SCDs did not occur during physical activity.[6] Race and gender suggest some minor changes in risk stratification. Blacks are slightly more at risk than Whites in various epidemiological studies.[1,10-13] Epidemiological research has suggested that males are at greater risk than females.[8] However, the rate of sports participation is greater in males compared to females, making an unstratified sample difficult in comparison.

Other risk factors for cardiac conditions include history of syncope, or unexplained collapse, and family history. A difficulty with cardiac conditions is that the initial presentation includes seizure-like activity and unconsciousness. This increases diagnostic difficulty if there was no family or personal history of collapse because some clinicians may assume it was a seizure, and a detailed history is not possible if the patient is unconscious. At a minimum, asking questions related to these factors as part of the preparticipation evaluation is an effective screening process.[8-13]

Cardiac Screening for Prevention of Sudden Cardiac Death

Health care professionals must strive, at 2 distinct times, to limit the potential of death from a sudden cardiac condition. First, the preparticipation evaluation should serve as an efficient and thorough risk screening. Second, once an episode occurs, a simple and effective EAP must be in place.[8] Many strategies and recommendations for practice exist regarding the prevention of SCD. Because most death occurs as a result of structural abnormality, imaging via echocardiogram is considered by many as a gold standard in preseason screening.[14-16] This is effective in diagnosing many with HCM, but true sensitivity and specificity have yet to be determined for all causes.[9] The price of individual testing via echocardiogram makes it unattainable for many.[15] Other screening strategies include preseason resting electrocardiogram (EKG) analysis and review as part of the process.[8,9,11,12] Although effective, this assessment is somewhat subjective according to the practitioner and is based on electrical activity. Electrical and structural dysfunction in the heart are sometimes unrelated, which complicates specific recommendations. Some athletes gain ventricular thickness secondary to normal adaptation to intense training, known as athletic heart. Those with athletic heart are not at risk of SCD but can sometimes be diagnosed with HCM and be excluded from participation needlessly. Proponents of echocardiogram screening advocate in favor of disqualifying too many because they are saving lives for some with HCM.[17] More evidence regarding the effectiveness of electrocardiogram in preparticipation screenings is discussed in Chapter 11.

It is widely accepted that preseason screening for cardiac pathology is important in preventing SCD.[8] However, a consensus regarding best practice for screening has yet to be established. The American Heart Association (AHA) history questions are standard, but because symptoms are often not present until a major episode, their effectiveness is limited.[16] The effect of implementing a rigorous and mandatory screening protocol in the Veneto region of Italy resulted in a drastic incidence decrease from 4.19 to 0.21/100,000 athletes.[18] Standard EKGs and exercise restrictions have reduced incidence but may limit participation for those without contraindication to exercise.[15] A lack of consistency in interpretation of resting EKG analysis has also compromised the efficiency of a more cost-effective screening method.[19] Drezner et al[9] attempted to limit inconsistency with a template of step-by-step interpretation for physicians. Recommendations supported to date include a minimum of the 12-question AHA questionnaire, auscultation, and physical examination.[8,11,12,16] Further screening that is recommended is routine EKG read by a trained physician.[8,9] Follow-up echocardiogram is supported only when other methods suggest pathology or when resources are provided at a minimum cost.[7,15,18] In a recent study, history and physical examination identified 40% of potentially fatal conditions, and EKG was deemed appropriate in confirming or identifying more pathologies.[17] At a minimum, anyone participating in organized athletics should receive basic screening, including the cardiac screening questionnaire from the AHA,[16] blood pressure, pulse, and auscultation as part of his or her physical examination.[8,11,12,15]

Emergency Planning for Sudden Cardiac Death

The second potential for saving lives from cardiac pathology occurs once a patient collapses. If a cardiac episode presents, timing is key. EAPs that have been reviewed and practiced lead to better outcomes.[8,11,12,19] Three actions that save lives in these instances include early emergency medical services activation, cardiopulmonary resuscitation, and automated external defibrillator application.[8,11,12,19] The rate of survival decreases 10% for every minute of delay in treatment in cardiac arrest. Education and training for athletes, coaches, and strength staff can help expedite recognition and implementation of life-saving techniques.[8,11,12] Recent incidence data on SCD suggest that current practices have been successful at decreasing the number of deaths. In a study based in Minnesota, SCD was infrequent, and a prompt EAP was responsible for saving 33% of potentially fatal episodes.[11] Another study demonstrated 85% effectiveness for high school athletes and 61% survival in others given quick access to automated external defibrillators housed in high schools.[12] However, most instances were not a result of sport participation but involved bystanders (coaches, teachers, and fans).[11,12,19] Experts agree on consistent recommendations regarding expedited recognition and treatment for cardiac episodes. Although limited evidence is available to support these recommendations, sports medicine professionals do not disagree with these standards. Large cohort studies are underway to demonstrate the best prevention methods for SCD.

EXERTIONAL SICKLING

Exertional sickling occurs when muscle cells are deprived of oxygen during physical activity because the red blood cells of the athlete are deformed. Athletes at risk of exertional sickling are carriers of sickle cell trait. It is an inherited condition found predominantly in Black, Hispanic, and Mediterranean populations.[20] When intense or long-term exercise ensues, sickle cell trait causes red blood cells to take on an abnormal sickle shape (Figure 7-1). When this occurs, logjams or blood clots can occur in the blood vessels, depriving cells of oxygen or nutrients. Ultimately, rhabdomyolysis occurs due to muscle breakdown, which stresses the kidneys, heart, and blood vessels.[8,20] If not corrected, renal failure, hyperkalemia, myocardial infarction, stroke, and pulmonary edema are possible and often fatal. Athletic trainers must quickly recognize the signs and symptoms of exertional sickling and apply life-saving treatment promptly to prevent fatality.[8,20]

Incidence of Exertional Sickling

The number of deaths from exertional sickling are startling. In collegiate athletics, there were 10 deaths in 11 years.[21] The incidence in football, including high school, is .08/100,000 participants.[20] Sixty-four percent of these football deaths occurred during off-season conditioning activities. Between 2000 and 2007, there were 9 exertional sickling fatalities known in athletes aged 12 to 19 years.[21] According to Harmon et al,[22] 42% of football deaths resulted from exertional sickling

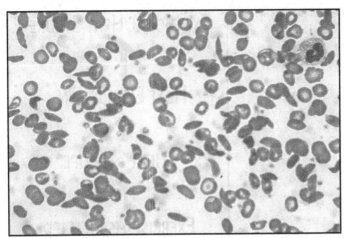

Figure 7-1. Red blood cells with and without sickle shape. (Reprinted with permission by Ed Uthman, Houston, Texas [Sickle Cell Anemia Uploaded by CFCF; CC BY 2.0, http://creativecommons.org/licenses/by/2.0] via Wikimedia Commons.)

between 2004 and 2008. Sickle cell–positive athletes were 37 times more likely to die in Division I football compared to nonsickle cell athletes.[22]

Exertional sickling is not exclusive to football athletes; it has taken the lives of distance runners and basketball players, among others.[8] Two high school female basketball players are known to have succumbed to this pathology following intense conditioning. According to Kark and Ward,[23] the military reported that sickle cell–positive recruits were 30 times more likely to die during basic training compared to nonsickle cell–positive recruits. All known deaths from exertional sickling have involved intense conditioning activities.

Risk Factors of Exertional Sickling

Risk factors associated with exertional sickling are related to the demand for oxygen and the body's ability to adapt to physical and environmental stressors. The first and main risk factor is having the sickle cell trait. Most newborns in the United States are screened for sickle cell carrier status.[24] In 1999, only 4 states (Montana, North Dakota, South Dakota, and Utah) were not testing at-risk populations.[24] If an athlete is not a carrier, he or she will not exhibit red blood cell sickling. Blacks have the highest prevalence but are not the only potential sickle cell–positive athletes. Roughly 8% of Blacks are sickle cell positive, whereas Whites are normally less than .05% carriers.[8,20] Epidemiological data from California demonstrated that 7.1% of Blacks, 0.5% of Hispanics, 0.03% of Middle Easterners, and 0.0075% of Asians were sickle cell trait carriers.[24]

Intense conditioning exercise, especially an intensity that the athlete is not accustomed to, is another major risk factor. Physiological stress includes anything that creates an imbalance in the supply and demand for oxygen at the working muscles. Altitude; asthma, or bronchoconstriction; hyperthermia; metabolic acidosis; and dehydration, individually or in combination, can create the discouraging onset of exertional sickling.[8,20,23] Exercise in the heat and humidity are known to contribute to the onset of exertional sickling because it normally causes hyperthermia and dehydration.[20] These are all known to contribute to local or systemic hypoxemia for working muscles, potentially leading to a sickling episode. Athletic trainers should strive to assure prevention steps for all of these during activity for those known to be sickle cell positive.[8,20]

Exertional Sickling Prevention

The strategies to prevent exertional sickling in organized sport have only been present for about 10 years. It was not until 2010 that the NCAA required screening for Division I athletes, and it

Figure 7-2. Continuum of severity for exertional heat illness.

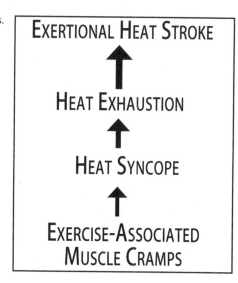

was later for all NCAA athletes.[25] Most high school student-athletes and collegiate newcomers have been screened at birth, which offsets the cost of collegiate athletic programs having to pay for all new athletes to be screened.[22] However, this depends on the state or country where they were born. In 2007, the US Preventive Services Task Force concluded with strong recommendation to screen for sickle cell trait at birth, but some states have yet to adopt mandatory screening.[24] Not all student-athletes may be able to document their results from birth. Other policies related to exertional sickling prevention involve education and altering activity for athletes who are sickle cell positive. Athletic trainers are responsible for informing athletic administrators, coaches, parents, athletes, and other medical professionals of an athlete's status and providing education on how to best condition an athlete who is a carrier for the sickle cell trait.[8,20] Furthermore, the athletic trainer should establish a protocol for management and treatment if there is an episode. It is imperative with exertional sickling that the athlete has the unquestioned authority to remove his- or herself from activity if initial signs or symptoms are noted.[8,20]

Documented cases of exertional sickling are consistently brought on by lapses in judgment or education.[8] This means that administrators, medical staff, coaches, or athletes were not effective at following recommendations when an exertional sickling death occurred, either in planning or at the time of sickling event. It appears that education and training have led to a reduction in the incidence of exertional sickling (3 deaths in 2010 and 0 in 2011-2012 in high school or college).[1,8] Long-term epidemiological studies are encouraged, prior to removing exertional sickling from the current list of causes of sudden death related to physical activity.

Exertional Heat Stroke

EHS is a potentially fatal condition that warrants prompt recognition and immediate whole-body cooling. EHS is diagnosed when core body temperature exceeds 104°F and central nervous system dysfunction occurs (collapse, altered consciousness, combative persona, etc). EHS represents the pinnacle of severity in the continuum of heat illness, but there is not necessarily a progression of heat illness to reach the most severe (Figure 7-2).[8] There are cases of EHS in which collapse is the first outward sign or reported symptom from the patient. Although death from EHS is preventable, complete prevention of EHS may never be achieved.

TABLE 7-1
TYPES OF RISK FACTORS

EXTRINSIC RISK FACTORS	INSTRINSIC RISK FACTORS
• High ambient temperature, solar radiation, and high humidity	• High intensity of exercise and/or poor physical conditioning
• Athletic gear or uniforms	• Sleep loss
• Peer or organizational pressure	• Dehydration or inadequate water intake
• Inappropriate work-to-rest ratios based on intensity, wet bulb globe temperature, clothing, equipment, fitness, and athlete's medical condition	• Use of diuretics or certain medications (ie, antihistamines, diuretics, antihypertensives, attention deficit hyperactive disorder drugs)
• Predisposing medical conditions	• Overzealousness or reluctance to report problems, issues, or illnesses
• Lack of education and awareness of heat illnesses among coaches, athletes, and medical staff	• Inadequate heat acclimatization
• No emergency plan to identify and treat exertional heat illnesses	• High muscle mass to body fat ratio
• Minimal access to fluids before and during practice and rest breaks	• Presence of a fever
• Delay in recognition of early warning signs	• Skin disorder

Table created using reference 29.

Incidence of Exertional Heat Stroke

Despite recent changes in policies regarding preseason heat acclimatization for NCAA and secondary school athletics, there has been an unfortunate increase in sport-related EHS fatalities. In the past 60 years, there have been 127 recorded deaths from EHS according to the National Center for Catastrophic Sport Injury Research.[26,27] More alarming than this average of just more than 2/year is that there were 12 EHS fatalities between 2005 and 2009. Since 1990, the incidence of EHS fatality was 0.16/100,000 participants, represented by 30 high school and 8 collegiate deaths.[26,27]

Analysis of EHS fatalities has produced moderate associations with certain risk factors. An important note about EHS is that individual risk factors compound environmental risk factors. Extremes of temperature and humidity contribute largely to EHS onset.[28] Preseason or early portions of a season account for almost all EHS fatalities, and only one fatality was a result of game participation. Eighty-three percent of these occurred during multiple practice days, and 44% occurred on the initial day of activity.[26]

The most recent NATA Position Statement on Exertional Heat Illnesses[29] suggests that a thorough preparticipation evaluation should include a risk assessment of EHS. However, little evidence suggests that EHS risk can be identified during a screening. Most risk factors for EHS are transient, such as hydration status, presence of an illness, sleep loss, and psychological stress (Table 7-1). However, when combined, the risk factors exacerbate each other and increase EHS risk. For example, an athlete who is unacclimatized to the heat and is psychologically stressed is at risk for EHS. However, an athlete who has not gotten sleep, has an upper respiratory infection, is dehydrated, and is overzealous, combined with the lack of acclimatization and personal stress, is at much greater risk. EHS normally occurs when a myriad of predispositions contribute to the onset. Table 7-1 is an updated list of risk factors for EHS.[29]

One important consideration for EHS risk is the fact that extrinsic and intrinsic factors are involved. Table 7-1 is separated into these categories for clear representation of these factors. Steps should be taken to prevent each factor individually. Intrinsic factors can be addressed with education (eg, teaching athletes and coaches the importance of hydration and that regular water breaks aid in preventing dehydration and EHS).[8,29] Athletes should know how to self-check their hydration status and, perhaps, their sweat rate. When athletes are educated on these factors, there is little excuse for athletes to report to activity in a hypohydrated state. If they do, the athletic trainer and coaches should be on the same page in terms of limiting activity on that day or for that particular session. Athletic trainers and coaches should agree that one activity session or practice will not be responsible for the outcome of a season and that the medical best interest of student-athletes should pervade.

Prevention of Exertional Heat Stroke

The responsibility of establishing and following preventive measures for extrinsic risk factors falls on coaches or athletic activity associations. The most effective method to reduce the incidence of EHS is to mandate heat acclimatization for every athlete.[29,30] For example, a state secondary school athletic association should mandate that preseason practices include gradual increase in duration, intensity, and amount of equipment worn. Furthermore, when more than one practice is held within a day, they must be separated by at least 4 hours.[30] It is up to the coaching staff and athletic trainer to ensure that good practices are in place prior to the season and that they are followed. When athletic associations establish guidelines, it is important that they regard all potential extrinsic EHS risk factors as important. This will foster a safer environment for all athletes during participation.

True prevention of EHS is difficult to gauge. Sports medicine professionals need to improve injury and outcome documentation. In terms of all heat illnesses, the NCAA's online injury reporting system has improved reporting. Now that research has been published on incidence and prevalence of heat illness during athletic activity, there is a starting point. From this baseline, continual tracking of pathology will determine whether prevention measures are effective. Military branches have good data on prevalence and preventive strategies. However, the military data show almost no trends in prevention despite strict and consistent measures implemented.[31] One of the major detriments to EHS research is the inadequate reporting and records of EHS cases. Cases of EHS are mostly known when they end in death. However, if a patient is treated appropriately and he or she survives, it often gets documented as severe heat exhaustion. Research is steadily increasing for the incidence and prevention of heat illness.

CATASTROPHIC HEAD AND SPINE INJURIES

Injuries affecting the head and spine are inherent risks during collision sport participation, especially in American football, rugby, and ice hockey. Also, in activities such as cheerleading, diving, and gymnastics where athletes are airborne before contacting other athletes, equipment or surfaces increase potential head and spine trauma. American football has received the most attention in relation to concussion and the long-term effects of repeated blows to the head. The discussion here focuses on the incidence of sport-related head fatalities and catastrophic (fatal cases and career-ending injuries) spinal injuries. The incidence, mechanisms, and risk factors for concussion have been described in Chapter 6.

Determining rates of head and spine injuries is essential for keeping athletes safe during sport participation. More importantly, data after prevention strategies have been implemented provide the best evidence for preventing these injuries. For example, a rule change, such as the spearing rule in American football in 1976, should be analyzed to determine its effect on sport safety. Pre- and postinjury rates and the odds of injury at various levels of sport (high school, college, professional) are more important to have.

Monitoring head and spine injury data can demonstrate the effectiveness of prevention strategies. The best example of how surveillance data have been used as a prevention strategy to reduce the risk of head and spine injuries comes from American football. The National Football Head and Neck Injury Registry has tracked head and neck injuries since the 1950s. Prior to the 1970s, many catastrophic injuries in football involved head injuries due to the limited protection that the helmet provided. When helmets were modernized in 1970, there was a large increase in cervical neck injuries directly related to athletes using the crown of their helmet to tackle opponents. Rules prohibiting spearing in 1975 drastically reduced the number of cervical spine injuries, and injuries were further reduced in the mid-2000s with an additional rule change that removed the word *intentional* before spearing to include any form of spearing. The magnitude in which catastrophic cervical spine injuries were reduced after intentional spearing was banned is roughly 80%.[32] In 1976, there were 34 incidents causing quadriplegia. That was reduced to 10/year in the 1980s and then 6/year in the 1990s.[33]

INCIDENCE OF HEAD AND SPINE INJURIES

Death due to head injuries is the second-leading sport-related cause of death in American football. It accounted for 62 football deaths (0.26/100,000 participants) between 1990 and 2010.[34] One can see the evolution of player safety in high school and college football by examining the average number of deaths from head trauma. Between 1945 and 1975, there were an average of 9.5 deaths/year. A spike in deaths occurred between 1965 and 1969, when the average increased to 17.5 deaths/year.[35] The number of deaths from brain injuries dropped dramatically in the 1980s, primarily due to new standards for safety equipment and rule changes, such as no spearing and the fair catch. Helmet technology has continued to improve since 1978, when certification of equipment by the National Operating Committee on Standards for Athletic Equipment became required at the collegiate level, followed by the high school level in 1980.

Sport is the fourth most common cause of spinal injury in the United States, followed by motor vehicle accidents, violence, and falls.[36] In football, there have been 269 cases of permanent neurological injuries related to spinal cord injuries over the past 30 years. Of those, 70% were defensive players in the process of blocking or tackling. The mechanism of injury most associated with spinal cord injuries is spearing[37] (Figure 7-3).

The rate of cervical spine injuries has decreased dramatically.[35,37-40] From 1977 to 2002, the incidence of cervical spine injury went from 2.24/100,000 players and 10.66/100,000 players in high school and college, respectively, to .33/100,000 players and 1.33/100,000 players, respectively.[39] The incidence of cervical spine injuries increases with higher levels of play. Collegiate players are 1.5 times more likely than high school players to suffer a catastrophic spine injury.[39] Over the past 11 seasons in the National Football League, there have been 2208 injuries involving the spine and axial skeleton. Of those, 987 (44.7%) involved the cervical spine, resulting in missed time of approximately 80 days/injury.[41] At the youth level, evidence is not as well documented, but based on the available data, spine injuries in youth athletes account for 7% to 10% of injuries.[42]

Other collision sports have similar incidences of spinal injuries to American football. Rugby has an incidence of anywhere from 1 to 2/100,000 to 10/100,000 players, but recent evidence suggests that the incidence is 1.73 cervical spinal injuries/100,000 players/year.[43] In addition, ice hockey has an incidence rate of 2 to 5/100,000 player-hours.[44]

Figure 7-3. Teaching proper tackling techniques at the youth football level.

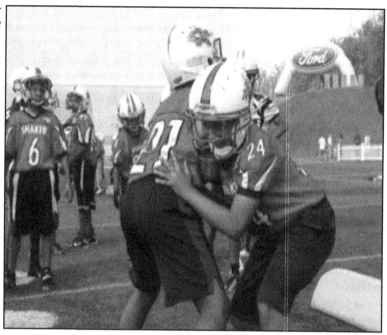

Epidemiological data analyzing catastrophic injuries has shown that 63.3% and 71.2% of direct catastrophic injuries occurring in female athletes occur in cheerleaders at the high school and college level, respectively. Of the 183 catastrophic injuries occurring in female athletes at the high school and college levels from 1982 to 2012, 120 (65.5%) of them occurred in cheerleaders and 19.3% involved the head or neck.[1] The rate of catastrophic injuries in cheerleaders per 100,000 athletes is 5 times higher in collegiate than high school cheerleaders.[45] Seventy-five percent of the catastrophic injuries occurring in cheerleaders are the result of a fall.[1] Furthermore, Boden et al[45] examined the relationship between catastrophic injuries in cheerleaders and the surface on which they were performing. Results indicate that hard, nonimpact, absorbing surfaces (concrete, asphalt, and gym floors) were a factor in 72% of the catastrophic injuries.[46]

Gymnastics is the second leading cause of catastrophic injury in female athletes,[1] and of 38 reported cases of accidents involving gymnasts, 35 involved the cervical spine.[47] Analyzing injuries that resulted in paralysis between 1985 and 1997, 10% of the sport-related accidents occurred in gymnastics.[48] Catastrophic head and spine injuries are also prevalent in diving, typically due to individuals diving into shallow water (1 to 2 m deep). Diving accidents account for 7% to 9.5% of all catastrophic spine injuries.[49-51] Males are at a much greater risk than females for diving-related cervical spine injuries.[49] When combined with gymnastics, diving accounts for 14.5% of catastrophic spine injuries.[48]

Risk Factors of Head and Spine Injuries

Head and cervical spine injuries are a result of a blow to the head or body that causes a whiplash effect at the head. Specifically with head injuries, the whiplash motion causes a coup or countercoup brain injury. With cervical spine injuries, the primary mechanism is forced hyperflexion of the neck, which causes an axial load on the spine, resulting in injury. This occurs most frequently in football when a tackler uses the crown of his head as the point of first contact, known as spearing.[35] In sports, such as diving, cheerleading, and gymnastics, axial loading resulting in a possible catastrophic outcome can occur from any fall greater than an individual's height while the neck is flexed.

Not all risks in collision sports are modifiable because collisions are inherent in these sports (American football, rugby, and ice hockey). Protective equipment, such as a helmet in American football and ice hockey, protects against traumatic injuries but not against internal brain injuries caused by blows to the head, body, or both. Also, when athletes wear protective equipment, they often feel invincible and are more likely to take risks that may contribute to the increased risk of catastrophic injury.[35] In rugby, athletes wear no form of head protection, so they are at increased risk of head injury and facial trauma.[52-54]

The spearing and hyperflexion risk factors are modifiable. Rule changes have decreased the rates of head and spine injuries. Eliminating spearing, intentional or unintentional, in American football, has reduced the incidence of cervical spine injuries. Also, penalizing athletes for intentional blows to the head or checking from behind in ice hockey assists in teaching athletes the proper technique and reduces the risks of head and spine injuries.[55]

A history of head and neck injuries may be another risk factor. Precautions should be taken in athletes with a previous history of concussion or other head injury and athletes with diagnosed cervical stenosis. Evidence shows that 25% of athletes with a brain fatality had a previous history of concussion, with 16% of those suffering from second-impact syndrome after sustaining a concussion within 1 month of death.[35,52] Although it has been documented that history of a concussion may predispose an athlete to a more serious head injury, additional research needs to investigate exact mechanisms.[35,56] In addition, athletes with conditions such as cervical stenosis have an increased risk of cervical spine injury during sports in which they may sustain an axial load on the spine due to the narrowing of the neural foramina in the cervical vertebrae.[35,57]

Prevention of Head and Spine Injuries

The preparticipation examination is an important tool for determining if an athlete is predisposed to a head or spine injury. Assessing the athlete's prior history of head and neck injuries and recovery from such injuries provides sports medicine professionals with an indication of the athlete's predisposition for future, potentially catastrophic injuries of the head and neck. The preparticipation physical examination may disqualify an athlete from participation if there are contraindications that dramatically increase the likelihood of them suffering a catastrophic head and neck injury. Examples of disqualifications include spinal stenosis with neurological impairments, prior history of head or spine injury with incomplete neurological recovery, degenerative disease, and other conditions that may predispose athletes to head or spine injury.

Proper education is essential in reducing the incidence of head and spine fatalities. Teaching athletes the proper technique for tackling in American football and rugby and checking in ice hockey and lacrosse should begin at the youth level and continue throughout to ensure that athletes minimize their risk of catastrophic injury. Athletes should be taught to keep their head up and use their shoulders to contact their opponents. This takes the head out of the hit in collision sports. Teaching athletes the proper technique, beginning at a young age, helps them develop the motor control necessary to play the sport safely.

In sports that do not involve tackling but have a high incidence of catastrophic head and neck injuries, such as diving, cheerleading, and gymnastics, proper technique and safety practices need to be taught at a young age (-3). Proper and attentive spotting during practice and competition reduces the risk of catastrophic outcome. Also, more advanced techniques such as pyramids and basket tosses should only be performed by experienced athletes who are capable of performing these skills safely.[55] Specific to cheerleading, various organizations have limited the height in which pyramids can be performed (2 levels high at the high school level and 2.5 times the body height at the collegiate level).[55]

LIGHTNING STRIKES

Lightning is consistently a leading cause of weather-related death in the United States. Sport participation and recreational activity lightning deaths account for 15% and 25% to 30% of the fatalities respectively.[58,59] Due to the number of sports played outside during the stormy seasons from early spring into the fall and the frequency of lightning-producing storms combined with population density in certain areas of the United States, athletes and spectators are at risk for sustaining a lightning-related injury.[58,59] It is important for athletic trainers to be cognizant of the risks associated with lightning and take steps to reduce risk of lightning-related fatalities.

Incidence of Lightning Injuries

Lightning fatalities are often not reported as sport related, making it difficult to understand the scope of the problem. Between 1940 and 2011, the National Oceanic and Atmospheric Administration reported 9207 deaths attributed to lightning strikes.[60] Although the underreporting of lightning-related injuries and deaths has been documented,[61] evidence suggests that an average of 42 deaths per year are attributed to lightning and that lightning-associated injuries surpass the number of fatalities by a factor of 10.[59] In addition, roughly 50% of the lightning-related fatalities occur during sport participation.[62,63] Furthermore, 90% of lightning-related fatalities occur between May and September, with 45% and 80% of deaths and injuries occurring during the hours of 10 o'clock AM and 7 o'clock PM. Coincidentally, this time period, including the time of year and day, directly correlates with the time of sporting events.[59,64,65] Geographically, the Southeast and Midwest United States account for 75% of the lightning-related deaths, with Florida and Texas accounting for the most commonly afflicted states.[65,66]

Injury or death associated from a lightning strike occurs by 1 of 6 mechanisms (Table 7-2). The most common mechanism is ground current or step voltage, accounting for 50% to 55% of all lightning-related injuries and fatalities, and is closely followed by a side flash (30% to 35% of fatalities).[59] For sporting events, ground current/step voltage is particularly dangerous due to the electric current's ability to travel through the ground, affecting anyone within a radius of the current.[59]

Risk Factors and Prevention of Lightning Injuries

Risk factors associated with lightning-related death are time of year, geographical location, time of day, availability of lightning safe structures, and proximity of the storm. These risk factors are modifiable in that with appropriate prevention strategies and proper education, the likelihood of a lightning-related injury or fatality can be greatly reduced. Suspension of play and evacuation of the playing field when an impending storm approaches is the best way in which to reduce the risk of injury or fatality. Athletes, coaches, and spectators should be moved to lightning-safe structures. NATA's position statement on lightning safety identifies safe locations as fully enclosed buildings complete with wiring and plumbing and metal enclosed vehicles, such as cars, buses, and vans. Open buildings, such as dugouts, pavilions, tents, and picnic shelters, are not considered lightning-safe locations due to their open nature.[59]

Implementing appropriate prevention strategies in regard to lightning safety during sport and physical activity reduces the number of lightning injuries and deaths per year. The most important prevention strategy is proper education. Educating athletes, coaches, and spectators on safe and unsafe locations to take refuge during a lightning-producing storm is an effective means of reducing the number of lightning-related injuries and deaths. Having a written lightning policy in an institution's EAP that identifies the criteria for suspension/resumption of play during a lightning-producing storm and describes the evacuation of athletes and spectators from the field

	TABLE 7-2 MECHANISMS OF LIGHTNING-RELATED FATALITIES IN SPORT AND PHYSICAL ACTIVITY	
LIGHTNING MECHANISM	**DESCRIPTION OF MECHANISM**	**PERCENTAGE OF FATALITIES ASSOCIATED**
Direct strike	Lightning bolt directly hits the victim before coming in contact with anything else	3% to 5%
Contact injury	The victim is in physical contact with something (a fence, pole, etc) that is in the pathway of lightning current	3% to 5%
Side flash	When lightning strikes an object in proximity to the victim and a portion of the energy/current jumps to the victim	30% to 35%
Ground current/ step voltage	Lightning striking the ground and during the radial outward flow of current the victim is in a position where one foot is closer to the strike than the other. The current then travels up the closer leg and down the farther leg and then continues it's movement of current in the ground	50% to 55%
Upward leader	Occurs when a lightning channel develops originating at the ground and traveling toward the cloud	10% to 15%
Concussive	Blunt trauma related to the lightning causing violent muscle contractions, and explosive/implosive forces. This can cause victims to be thrown through the air and/or sustain other traumatic injuries	Unknown
Table created using reference 59.		

of play to lightning-safe locations is critical to managing athletic events. Daily weather monitoring through local reports from the National Weather Service or by lightning detectors are components recommended as part of the prevention strategy.[59]

Assessing the effectiveness of lightning prevention strategies can be done by obtaining data relevant to lightning-related injuries or deaths occurring during sport or physical activity. This could provide vital information to determine if appropriate prevention strategies are in place and being followed to prevent a catastrophic injury from occurring due to lightning. Investigating lightning-related deaths during sport and which preventive strategies are in place could determine effectiveness and if other steps could have prevented loss of life.

Lightning accounts for many weather-related fatalities annually, with those participating in sporting events most at risk of a lightning-related injury or death. Although lightning consistently accounts for the top 2 reasons a person dies during a weather-related event, proper steps can be taken to help minimize this risk during sport participation. Athletic trainers need to ensure that there is a written lightning policy in their institution's EAP that explains proper prevention strategies, evacuation plans, and suspension/resumption of activity for each specific sport venue hosting outdoor sporting activities.

Bringing It Together

- Adequate preparticipation screenings are the first step in preventing catastrophes.
- The incidence of medically related sudden death is roughly 1 death for every 25,000 athlete participation years.[1]
- SCD, although rare, continues to be the most common reason for sudden death in sport. Success has been documented with the use of screening questions and routine EKGs. Further success is demonstrated with more advanced testing; however, debate continues over ideal screening in athletic populations.
- Exertional sickling represents a potentially fatal condition only when proper guidelines are not followed. Those who carry the sickle cell trait should be allowed alternate training and accommodations during intense workouts, but they can safely compete provided athlete, coach, and athletic trainers are on the same page regarding prevention and management. Risk factors for exertional sickling involve intense exercise in a short period of time, heat stress, dehydration, asthma, and altitude.
- EHS risk increases with environmental heat strain, intense workouts, protective equipment, and previous heat exposure. Heat acclimatization and adequate rest based on environmental conditions protect athletes from this condition effectively.
- Catastrophic head and spine injuries are relatively common in a wide variety of athletics, especially when improper tackling or stunt techniques are used by athletes. Preventive measures include proper technique education, rule and penalty impositions, and ensuring that stunt performance is done when athletes are adequately prepared.
- Lightning is the leading cause of weather-related injury in the United States. The afternoon hours in the summer months in the southern states represent risk factors for lightning injury. Prevention from injury and death from lightning requires close proximity of substantial shelter and monitoring of lightning proximity.

Review Questions

1. List the predisposing risk factors (intrinsic and extrinsic) for the causes of sudden death in athletes discussed in this chapter.
2. What is axial loading, and why is it a risk factor for spinal injury? What sports besides football have this risk?
3. What sport has the highest incidence of exertional sickling deaths?
4. What qualifies as appropriate shelter for a lightning storm?
5. What is the gold standard for diagnosing HCM?
6. What steps should coaches take to allow athletes to acclimatize to high heat and humidity?

LEARNING ACTIVITIES

1. Look up incidence of deaths using the following databases. What are the top 5 reasons for sudden death in sport in the last 5 years?

   - Datalys Center: Sports Injury Research and Prevention: http://datalyscenter.org/
   - Korey Stringer Institute: www.ksi.uconn.edu
   - National Center for Catastrophic Sport Injury Research: http://nccsir.unc.edu/

2. Write a sport-related rule that could reduce the incidence of fatalities and explain your rationale behind the rule change. What evidence and injury data justifies the need for your rule change?

3. Develop a policy that would prevent a potentially fatal condition. What else do you have do consider besides the evidence?

4. What recent safety measures or equipment have been introduced or modified in sport to keep athletes safe? Pick one sport. What additional safety measures would you take in terms of equipment?

5. Design a database to track sudden death in sport for all causes of death. What information would you need to have about each case?

REFERENCES

1. Mueller FO, Kucera KL, Cox LM, Cantu RC. Catastrophic sports injury research thirtieth annual report: fall 1982-spring 2012. National center for catastrophic injury research. http://nccsir.unc.edu/files/ 2014/06/ NCCSIR-30th-Annual-All-Sport-Report-1982_2012.pdf. Accessed August 21, 2014.
2. Windsor JS, Firth PG, Grocott MP, Rodway GW, Montgomery HE. Mountain mortality: a review of deaths that occur during recreational activities in the mountains. *Postgrad Med J.* 2009;85(1004):316-321.
3. Franklin BA, Bonzheim K, Gordon S, Timmis GC. Snow shoveling: a trigger for acute myocardial infarction and sudden coronary death. *Am J Cardiol.* 1996;77(10):855-858.
4. Schwabe K, Schwellnus M, Derman W, Swanevelder S, Jordaan E. Medical complications and deaths in 21 and 56 km road race runners: a 4-year prospective study in 65 865 runners--SAFER study I. *Br J Sports Med.* 2014;48(11):912-918.
5. Shortreed SM, Peeters A, Forbes AB. Estimating the effect of long-term physical activity on cardiovascular disease and mortality: evidence from the Framingham Heart Study. *Heart.* 2013;99(9):649-654.
6. Harmon KG, Asif IM, Klossner D, Drezner JA. Incidence of sudden cardiac death in National Collegiate Athletic Association Athletes. *Circulation.* 2011;123(15):1594-1600.
7. Maron BJ, Haas TS, Murphy CJ, Ahluwalia A, Rutten-Ramos S. Incidence and causes of sudden death in U.S. college athletes. *J Am Coll Cardiol.* 2014;63(16):1636-1643.
8. Casa DJ, Guskiewicz KM, Anderson SA, et al. National Athletic Trainers' Association position statement: preventing sudden death in sports. *J Athl Train.* 2012;47(1):96-118.
9. Drezner JA, Ackerman MJ, Cannon BC, et al. Abnormal electrocardiographic findings in athletes: recognizing changes suggestive of primary electrical disease. *Br J Sports Med.* 2013;47(3):153-167.
10. Boden BP, Breit I, Beachler JA, Williams A, Mueller FO. Fatalities in high school and college football players. *Am J Sports Med.* 2013;41(5):1108-1116.
11. Roberts WO, Stovitz SD. Incidence of sudden cardiac death in Minnesota high school athletes 1993-2012 screened with standardized pre-participation evaluation. *J Am Coll Cardiol.* 2013;62(14):1298-1301.
12. Drezner JA, Toresdahl BG, Rao AL, Huszti E, Harmon KG. Outcomes from sudden cardiac arrest in US high schools: a 2-year prospective study from the National Registry for AED Use in Sports. *Br J Sports Med.* 2013;47(18)1179-1183.
13. Kenney WL, Craighead DH, Alexander LM. Heat waves, aging and human cardiovascular health. *Med Sci Sports Exerc.* 2014;46(10):1891-1899.
14. Heidbuchel H, Papadakis M, Panhuyzen-Goedkoop N, et al. Position paper: proposal for a core curriculum for a European Sports Cardiology qualification. *Eur J Prev Cardiol.* 2013;20(5):889-903.

15. Menafoglio A, Di Valentino M, Segatto JM, et al. Costs and yield of a 15-month preparticipation cardiovascular examination with ECG in 1070 young athletes in Switzerland: implications for routine ECG screening. *Br J Sports Med.* 2014;48(15):1157-1161.

16. Maron BJ, Thompson PD, Puffer JC, et al. Cardiovascular preparticipation screening of competitive athletes. A statement for health professionals from the Sudden Death Committee (clinical cardiology) and Congenital Cardiac Defects Committee (cardiovascular disease in the young), American Heart Association. *Circulation.* 1996;94(4):850-856.

17. Price DE, McWilliams A, Asif IM, et al. Electrocardiography-inclusive screening strategies for detection of cardiovascular abnormalities in high school athletes. *Heart Rhythm.* 2014;11(3):442-449.

18. Corrado D, Basso C, Pavei A, Michieli P, Schiavon M, Thiene G. Trends in sudden cardiovascular death in young competitive athletes after implementation of a preparticipation screening program. *JAMA.* 2006;296(13):1593-1601.

19. Drezner JA, Rogers KJ, Horneff JG. Automated external defibrillator use at NCAA Division II and III universities. *Br J Sports Med.* 2011;45(15):1174-1178.

20. National Athletic Trainers' Association. Consensus statement: sickle cell trait and the athlete. http://www.nata.org/sites/default/files/SickleCellTraitAndTheAthlete.pdf. Accessed April 20, 2014.

21. Eichner ER. Sickle cell considerations in athletes. *Clin Sports Med.* 2011;30(3):537-549.

22. Harmon KG, Drezner JA, Klossner D, Asif IM. Sickle cell trait associated with a RR of death of 37 times in National Collegiate Athletic Association football athletes: a database with 2 million athlete-years as the denominator. *Brit J Sports Med.* 2012;46(5):325-330.

23. Kark JA, Ward FT. Exercise and hemoglobin S. *Semin Hematol.* 1994;31(3):181-225.

24. Ashley-Koch A, Yang Q, Olney RS. Sickle hemoglobin (HbS) allele and sickle cell disease: a HuGE review. *Am J Epidemiol.* 2000;151(9):839-845.

25. Klossner D. *2013-2014 NCAA Sports Medicine Handbook.* Indianapolis, IN:, NCAA; 2013.

26. Kerr ZY, Roos K, Mueller FO, Casa DJ. Fatal and catastrophic injuries in athletics: epidemiologic data and challenging circumstances. In: Casa DJ, Stearns RL, eds. *Emergency Management for Sport and Physical Activity.* Burlington, MA: Jones and Bartlett Learning; 2014:17-30.

27. Kerr ZY, Marshall SW, Comstock RD, Casa DJ. Exertional heat stroke management strategies in United States high school football. *Am J Sports Med.* 2014;42(1):70-77.

28. Cooper ER, Ferrara MS, Broglio SP. Exertional heat illness and environmental conditions during a single football season in the southeast. *J Athl Train.* 2006;41(3):332-336.

29. Casa DJ, DeMartini JK, Bergeron MF, et al. National Athletic Trainers' Association Position Statement: Exertional Heat Illnesses. *J Athl Train.* 2015;50(9):986-1000.

30. Casa DJ, Csillan D; Inter-Association Task Force for Preseason Secondary School Athletics Participants, et al. Preseason heat-acclimatization guidelines for secondary school athletics. *J Athl Train.* 2009;44(3):332-333.

31. Wallace RF, Kriebel D, Punnett L, et al. Risk factors for recruit exertional heat illness by gender and training period. *Aviat Space Environ Med.* 2006;77(4):415-421.

32. Torg JS, Guille JT, Jaffe S. Current concepts review: injuries to the cervical spine in American football players. *J Bone Joint Surg Am.* 2002;84(1):112-122.

33. Boden BP, Tacchetti RL, Cantu RC, Knowles SB, Mueller FO. Catastrophic cervical spine injuries in high school and college football players. *Am J Sports Med.* 2006;34(8):1223-1232.

34. Torg JS, Vegso JJ, O'Neill MJ, Sennett B. The epidemiologic, pathologic, biomechanical, and cinematographic analysis of football-induced cervical spine trauma. *Am J Sports Med.* 1990;18(1):50-57.

35. Gill SS, Boden BP. The epidemiology of catastrophic spine injuries in high school and college football. *Sports Med Arthrosc.* 2008;16(1):2-6.

36. McCrory P, Johnston K, Meeuwisse W, et al. Summary and agreement statement of the second international conference on concussion in sport, Prague 2004. *Phys Sportsmed.* 2005;33(4):29-44.

37. Swartz EE, Boden BP, Courson RW, et al. National Athletic Trainers' Association position statement: acute management of the cervical spine-injured athlete. *J Athl Train.* 2009;44(3):306-331.

38. Rihn JA, Anderson DT, Lamb K, et al. Cervical spine injuries in American football. *Sports Med.* 2009;39(9):697-708.

39. Cantu RC, Mueller FO. Catastrophic spine injuries in American football, 1977-2001. *Neurosurgery.* 2003;53(2):358-362.

40. Boden BP, Tacchetti RL, Cantu RC, Knowles SB, Mueller FO. Catastrophic cervical spine injuries in high school and college football players. *Am J Sports Med.* 2006;34(8):1223-1232.

41. Mall NA, Buchowski J, Zebala L, Brophy RH, Wright RW, Matava MJ. Spine and axial skeleton injuries in the National Football League. *Am J Sports Med.* 2012;40(8):1755-1761.

42. Adickes MS, Stuart MJ. Youth football injuries. *Sports Med.* 2004;34(3):201-207.

43. Trewartha G, Preatoni E, England ME, Stokes KA. Injury and biomechanical perspectives on the rugby scrum: a review of the literature. *Br J Sports Med.* 2015;49(7):425-433.

44. Tator CH, Provvidenza C, Cassidy JD. Spinal injuries in Canadian ice hockey: an update to 2005. *Clin J Sport Med*. 2009;19(6):451-456.

45. Boden BP, Tachetti R, Mueller FO. Catastrophic cheerleading injuries. *Am J Sports Med*. 2003;31(6):881-888.

46. Gill SS, Boden BP. The epidemiology of catastrophic spine injuries in high school and college football. *Sports Med Arthrosc*. 2008;16(1):2-6.

47. Silver JR, Silver DD, Godfrey JJ. Injuries of the spine sustained during gymnastic activities. *Br Med J (Clin Res Ed)*. 1986;293(6551):861-863.

48. Schmitt H, Gerner HJ. Paralysis from sport and diving accidents. *Clin J Sport Med*. 2001;11(1):17-22.

49. Chan-Seng E, Perrin FE, Segnarbieux F, Lonjon N. Cervical spine injuries from diving accident: a 10-year retrospective descriptive study on 64 patients. *Orthop Traumatol Surg Res*. 2013;99(5):607-613.

50. Borius PY, Gouader I, Bousquet P, Draper L, Roux FE. Cervical spine injuries resulting from diving accidents in swimming pools: outcome of 34 patients. *Eur Spine J*. 2010;19(4):552-557.

51. Aito S, D'Andrea M, Werhagen L. Spinal cord injuries due to diving accidents. *Spinal Cord*. 2005;43(2):109-116.

52. Gardner A, Iverson GL, Levi CR, et al. A systematic review of concussion in rugby league. *Br J Sports Med*. 2015;49(8):495-498.

53. Gardner AJ, Iverson GL, Williams WH, Baker S, Stanwell P. A systematic review and meta-analysis of concussion in rugby union. *Sports Med*. 2014;44(12):1717-1731.

54. Fuller CW, Taylor A, Raftery M. Epidemiology of concussion in men's elite Rugby-7s (Sevens World Series) and Rugby-15s (Rugby World Cup, Junior World Championship and Rugby Trophy, Pacific Nations Cup and English Premiership). *Br J Sports Med*. 2015;49(7):478-483.

55. Boden BP, Jarvis CG. Spinal injuries in sports. *Neurol Clin*. 2008;26(1):63-78.

56. Eismont FJ, Clifford S, Goldberg M, Green B. Cervical sagittal spinal canal size in spine injury. *Spine (Phila Pa 1976)*. 1984;9(7):663-666.

57. Bailer AJ, Bena JF, Stayner LT, Halperin WE, Park RM. External cause-specific summaries of occupational fatal injuries. Part II: an analysis of years of potential life lost. *Am J Ind Med*. 2003;43(3):251-261.

58. Holle RL, López RE, Navarro BC. Deaths, injuries, and damages from lightning in the United States in the 1890s in comparison with the 1990s. *J Appl Meteorol*. 2005;44(10):1563-1573.

59. Walsh KM, Cooper MA, Holle R, et al. National Athletic Trainers' Association position statement: lightning safety for athletics and recreation. *J Athl Train*. 2013;48(2):258-270.

60. Thomson EM, Howard TM. Lightning injuries in sports and recreation. *Curr Sports Med Rep*. 2013;12(2):120-124.

61. López RE, Holle RL, Heitkamp TA, Boyson M, Cherington M, Langford K. The underreporting of lightning injuries and deaths in Colorado. *Bull Am Meteorol Soc*. 1993;74(11):2171-2178.

62. National Weather Service. Lightning fact page. http://www.lightningsafety.noaa.gov. Accessed April 15, 2014.

63. National Weather Service. Lightning fatalities. www.nws.noaa.gov/om/hazstats.shtml. Accessed April 15, 2014.

64. Lopez R, Holle R, Heitkamp T. Lightning casualties and property damage in Colorado from 1950 to 1991 based on storm data. *Forecast*. 1995;10(1):114-126.

65. Curran EB, Holle RL, Pez EL. Lightning casualties and damages in the United States from 1959 to 1994. *J Clim*. 2000;13(19):3448.

66. Adekoya N, Nolte KB. Struck-by-lightning deaths in the United States. *J Environ Health*. 2005;67(9):45-50.

8

Musculoskeletal Injuries in Sport

Ashley S. Long, PhD, LAT, ATC

CHAPTER OBJECTIVES

- Understand the incidence of musculoskeletal injury in youth, college, and professional sports.
- Emphasize the increased risk of injury during game participation and risk factors contributing to increased incidence of injury in specific sports.
- Describe the emerging evidence of anterior cruciate ligament (ACL) and rotator cuff injury descriptive epidemiology and risk factors.
- Address sport-specific motions and their influence on musculoskeletal injury.

INTRODUCTION

Rates of musculoskeletal injury vary greatly depending on age, sport, gender, type, or participation level. Predicting and preventing injury are key components of the duties of an athletic trainer, physical therapist, or orthopedic surgeon. Knowledge of specific risks can be helpful in preventing injury or determining return to play after an injury.

Athletes and parents wish to minimize the likelihood of injury. Musculoskeletal injuries comprise 79% of injuries seen by team physicians.[1] Avoiding factors that contribute to particular injuries, such as ACL tears or lateral epicondylitis, can reduce the incidence of those conditions. Also, athletes and parents should have accurate information on the safety of sports so that they can make an informed choice about participation. Sports epidemiology provides athletic trainers, coaches, parents, administrators, and athletes with evidence upon which to base these decisions.

Athletic trainers play an integral role in the collection of data for the epidemiological examination of sports injuries. Their daily documentation reflects the true relationship between injury and sports participation. These notes become the epidemiological data upon which the athletic training profession relies.

Adams M, Swiger W.
*Epidemiology for Athletic Trainers: Integrating
Evidence-Based Practice (pp 137-165).*
© 2016 Taylor & Francis Group.

INCIDENCE IN YOUTH, COLLEGE, AND PROFESSIONAL SPORTS

The incidence of sport can vary depending on many factors, but competition level can have a great impact on the quantity and type of injury. Youth, college, and professional sports have unique demands and incidences of injury. Characteristics of players between competition levels vary greatly on variables, such as body composition, strength, physical maturation, skill, etc. An understanding of the uniqueness of each level is essential to providing preventive measures.

Youth Sports

It is well accepted that participation in youth sports is beneficial to the social, emotional, and physical development of young people.[1] Participation in youth sports is continuously growing. The 2008 report by the National Council of Youth Sports indicated more than 60 million participants, with girls continually beginning participation at a younger age.[2] Unfortunately, at least 4.3 million sport-related injury (SRI) episodes occur each year to school-aged children in the United States.[3] There are few reports of the incidence of overuse injuries in children, but overall estimates of overuse injuries vs acute injuries range from 45.9% to 54%.[4] The prevalence of overuse injury in youth athletes varies depending on sport, ranging from 37% in skiing and handball to 68% in running.[4]

Furthermore, the recent phenomenon of competition, intense training, early specialization, and an increased volume of practices and competitions have led to overuse injuries and burnout in young athletes. It has been reported that high school athletes have an injury rate of 1.71/1000 athlete-exposures (AEs).[5] The High School Reporting Information Online Sport-Related Injury Surveillance Study[5] revealed that the overall injury rate in the 2012 to 2013 year was 2.16/1000 AEs. This means that an estimated 1.3 million injuries occur in US high schools annually.[5] There is a lack of literature on the incidence of overuse injuries in children, but overall estimates of overuse vs acute injuries range from 45.9% to 54%.[4]

Health care providers of youth athletes should be highly concerned by injuries that effect musculoskeletal growth and development, such as apophysitis and physeal stress injuries. These are specific to this population and occur at common sites in the body, such as the tibial tuberosity and calcaneus. Injury is more likely to occur during an adolescent growth spurt because of the change in bone physiology and biomechanical characteristics.[4]

Apophysitis commonly presents with a gradual onset of pain, no specific mechanism of injury, and, generally, localized pain at the apophysis. Because the injury occurs at the site where the muscle attaches to the bone, this is a weak point of the muscle-tendon-bone attachment and is vulnerable to injury from repeated stress. A youth athlete presenting with pain specific to the site of an apophysis who has participated in repetitive stress of the area, and particularly if the volume and intensity of his or her participation has increased, should be examined for apophysitis.

Approximately 15% of fractures in children involve the physis.[6] Physeal injuries can be acute or chronic but are a concern because of the possible disturbance of bone growth that can occur. Cartilage in this area is weak compared to adults. Forces to an extremity may result in structural failure through the physis. A force to the extremity that may cause a ligament sprain or joint dislocation in an adult may result in the disruption of a growth plate in a developing child.[7] There is a decrease in physeal strength during pubescence and a strong association between peak fracture rate and the period of peak height velocity.[8]

Risk factors in youth athletes, particularly concerning overuse injuries, have been identified. Prior injury is a strong predictor. This underlines the importance of a comprehensive sports preparticipation examination and the availability of qualified personnel to prevent and treat recurring injury. Also, the period during a growth spurt can have a large effect on physical properties of bone. Skilled monitoring of youth athletes should be particularly vigilant during

	TABLE 8-1	
	INJURY RATE AND NATIONAL ESTIMATES OF HIGH SCHOOL ATHLETES BY GENDER AND SPORT	
GENDER AND SPORT	**INJURY RATE (PER 1000 AES)**	**NATIONALLY ESTIMATED NO. OF INJURIES**
Boys' football	3.87	616,209
Boys' soccer	1.52	149,049
Girls' soccer	2.29	190,382
Girls' volleyball	0.89	44,064
Boys' basketball	1.47	85,819
Girls' basketball	1.83	83,107
Boys' wrestling	2.33	85,485
Boys' baseball	0.88	49,747
Girls' softball	1.15	58,124
Abbreviation: AE, athlete-exposure.		

times of rapid growth. Female youth athletes with a history of amenorrhea pose a significant risk factor for stress fractures. Furthermore, high training volumes have been associated with overuse injury in a variety of sports. Finally, other factors that may contribute but that lack empirical evidence include ill-fitted equipment and overscheduling with inappropriate recovery time.[4]

Sport Affiliation

Various sports are available to youth athletes. For most sports, some epidemiological data are available, but the amount of literature is less compared to that for adult athletes. The demands of each sport determines the forces placed upon the body, as well as the type and incidence of injury. For example, the highest rates of injury per 1000 hours of AE include ice hockey (range, 5 to 34.4), rugby (range, 3.4 to 8.7), and soccer (range, 3.2 to 7.9) for boys and soccer (range, 2.5 to 10.6), basketball (range, 3.6 to 4.1), and gymnastics (range, 0.5 to 4.1) for girls.[9] Comparison across studies can be difficult when attempting to compare sports, but studies examining multiple sports can be helpful. Powell et al[14] reported the highest overall injury rate per 1000 AEs in football, followed by wrestling, basketball, soccer, and baseball. Among girls, the highest injury rate occurred in soccer, followed by basketball, field hockey, softball, and volleyball.

Many youth participants are now engaging in early sport specialization. This may be defined as intense, year-round training and competition in a single sport. It is widely believed that early sport specialization may increase rates of overuse injury, and many researchers continue to examine the relationship between intense exclusive participation in one sport and injury incidence. Parents, coaches, athletic trainers, and youth athletes may benefit from diversifying sport training. This diversification may be more effective in developing future competitive skills in the primary sport.[4]

The high school injury rates for the most common sports are listed in Table 8-1. Practice and competition injuries are presented separately and by level of competition (middle vs high school; Table 8-2). Notice that the risk of injury during practice is higher than the competition rate for middle schoolers but that the reverse is true of high school athletes. Injuries are more likely in competition than in practice for older adolescents. Football has the highest injury rate, and swimming has the lowest.

TABLE 8-2

INJURY RATE FOR SPECIFIC SPORTS IN MIDDLE AND HIGH SCHOOL ATHLETES DURING PRACTICES AND GAMES

SPORT/LEVEL	OVERALL INJURY RATE/1000 AES	PRACTICE	GAME
Football			
Middle school	16.030	7.421	15.026
High school	3.87	2.08	12.53
Baseball			
Middle school	7.373	3.762	2.223
High school	0.88	0.66	1.3
Softball			
Middle school	7.090	3.1	1.001
High school	1.15	.73	1.96
Girls' basketball			
Middle school	9.151	3.625	3.036
High school	1.83	1.24	3.13
Boys' basketball			
Middle school	8.867	3.843	2.229
High school	1.47	1.04	2.44
Girls' soccer			
Middle school	7.964	3.217	3.110
High school	2.29	0.92	5.54
Boys' soccer			
Middle school	7.445	2.897	2.859
High school	1.52	0.78	3.28
Girls' swimming			
Middle school	1.315	.801	0
High school	0.38	0.43	0.14
Boys' swimming			
Middle school	0.706	0.238	0
High school	0.19	0.21	0.08
Wrestling			
Middle school	10.256	6.903	3.205
High school	2.33	1.88	3.54
Abbreviation: AE, athlete-exposure.			

(continued)

TABLE 8-2 (CONTINUED)			
INJURY RATE FOR SPECIFIC SPORTS IN MIDDLE AND HIGH SCHOOL ATHLETES DURING PRACTICES AND GAMES			
SPORT/LEVEL	OVERALL INJURY RATE/1000 AES	PRACTICE	GAME
Girls' volleyball			
Middle school	4.638	1.734	0.179
High school	0.89	1.08	0.78
Boys' volleyball			
Middle school	5.167	2.335	0.475
High school			
Abbreviation: AE, athlete-exposure.			

Gender

Evidence examining gender differences in injury incidence of youth sport participants is mixed. Fridman et al[10] examined injury rates of youths presenting to the emergency department over a 3-year period. They reported that males suffered the majority of SRIs (71.1%), and, in 11 of 13 sports analyzed, males reported a greater number of injuries.[10] Also, it has been reported that there are no significant gender differences in youth soccer injury.[11] Several studies of youth soccer athletes also show no differences between genders in the incidence of injury.[12-14] Others report higher rates for girls compared with boys in sports such as cross-country running, gymnastics, skiing, snowboarding, and soccer.[15]

Boys and girls are similar in many aspects of musculoskeletal injury. Messina et al[16] prospectively reported the injury rate as 0.56 among boys and 0.49 among girls, and the risk of injury per AE was not statistically different between genders. Both groups displayed sprains as the most common injury, as well as the ankle as the most common injury site. Female high school basketball athletes displayed a risk of ACL injury 3.79 times greater than their male counterparts.[16]

Females consistently show an increased incidence of knee injury compared to males.[17,20] Many variables of the gender discrepancy have been postulated and may include differences in hormone levels, increased female joint laxity, anatomical differences, and differences in motor control.[18] Perhaps differences in specialized training for boys vs girls and access to knowledgeable, quality coaching may also contribute to injury differences.

Male and female athletes gradually, and sometime suddenly, emerge into their adult bodies. Physical characteristics, such as larger mass, higher velocity of motion, and stronger muscular contraction contribute to teenage boys having a higher incidence rate than younger male youths in sports such as football, rugby, and soccer. The generation of greater force results in increased incidence of injury as young boys develop into teens. The literature is inconsistent regarding injury in various ages of youth female athletes. One study reports higher rates of injury in younger players compared to older players for girls' soccer.[19] However, other evidence highlights a higher incidence of injury in more advanced female athletes.[19,20] Higher participation level may be linked to increased injury incidence through an increased number of training hours, leading to increased risk of injury. Overall, high training volumes are consistently linked to an increase in the risk of overuse injury for both genders.[4]

Amenorrhea and the female athlete triad syndrome affect female athletes and their resistance to injury. These conditions are unique to female athletes. For example, a significant risk factor for stress fracture in female youth athletes is a history of amenorrhea.[4] Primary amenorrhea is diagnosed with the absence of menses by age 16. Secondary amenorrhea is typically defined as the absence of at least 3 to 6 consecutive menstrual cycles in a female who has begun menstruating. The prevalence of secondary amenorrhea in youth athletes is unknown, but primary and secondary can be a concern with female youth athletes. Adolescents may have irregular periods, but cessation of menses for longer than 3 months after regular cycles have begun is considered abnormal. Female athletes who begin participation before menarche occurs may experience a later menarche and have an increased incidence of dysfunction when compared to those who begin after.[21] Amenorrhea may lead to low bone mineral density, which may lead to bone injury. Irregular menstrual pattern and decreased body weight, together, have been shown to predict low lumbar bone density in young athletes.[22]

Standards of Care in Youth Sports

The American Medical Society for Sports Medicine published a position statement titled, "Overuse Injuries and Burnout in Youth Sports," as a resource for clinicians.[4] The paper identified risk factors and provided evidence-based recommendations on overuse injury prevention.[4]

- Rapid growth periods: Injuries are most common during rapid growth periods. Awareness of the growth phases and attention paid to individual athletes can bring increased awareness to an individual athlete's susceptibility to injury.

- Biomechanics: If biomechanical abnormalities are present, this may predispose youth athletes to injury. Developing bones and muscles of youth participants cannot handle forces from sport to the same degree as adult structures. Therefore, athletes with poor mechanics can put themselves in particular danger for apophysitis, stress fractures, or tendonitis.

- Overtraining: Defined as a "series of psychological, physiologic, and hormonal changes that result in decreased sports performance."[23] Look for signs of overtraining in youth athletes, such as chronic muscle or joint pain, personality changes, elevated resting heart rate, decreased sports performance, fatigue, lack of enthusiasm, or difficulty with successful completion of daily routine activities.

- Participation in endurance events: The American Academy of Pediatrics has determined that triathlons for youth athletes are reasonably safe as long as the events are modified to be appropriate for the age of the participants.

- Early specialization: Youth athletes are placed at higher risk for overuse musculoskeletal injuries and burnout if there is no break from athletics during the year. Single-sport, year-round training and competition is growing in popularity and should be approached with caution.

The recommendations from the American Medical Society for Sports Medicine were based on the true purpose of youth sport: "To promote lifelong physical activity, recreation, and skills of healthy competition that can be used in all future endeavors."[24]

- Proper training program: Insist upon a sound training regimen that includes repetition but not to the point of harm. Regarding distance events, such as marathons, a clearly devised weekly plan is warranted.

- Limit training: The American Academy of Pediatrics Council on Sports Medicine and Fitness recommends limiting one sporting activity to a maximum of 5 days/week with at least 1 day off from any organized physical activity.[24] Also, youth athletes should be given at least 2 to 3 months off per year from their primary sport. During this time, they should allow injuries to heal, relax their mind, and condition from an injury prevention perspective. Athletes should not increase the volume of training by more than 10% each week. If participating in more than one team at one time, the guidelines listed should still be followed.

- Variety of activity: Specialization can lead to injury and burnout. Youth athletes should be encouraged to become well rounded and participate in a variety of activities, not just one sport. Make workouts interesting and fun, and incorporate cross training.

College Sports

There are many differences between youth, adolescent, and college athletes. Although it should not be assumed that college athletes are fully developed, the largest percentage of changes in their bodies have already occurred. Epiphyseal plates have, for the most part, closed, and the window for the highest prevalence of epiphyseal growth plate injuries—ages 10 to 16 years—has passed. Children have increased elastic soft tissue and greater potential for remodeling than adults. College-aged athletes are generally allowed to participate in a full spectrum of training, including heavy weight lifting and plyometrics without the more careful consideration that goes into adolescent guidelines.

Although the physical characteristics may appear to be more robust for coping with stresses, other external factors may influence musculoskeletal injury in college athletes. In college, the seasons are longer, and, in some sports, training and competition can last year-round, resulting in increased risk and exposure. The intensity increases, expectations are greater for performance, and the demands can be overwhelming. Travel associated with competition can be taxing and call for days on the road. Fatigue can influence injury susceptibility. Football players in the National College Athletic Association's (NCAA's) Division I Bowl Subdivision (formerly Division I-A) reported spending an average of 44.8 hours/week at their sport, the equivalent of a full-time job. Division I baseball players reported spending 40 hours/week on their sport, whereas men's basketball players reported an average of 36.8 hours/week.[25] These time commitments, in addition to schoolwork, can place a tremendous toll on the athlete's mind and body.

In 2007, the NCAA and National Athletic Trainers' Association partnered to publish 25 years of data collected on athletic injuries at the collegiate level. The NCAA Injury Surveillance System (ISS) is a valuable source from which to glean epidemiologic data. The ISS provides a resource for scientific examination of injury prevention. Tables 8-3 and 8-4 summarize these NCAA injury data.

Sport Affiliation

Characteristics of specific sports can pose demands that result in injury to specific areas and structures of the body. Thankfully, researchers working with the NCAA have collected years of epidemiologic data that provide insight into injury rates during various points during the season, as well as differences between practices and competitions.

Evidence suggests that high-contact sports are more commonly associated with a higher incidence of acute injury[26-30], while non-contact sports are associated with a greater amount of overuse injuries.[30,31] The high-impact sports generally yield the highest rate of injury due to the contact characteristics of the games. Specific sports can have notable risk factors. Table 8-5 shows college sport-specific injury risk highlights.

Gender

Female athletes experience overuse injuries at higher rates than males.[30,32] Specifically, Yang et al[30] reported that females have a rate of 24.6/10,000 AEs compared to 13.2/10,000 AEs in males. However, acute injury occurs more frequently in male athletes.[30] A possible explanation for the gender differences could be attributed to structural and biomechanical differences.[30] Females' lower extremities comprise 51.2% of their total height, compared to 56% in males.[33] Females have a wider pelvis and larger Q-angle, which are well known for predisposing female athletes to patellofemoral pain syndrome. The muscle mass of males and females prior to puberty is comparable; however, as testosterone begins to influence growth during puberty, males accumulate

Table 8-3

Total Injury Rate for Practices and Games Preseason, During Competitive Season, and Postseason by NCAA Sport

NCAA SPORT	GAME INJURY RATE/1000 AES	PRACTICE INJURY RATE/1000 AES	NO. OF TIMES HIGHER INJURY RATE IS IN GAME COMPARED TO PRACTICE	OUT-OF-SEASON PRACTICE		OUT-OF-SEASON GAMES	
				PRESEASON INJURY RATE/1000 AES	POSTSEASON INJURY RATE/1000 AES	PRESEASON INJURY RATE/1000 AES	POSTSEASON INJURY RATE/1000 AES
Football	36	4	9	7.24	1.35	7.55	23.71
Baseball	5.78	1.85	3	2.97	0.7	3.24	4.17
Softball	4.3	2.7	1.6	3.65	0.81	2.65	2.39
Men's basketball	9.9	4.3	2	7.5	1.5	12.1	6.4
Women's basketball	7.68	3.99	2	9.53	5.52	6.75	1.49
Field hockey	7.87	3.7	2	6.37	1.63	6.49	7.19
Women's gymnastics	15.19	6.07	2.5	7.9	2.11	15.84	10.82
Men's ice hockey	16.27	1.96	>8	5.05	1.27	11.59	11.91
Women's lacrosse	7.15	3.3	>2	4.29	1.10	5.74	5.20
Men's lacrosse	12.58	3.24	4	4.89	1.55	17.74	7.54

(continued)

TABLE 8-3 (CONTINUED)

TOTAL INJURY RATE FOR PRACTICES AND GAMES PRESEASON, DURING COMPETITIVE SEASON, AND POSTSEASON BY NCAA SPORT

NCAA SPORT	GAME INJURY RATE/1000 AES	PRACTICE INJURY RATE/1000 AES	NO. OF TIMES HIGHER INJURY RATE IS IN GAME COMPARED TO PRACTICE	OUT-OF-SEASON PRACTICE		OUT-OF-SEASON GAMES	
				PRESEASON INJURY RATE/1000 AES	POSTSEASON INJURY RATE/1000 AES	PRESEASON INJURY RATE/1000 AES	POSTSEASON INJURY RATE/1000 AES
Men's soccer	18.75	4.34	4	7.89	1.62	19.02	14.58
Women's soccer	16.4	5.2	3	9.52	1.45	19.65	11.67
Women's volleyball	4.58	4.10	Comparable	6.19	1.17	3.26	2.67
Men's wrestling	26.4	5.7	4	8.3	1.8	39.1	21.9

TABLE 8-4

TOP 5 GAME INJURY RATES/1000 AEs BY NCAA SPORT

SPORT	ANKLE LIGAMENT SPRAIN	KNEE INTERNAL DERANGEMENT	CONCUSSION	UPPER LEG CONTUSION	UPPER LEG MUSCLE-TENDON STRAIN	SHOULDER MUSCLE-TENDON STRAIN	LOWER LEG CONTUSION	PATELLA/PATELLAR TENDON INJURY	UNSPECIFIED	FINGER FRACTURE	LOWER BACK MUSCLE-TENDON STRAIN	PELVIS, HIP MUSCLE-TENDON STRAIN	NOSE FRACTURE	SHOULDER AC JOINT	SHOULDER LIGAMENT SPRAIN
Football	5.39	6.17	2.34	1.27	1.24										
Baseball	0.43	0.21	0.19		0.63	0.37									
Softball	0.44	0.37	0.25	0.34	0.22		0.14								
Men's basketball	2.33	0.66	0.32					0.21							
Women's basketball	1.89	1.22	0.5					0.19	0.21						
Field hockey	0.76	0.57	0.52		0.39					0.36					
Women's gymnastics	2.48	3.04			0.43				0.43		0.49				
Men's ice hockey		2.20	1.47	1.02								0.73		1.45	

Abbreviations: AC, acromioclavicular; AE, athlete-exposure.

(continued)

Table 8-4 (Continued)
Top 5 Game Injury Rates/1000 AEs by NCAA Sport

SPORT	ANKLE LIGAMENT SPRAIN	KNEE INTERNAL DERANGEMENT	CONCUSSION	UPPER LEG CONTUSION	UPPER LEG MUSCLE-TENDON STRAIN	SHOULDER MUSCLE-TENDON STRAIN	LOWER LEG CONTUSION	PATELLA/PATELLAR TENDON INJURY	UNSPECIFIED	FINGER FRACTURE	LOWER BACK MUSCLE-TENDON STRAIN	PELVIS, HIP MUSCLE-TENDON STRAIN	NOSE FRACTURE	SHOULDER AC JOINT	SHOULDER LIGAMENT SPRAIN
Women's lacrosse	1.62	1.00	0.70		0.52								0.18		
Men's lacrosse	1.43	1.14	1.08	1.00	0.94										
Men's soccer	3.19	2.07	1.08	1.21	1.54										
Women's soccer	3.01	2.61	1.42		1.14		0.75								
Women's volleyball	1.44	0.46	0.15			0.17					0.16				
Men's wrestling	1.97	6.03	1.27			1.45									0.87

Abbreviations: AC, acromioclavicular; AE, athlete-exposure.

TABLE 8-5

SPORT-SPECIFIC INJURY FACTS FOR SELECT NCAA SPORTS

SPORT	INJURY RISK CHARACTERISTICS
Football	• Highest ratio of acute (17.8%) vs overuse (5.2%) injuries in college athletes[30]
Baseball	• Relatively low incidence of injury • Division I baseball players have a significantly higher incidence of injuries compared to Divisions II and III
Softball	• Increased demands of sliding and high speed of the ball contribute to lower-extremity contusions and strains • Repetitive motion stresses shoulder complex
Field hockey	• 66% of game injuries occurred inside of the 25 yard line, closest to each goal • Contact with the ball or stick is dangerous and causes a considerable amount of injury • NCAA Field Hockey Committee recommended that players wear protective eyewear
Women's gymnastics	• 70% of injuries result from landings
Men's ice hockey	• Player contact was cited as the mechanism of injury for 47.7% of game injuries • Contact with the boards or glass was involved in 22% of injuries[108]
Women's lacrosse	• 44% of game injuries resulted from no direct contact • Participation increased by > 100% between 1988 and 2004[109]
Men's lacrosse	• 60% of all injuries in games were attributed to a contact mechanism • 50% of those injuries occurred within the 25 yard line • Dive rule prohibited offensive players from leaving the ground to shoot the ball and landing inside the crease, reducing injuries • Changes to the helmet make it lighter, less bulky, and allow for increased mobility and vision
Women's volleyball	• Mechanism most commonly reported is a player landing on another player's foot • 23% of ankle injuries result in ≥ 10 days out of activity[110]
Men's wrestling	• Takedown and the down position after a restart have the most risk of injuries for a wrestler competing defensively[111]

Abbreviations: NCAA, National Collegiate Athletic Association.

TABLE 8-6
ANTERIOR CRUCIATE LIGAMENT INJURY RATES PER 1000 ATHLETE-EXPOSURES COMPARING MALES AND FEMALES BY SPORT

SPORT	FEMALE	MALE
Softball/baseball	0.08	0.02
Basketball	0.23	0.07
Ice hockey	0.03	0.06
Lacrosse	0.17	0.12
Soccer	0.28	0.09
Wrestling	N/A	0.11
Abbreviation: N/A, not applicable.		

a greater total muscle mass into adulthood. The total cross-sectional area of muscles in women is 60%, compared to 80% in males.[34] As a result, males are generally able to produce greater strength and power. Sport and sport injury are greatly influenced by forces created by the generation of physical power. Females also have greater general joint laxity compared to males. Finally, females have a larger percentage of body fat (22% to 26%) compared to males (12% to 16%).[35]

When examining the total number of overuse injuries, the incidence is higher in females (61.7%) than males (38.3%).[26] Hootman et al[26] examined injury rates of 16 college sport teams and found that 4 women's teams—field hockey, soccer, softball, and volleyball—had the highest rates of overuse injury of the investigation. Females have higher rates of noncontact ACL injury (Table 8-6),[26] patellofemoral pain, and stress fractures of the pelvis and hip.[36,37] Other researchers have concluded that, for sex-comparable sports, the differences between genders is reduced.[30] Ristolainen et al[27] found no gender differences in the incidence of acute and overuse injuries in cross-country skiers, swimmers, distance runners, and soccer players. Even when calculating injury rate by 1000 training hours, 1000 competition hours, or all hours combined, there were no gender differences.[27] Overall, gender-related differences for acute and overuse injuries in top-level athletes between the sexes have been found to be small.

Type and Timing of Participation

There is generally a contract between game and practice injury rates across sports. The higher number of injuries in preseason practices and spring practices may be due to varying dynamics and focuses. Athletes may not be as conditioned and, therefore, not physically prepared for the intensity and demands of the sport. Also, preseason is a typical time for overloading the body. Players transition from little activity to long hours of participation. Finally, players may be playing with increased intensity in an effort to become a member of the team as this is often a time of trying out for the squad.[38]

Professional Sports

Professional athletes have the benefit of experience and training that leads to development of strength, power, skill, and control. Although participating in professional sports is widely considered an opportunity and a privilege, it comes with greater costs. Injury at the professional level often results in financial implications not considered at amateur levels. Due to the need to maximize their income during their brief careers, professional athletes are susceptible to overuse and overtraining because they often push through musculoskeletal injuries and limit their recovery times.

Baseball

Many athletes participate in professional baseball, adding importance to the study of injury in this sport. The stress placed upon the upper extremity due to the biomechanics of the overhead throwing motion, excessive training, and demanding season schedule place baseball players, particularly pitchers, at great risk for injury. A majority of injuries in Major League Baseball are to the upper body.[39-41] Shoulder injuries account for significant time on the injury/disabled list, but pitchers, specifically, were more likely to miss playing days due to elbow and wrist injuries.[39]

Lower body injuries have been reported to account for 30% to 50% of all injuries in baseball players.[40] Although pitchers are more likely to sustain shoulder injury and greater time loss from elbow and groin injury, position players are more likely to sustain abdominal/groin and knee injuries.[39] Time loss from muscle strain and hip labral tear is considerable.[39]

Football

The physical nature of football, coupled with the high-impact forces and brief, but intense, format culminates into a high-risk endeavor. During training camp, the overall rate of injury is 17.3/1000 AEs.[42] Players were more likely to suffer injury during weeks 1 and 2 compared to 3 through 5. The injury rate is significantly higher during games than practices. The injury rate has been reported as 64.7/1000 AEs during games and 12.7/1000 AEs during practices.[42] The most common types of injuries during training camp are knee sprain (10.84/1000 AEs during games and 2.12/1000 AEs during practices), hamstring strain (4.07/1000 AEs during games and 1.79/1000 AEs during practices), and contusions (12.47/1000 AEs during games and 0.92/1000 AEs during practices).[42]

Quarterbacks have a unique role in football because they throw the ball. Whereas most other positions suffer from lower body injuries, quarterbacks have a higher risk of shoulder injury. Kelly et al[43] studied 1534 quarterback injuries using the National Football League Injury Surveillance System (NFLISS) and found a mean time loss of 22.1 days from acromioclavicular joint injuries and 14.1 days for shoulder contusions. Of these, 83.8% occurred during a game. Of all quarterbacks, 77.4% were injured during passing plays. Direct trauma was the predominant mechanism of injury, with less than 15% resulting from overuse.[43]

Another specific epidemiologic consideration is the effect of anabolic-androgenic steroids on musculoskeletal injuries. An association between increased risk of injury with steroid use may exist. Horn et al[45] surveyed a large sample of retired NFL players and found that steroid use during a professional football career may be associated with ligamentous and joint-related injuries. Significant association was found between anabolic steroid use and medial collateral ligament (MCL), ACL, meniscus, and ankle injury.[44] Pressures to perform, even when injured, continue to emerge in professional sports, such as baseball and football. Investigations into the long-term effects of analgesics, oral and injectable, are being requested by former players who believe that playing injured and under the influence of medication may have caused long-term health consequences.[45] Between 1997 and 2002, 31 Achilles tendon ruptures occurred in the NFL. Players generally took 9 to 12 months to return to play. Of the injured players, 32.3% never returned to play.[46] On average, players who ruptured their Achilles tendon had more than a 50% reduction in power following the injury.[46]

Playing surface has been shown to influence the rate of knee injury in professional football. Participation on AstroTurf yields higher injury rates for knee sprains compared to natural grass. However, a recent meta-analysis of the effect of field type on injury in soccer players demonstrated that the risk of sustaining an injury on artificial turf may be lowered compared to natural grass.[47] When comparing field type and position, backs on rushing plays and linemen on passing plays have shown to suffer a significantly higher rate of ACL sprains than other position players.[48]

Basketball

An epidemiological investigation into injuries suffered by National Basketball Association (NBA) players over 17 years points to key differences in acute vs overuse injuries.[49] Lateral ankle sprains were the most frequent orthopedic injury (13.2%), followed by patellofemoral pathology (11.9%), lumbar strains (7.9%), and hamstring strains (3.3%). No relationships were found between injury rate and player demographics, such as age, height, weight, or experience. Injuries were more likely suffered during games. Patellofemoral injury was the most likely to cause the greatest number of days lost in participation. True ligamentous injuries of the knee were rare.

More specifically, game-related injuries to the lateral meniscus have an injury rate of 1.01/10,000 AEs compared to the medial meniscus (0.57/10,000 AEs) in NBA athletes. Of the meniscal injuries, 59.7% involved the lateral meniscus, and 40.3% involved the medial meniscus. Injuries occurred more frequently in games, and injured players tended to miss an average of slightly more than 40 days.[50]

Finally, a comparison of injury risk between Women's NBA (WNBA) and NBA players was conducted.[51] With both leagues being followed over 6 seasons, the frequency and rate of game-related injuries were calculated. WNBA players had a higher injury rate of 24.9/1000 AEs compared to NBA players with 19.3/1000 AEs. Lower-extremity injuries are common in basketball. The WNBA players showed a significantly higher rate of lower-extremity injury at 14.6/1000 AEs compared to 11.6/1000 AEs in NBA players. Lateral ankle sprain was the most common diagnosis in either league. Although game-related knee injury was higher in WNBA players, the incidence of ACL injury in the NBA (0.8%) and WNBA (0.9%) was similar.[51]

Soccer

A study of more than 2000 first-team squads in professional European leagues revealed that a squad of 25 players can expect approximately 15 muscle injuries per season. Of all muscle injuries, 92% affected the 4 major muscle groups of the lower limbs: hamstrings (37%), adductors (23%), quadriceps (19%), and calf muscles (13%).[52] The majority of quadriceps strains (60%) affected the dominant leg, identified by preferred kicking leg. Muscle injuries constitute almost one-third of all time-loss injuries in men's professional soccer. Two of 3 muscle injuries were traumatic with an acute onset, although overuse injuries were more common among hip and groin injuries (42%). Researchers also reported that the incidence of calf muscle injury increased with the age of the players. Most muscle injuries occurred by noncontact mechanisms, with only 5% occurring during foul play.[52]

Another survey of Union of European Football Association (UEFA) injuries over 7 consecutive seasons revealed thigh strain as the most common injury type (17%). A team of 25, the average on a professional squad, can expect about 10 thigh muscle strains each season—7 affecting the hamstring and 3 affecting the quadriceps.[53] Other common injuries reported included adductor pain/strain (9%), ankle sprain (7%), and MCL injuries (5%).[53]

Giza et al[54] analyzed injury data from the first 2 seasons of the Women's United Soccer Association. The most common injuries were strains (30.7%), sprains (19.1%), contusions (16.2%), and fractures (11.6%). The most common location was the knee (31.8%), followed by the head (10.4%), ankle (9.3%), and foot (9.3%). Of the injuries, 60% were to the lower extremities, 82% were acute, 27.3% were strains, and 16.4% were contusions. There were acute ACL injuries during the 2 seasons (incidence of 0.09/1000 AEs).

AGE AS A RISK FACTOR

Age has an effect on rate and type of musculoskeletal injury. There are different susceptibilities at various stages in life. For example, children may acquire conditions specific to their growing bones and developing muscles, such as apophysitis and osteochondritides.[55] However, as people age, the composition and elastic properties of tissue decline, which contributes to increased frequency of certain injuries. Bone density decreases, making the bone more susceptible to injury. Risk factors for different stages of development should be acknowledged.

Youth and Adolescents

Children and adolescents experience a decrease in physeal strength during pubescence.[56] The cross-sectional area of muscle and isokinetic muscle strength have been shown to increase with age and training, with youth athletes having decreased size, strength, and composition of muscle.[57a]

In childhood, muscle and bone growth can affect injury incidence. Sullivan et al[57b] found that players younger than 10 years were rarely affected by injury (< 1 injury/100 participants), whereas the injury rate among older players was reported to be 7.7/100 players. There is an increase in the incidence of overuse injury in adolescents. This increase can be attributed to participation in year-long sport, early specialization, and participation in multiple sports simultaneously as athletes grow older.[24] Overuse injuries occur as a result of repetitive submaximal forces to the musculoskeletal system. Coupled with inadequate rest, injury can result. Injury can occur at the musculotendinous unit, bone, bursa, neurological system, and physes. Apophyseal and physeal stress injuries are of particular concern in youth athletes.[4]

Soft tissue injuries and fractures are common in younger patients because of involvement in physical activity, sports, and accidents. The increased exposure but incomplete development of the musculoskeletal system are likely reasons for increased soft tissue injury. Children aged 10 to 14 years accounted for more than half (56.6%) of SRIs evaluated in the emergency department. The majority (71.1%) of SRIs occurred in boys, and, overall, males had a greater number of injuries.[58] The Public Health Agency of Canada reported that 68% of SRIs occur in children aged 10 to 14 years.[59] Some injuries more commonly found in patients younger than 20 years include injury to the forearm/hand extensor tendon, thumb ulnar collateral ligament, forearm/hand flexor tendon, acromioclavicular joint, meniscus, ACL, posterior cruciate ligament, MCL, lateral collateral ligament, and peroneal tendon.

Middle Age

Matheson et al[64] examined overuse injury in older and middle-aged athletes. A study of 1407 cases revealed that common injury-associated activities with the younger group (mean age, 30.4 years) were running, fitness classes, and field sports, whereas racquet sports, walking, and low-intensity sports were more commonly associated with injury in the older group (mean age, 56.9 years). The frequency of tendinitis was similar in both age groups, but groups displayed increased frequency of other conditions. The younger group displayed a high frequency of patellofemoral pain syndrome and stress fracture/periostitis, whereas the older group displayed an increased frequency of metatarsalgia, plantar fasciitis, and meniscal injury.

Changes in physiology and anatomy caused by aging can increase the incidence of injury. Injuries such as Achilles tendon rupture, patellar tendon rupture, and quadriceps tendon rupture are most commonly seen in middle-aged men. Mallet finger is most commonly seen in middle-aged men and women. This pattern is likely due to degenerative changes in the tendons of patients who remain active.[60] Muscle mass decreases approximately 3% to 8% per decade after the age of 30 years.[61] The degenerative changes in the tendon that occur with aging include changes in the collagen and noncollagen matrices, decreased tensile strength, and a decrease in volume density. For example, shoulder pain was reported in 24% of high-level tennis players from ages 12 to 19 but increased to 50% for middle-aged participants.[62]

Older Adults

There are many negative effects of the aging process on the function of the musculoskeletal system. Bones become brittle and break more easily. Joints become inflamed, stiff, and deformed, causing painful motion. Older adults may experience more severe effects, including reduced activity tolerance, decreased height due to compressed intervertebral disks, altered posture, reduced reflexes, tremors, weakness from disuse, and contractures from prolonged limited range of motion (ROM). Luckily, physical activity and proper diet can slow or prevent many of these problems because bones and muscles adapt to the stresses placed upon them.

As people age, cartilage between bones gradually loses fluid and becomes thinner, therefore resulting in increased compressive forces on the bones. Joints grow stiffer and less flexible, with a decreased amount of fluid present to lubricate the joints. Calcification can occur in the joints, resulting in decreased ROM. Lean body mass decreases, partially because of loss of muscle tissue. Fat is increasingly deposited in the muscle tissue, muscle fibers shrink, and muscle tissue is replaced more slowly. Lost muscle tissue may eventually be replaced with fibrous tissue, which does not contribute to force generation. Eventually, changes in the muscle tissue, coupled with changes in the function of the nervous system, result in decreased muscular force generation, control, and contractile capability.[63] These adaptive mechanisms become less effective, and the body becomes more susceptible to injury.

Osteoarthritis was 2.5 times higher in older adults compared to a middle-aged group.[64] It could be speculated that decreased fluid in the joint, changing biomechanics, decreased extensibility and resilience, and degeneration of connective tissue contribute to the increased frequency of the injuries seen in older adults.

Fall prevention has been increasingly popular as the medical community has realized the frequency and financial burden associated with such incidences. Millions of adults, aged 65 years and older, experience a fall each year. Falls are the leading cause of fatal and nonfatal injuries, and it was estimated that, in 2012 alone, the direct medical costs from falls was $30 billion.[65] Exercise has been widely recommended as a fall-prevention method. This may be a double-edged sword. Although exercise is recommended for fall prevention and as a remedy for many health issues that arise commonly in the last decades of life, some speculate that soft tissue injuries will increase as older adults remain active later into the lifespan.[60] The safety margin of exercise dosage declines with age. Exertional injuries are common in older individuals and are connected to the degenerative process that occurs with aging. Acute injuries in older, active adults are most often associated with activities that require a high amount of coordination, reaction time, and balance. It is recommended that consideration be made regarding activity type and a proper match between ability and requirement be made. Muscle is the most commonly acutely injured tissue among active elderly athletes, and the lower extremities are the most widely affected.[66] The benefits of exercise and risk of injury must be weighed appropriately.

Activity

The duration of the activity influences the rate of injuries. In a comprehensive literature review, Abrams et al[67] determined that there is no association between age, sex, and skill level on injury rates in tennis players; however, the volume of play was associated with an increased risk of injury. Hootman et al[68] reported that men and women with high levels of duration of physical activity and cardiorespiratory fitness were associated with a significantly increased risk of musculoskeletal injury compared with gender-matched individuals with a low level of duration and fitness.

ANTERIOR CRUCIATE LIGAMENT INJURIES

The incidence of ACL injuries is estimated from surgical registries. These registries track information on the details of ACL surgery and monitor the outcomes. Although nonsurgical cases are missing, the registry can identify risk factors and methods of best practice. Rates of ACL reconstruction are estimated to be 34/100,000 for US citizens and 85/100,000 for those aged 16 to 39 years.[69] Data from the NCAA ISS reveal an average of 2000 ACL injuries in 15 designated collegiate sports per year. Percentagewise, the greatest number of ACL tears occur in women's soccer, women's lacrosse, women's gymnastics, and women's basketball.[70] If the ACL injury rate per 1000 AEs is examined, women's gymnastics ranks highest, followed by spring football, women's soccer, women's basketball, and fall football. ACL injuries are, most typically, noncontact in nature, with the exception of football, men's ice hockey, and men's wrestling.[70]

ACL injuries cause concern because of the time loss, pain, disability, and cost. More than 88% of athletes with an ACL injury will lose 10 or more days of participation.[26] Yet, in terms of incidence, ACL injuries are not epidemic. The probability of ACL injury would be considered rare (0.02 to 0.33/1000 AEs).[26]

Gender Differences

There is a plethora of evidence describing the increased incidence of ACL injury in female athletes compared to males. The NCAA ISS reported that the largest difference between the sexes in ACL injury is in basketball, with female injury being 3 times that of men, and in soccer, with female injury being twice that of men.[70] The gender disparity is also evident at the high school level. In basketball, the injury rate in younger females is the highest, with females injuring their ACLs at a rate 4 times higher than in males. The rate of noncontact ACL injuries in soccer was twice as high in female athletes compared to males.[70]

Risk Factors

Risk factors for ACL injury are considered internal or external. Examples of external risk factors include the type of competition, footwear, playing surface, and environmental conditions. Internal risk factors include anatomical, hormonal, and neuromuscular risk factors.[70]

Shoe-Surface Interaction

The coefficient of friction, or ratio of the force of friction between a shoe and a playing surface plus the amount of force pushing them together, is an important consideration when examining the influence of footwear on injury. Increasing the coefficient of friction and the force compressing the sole and surface together has the potential to increase the risk of suffering an ACL injury.[67] Biomechanical changes occur when there is a high coefficient of friction present between the shoe and playing surface. Changes such as lower knee flexion angle, lower external knee flexion moment, higher external knee valgus moment, and greater medial distance of the center of mass from the support limb have been observed during a sidestep cutting task.[72] This shoe-surface interaction can be affected by the characteristics of the shoes, the surface type, and the weather. Increasing the grab of the shoe to the surface may lead to an increased incidence of ACL injury. Moreover, athletes may make biomechanical adaptations to varying shoes, surfaces, and weather conditions that increase the risk for ACL injury due to the changed nature of movement. Conditions linked to an increase in ACL injury are sparse, narrow, long cleats; artificial turf and rubber surfaces; and hot and dry weather. More amicable conditions include numerous, wide, and short cleats; natural surfaces; and cold and wet weather.[72]

Environmental Conditions

Little research specifically examines the risk of ACL injury related to weather conditions. Orchard et al[73] examined environmental variables as risk factors for noncontact ACL injuries in male Australian football players and found that they were more common during periods of low rainfall and high evaporation. This combination results in a dry playing surface, which, theoretically, increases friction forces between the shoe surface and the playing surface.[73] Orchard et al[75] also observed a relative risk of 2.5 for suffering an ACL injury in dry weather conditions, with high water evaporation in the month prior.

Furthermore, epidemiological data reveal that injury incidence increases during games.[26,31,75-77] This could be due to the intensity of play increasing by the athlete and his or her competitors. It has been speculated that competition is more physically demanding, with greater risk taken by the participants, compared to practice activities.[38,78,79]

Anatomical

Anatomical dimensions are hypothesized to influence the gender differences in ACL incidence. Lower-extremity alignment, intercondylar notch size, and posterior tibial slope may increase strain on the ACL and predispose individuals to injury. Many studies have looked at specific structures of the lower extremities and their influence on ACL injury rates.[70]

Lower-Extremity Alignment

Lower-extremity alignment is recognized by the International Olympic Committee's current concept statement as an internal risk factor for ACL injury. Examining the position of the hip, knee, and ankle and noting abnormal posture can cue a clinician into increased ACL strain.[70] This being said, scarce literature supports alignment and its relationship to ACL injury, but it is still recommended as good clinical practice.

Intercondylar Notch Size

Geometric differences in the ACL have been examined heavily but are not well described. There is a lack of standardization in the methods used to obtain these data. Notch width of unilateral and bilateral ACL patients are smaller than notch widths of normal controls. Therefore, a strong relationship exists between small notch size and ACL injury.[80] Furthermore, there is evidence that the notch width of patients who have suffered bilateral ACL injury is smaller than those with unilateral injury to the ACL.[80] Notch size has also been shown to differ between genders, with females having a femoral intercondylar notch width smaller than that of males,[81] but some argue that there is no conclusive correlation between ACL size and notch dimension in relation to risk of ACL injury.[82] Comparatively, when normalizing for body mass index, women have a geometrically smaller ACL than men. The physical properties of the ACL may differ between the sexes, as well.[70] The female ACL is smaller than the male ACL. The female ACL shows lower mechanical properties compared to the male ACL. These differences are not simply due to the size of the ACL, but to the sex-based differences in the ACL itself. The female ACL has been found to have an 8.3% lower strain (relative change in shape or size due to external force) at failure, 14.3% lower stress (internal force associated with strain) at failure, 9.43% lower strain energy (energy stored during deformation) density at failure, and 22.49% lower modulus of elasticity (resistance to being deformed elastically) compared to the male ACL and considering factors such as age and anthropometric measurements.[83]

Posterior Tibial Slope

Increased anterior translation has been linked to a posteroinferior tibial slope (Figure 8-1).[80] Magnetic resonance imaging can be utilized to measure posterior tibial slope. One study revealed that subjects with ACL-deficient knees had a significantly greater slope of the lateral tibial plateau and a lower slope of the medial tibial plateau than the control group.[84]

Figure 8-1. Posterior tibial slope.

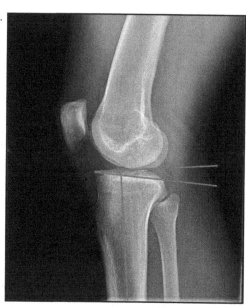

Hormonal

The presence of sex hormone receptors (estrogen, testosterone, and relaxin) on the human ACL presents the potential for sex hormones to affect its properties. No specific mechanism has been identified, but there are enough parallels with the structure physiology of collagen, muscle, and bone to suggest that hormones are factors.[70] Many areas are unexplored in this risk factor.

Structural and Mechanical Properties

Women have a lower joint resistance to translation and rotation, giving them greater tibiofemoral joint laxity than men. This multiplanar laxity cannot be wholly accredited to the mechanical properties of the ACL. Although their ACLs are smaller and have lower linear stiffness, there is also a bigger physiological mechanism that contributes to the sex differences in ACL injury. Women's ACLs have less elongation at failure and lower energy absorption and load at failure compared to men.[70]

Menstrual Cycle

There is a consensus in the literature that the risk for ACL tears changes over the course of the menstrual cycle.[85,86] The greatest risk exists during the preovulatory phase, and the lowest is during the postovulatory phase.[87,88] It is not estrogen alone, but likely the cyclic increase and decrease of estrogen and other hormones affecting estradiol that impact ACL injury risk.[70] Women vary widely in their hormonal composition. Some may experience greater effects of sex hormones on ligament biology than others. Future research is needed in this area, especially as ACL risk relates to the use of birth control pills.

Neuromuscular

Almost 80% of ACL injuries are noncontact. Common mechanisms include landing from a jump, cutting and changing direction, and decelerating. Anterior tibial translation, coupled with lower-extremity valgus at the knee, are important components of the mechanism of injury for noncontact ACL tears. Limited knee flexion with increased quadriceps and/or gastrocnemius activity is a key biomechanical situation that increases risk. Anterior translation, dynamic valgus of the lower extremity with the knee near extension, and most of the force on a single leg with the foot away from the center of mass have also been shown to be a biomechanical problem for the ACL.[70]

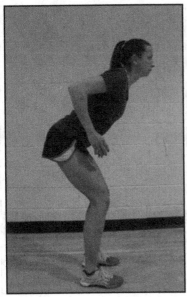

Figure 8-2. Extended knee during landing.

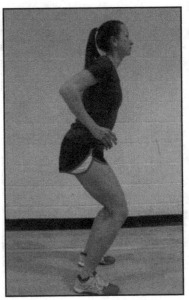

Figure 8-3. Extended hip during landing.

Neuromuscular imbalances, such as quadriceps dominance, have also been shown to contribute to risk. With greater propensity for quadriceps dominance and decreased hamstring recruitment, women are susceptible to neuromuscular risk factors when compared to men.[89] Isokinetic testing may be used as an objective clinical measure of risk.[90,91] Markers, such as females having one hamstring more than 15% weaker than the other or a flexion/extension ratio of less than 0.75, can significantly increase the risk of injury.[92]

Some neuromuscular training programs have produced quantifiable reductions in the risk of ACL injury for athletes and have been recommended, although a recent systematic review did not find the evidence compelling enough for universal implementation.[93] Two studies showed a decrease in ACL injury, 2 showed significant decreases in practices (not games) later in the season and in athletes with a history of ACL injury, 4 showed a trend toward reduction, and 2 showed an increase.[93]

Common components of neuromuscular training programs include stretching, awareness of high-risk positions, technique modification, aerobic conditioning, sports-specific agilities, proprioceptive and balance training, and plyometrics.[70] These components address specific risk factors, such as an extended knee (Figure 8-2) or hip (Figure 8-3) at the initial landing contact, knee valgus with tibiofemoral loading (Figure 8-4), balance deficits, and skill deficiency.[70] Proper alignment should be ensured (Figure 8-5).

Education and increased awareness of high-risk positons and situations can reduce the incidence of ACL injury.[94] Cutting, landing, and decelerating with the hip and knee in flexion, as well as rounding out cut maneuvers and using a 3-step quick stop are techniques that can attenuate the risk of ACL tear.[70] Programs using plyometric exercise and preseason components have been shown to be most beneficial, but more research into the most effective programs is warranted.[93]

ROTATOR CUFF INJURIES

The prevalence of partial- and full-thickness rotator cuff tears varies. Cadaver investigations and varied imaging techniques show rates ranging from 5% to 40% in the general population.[95]

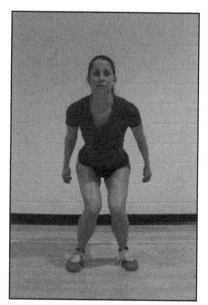

Figure 8-4. Proper landing alignment.

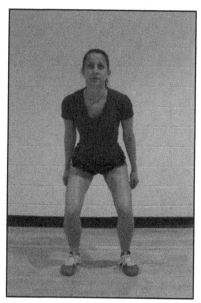

Figure 8-5. Knee valgus with tibiofemoral loading.

Rotator cuff epidemiology can be challenging because of the presence of asymptomatic tears and injury to the biceps tendon. Examination into asymptomatic individuals has, over time, revealed an increased incidence. Although micro- or macrotrauma can affect rotator cuff tear development, it is accepted that rotator cuff pathology occurs as a normal degenerative process. The current literature reports age differences, risk factors, and prevention strategies for evidence-based clinical application.[95]

Age and Overhead Activities

Rotator cuff injury is more common in those older than 40 years. Studies have shown that less than 1% of rotator cuff tears occur in patients younger than 20 years.[4] Shoulder symptoms in young, high-level tennis players, for example, are related to subtle instability of the glenohumeral joint, whereas the rotator cuff is more commonly involved in older players. Incidence of rotator cuff injuries in elderly patients is high. Yamaguchi et al[97] found average ages to be 48.7 years for patients with no rotator cuff tear, 58.7 years for those with a unilateral tear, and 67.8 years with bilateral tears in the general population. Those older than 66 years have a 50% chance of incurring bilateral tears. The results also showed that just more than 35% of patients with a full-thickness tear on one side had a full-thickness tear on the contralateral side. Ultrasound studies revealed a 50% likelihood of the presence of an asymptomatic rotator cuff tear in the contralateral shoulder in this age group.[97]

Degenerative changes have been acknowledged as a cause for rotator cuff tears. Etiologies may include extrinsic factors, such as subacromial and internal impingement, tensile overload, repetitive stress, or intrinsic factors, such as poor vascularity, alterations in material properties of the tissue, matrix composition, and aging. Ultrasonography has allowed for the examination of rotator cuffs across the age span. One study reported that out of a portion of the general population, tears were found in 0% in those younger than 50 years, 10.7% in those in their 50s, 15.2% in those in their 60s, 26.5% in those in their 70s, and 36.6% in those older than 80 years.[98] Asymptomatic rotator cuff injury is a challenge for epidemiologic study. Small tears are often asymptomatic. Symptomatic tears have been shown to be 30% larger than asymptomatic tears in the contralateral shoulder.[97]

Sports that require regular use of repetitive arm motion, such as throwing or tennis serve, have a greater risk for injuring the rotator cuff. An investigation into collegiate overhead athletes reported shoulder injuries in 30% of the athletes. Rotator cuff tendonitis was a common shoulder injury and accounted for 24% of the total shoulder injuries in 5 teams of overhead athletes. Besides subacromial impingement, the incidence rate of rotator cuff pathology was significantly higher than any other injury among overhead athletes.[99] Hand dominance and history of trauma have shown to be risk factors for rotator cuff pathology, as well.[95]

Prevention

Although age is a naturally occurring risk factor for rotator cuff pathology, sports participation places greater demand on this muscular unit. This is particularly true for throwing athletes. Specific intentional exercises can help prevent injury to the rotator cuff. Several principles guide the maintenance of a healthy shoulder, including maintenance of ROM, muscular strength, dynamic stabilization, neuromuscular control, and core and full-body strength.

Maintaining sport-specific ROM is important. Overhead athletes demonstrate increased ROM, ranging from 129 to 137 degrees of external rotation, 54 to 61 degrees of internal rotation, and 183 to 198 degrees of total internal and external rotation. Athletes should have equal, total shoulder range of internal-external rotation bilaterally, but they should be expected to present with greater external rotation and less internal rotation in the dominant shoulder.[101] Loss of total ROM is related to a greater risk of injury, so maintenance of a full, equal ROM should be evaluated and maintained with frequent, gentle stretching. A focus on stretching to maintain mobility, rather than to gain mobility, should be emphasized.

Overhead athletes must focus on the strength of the entire kinetic chain. Strengthening of the musculature of the shoulder, scapula, elbow, and wrist are essential for rotator cuff support. Throwing athletes, particularly, should focus on strengthening the external rotators, scapular retractors, and lower trapezius.[100] Basic exercises and sport-specific strengthening techniques of these muscles will assist in the healthy maintenance of the rotator cuff.

Good neuromuscular control of the glenohumeral and scapulothoracic joints is critical because stability is sacrificed for mobility in overhead athletes. The scapula provides a key attachment point for the musculature of the shoulder region that properly positions the glenohumeral joint for ideal movement. Scapular stability and strength are essential to maintaining the proper motion of the glenohumeral joint. Closed kinetic chain exercises are critical to maintaining or increasing the facilitation of cocontraction of the shoulder force couples.[101] Rhythmic stabilization, reactive neuromuscular exercises, and plyometric exercises should also be included.[102]

The body operates as a system of links. Overhead athletes desire to produce powerful motion, but this must be generated using the lower extremity and core. The ability to stabilize the core allows proximal stability with distal mobility of the upper extremity.[102] A deficit in the lower extremity or core can disrupt the overhead biomechanics and result in decreased performance or injury.

ACTIVITY-SPECIFIC INQUIRIES

Sport activities can place high demands on the body and increase risk of musculoskeletal injury. Particularly, repetitive motions that apply force to specific locations in the body can be injurious to athletes. Two activities that have a high incidence of injury are running and overhead activity. These are components of many widely played sports and can predispose athletes to injury over time.

Running

Exercise volume is a known factor influencing injury. For example, running distance is a significant risk factor for musculoskeletal injury. Overuse injuries are predominant in runners. Between 24% and 65% of runners report at least one injury annually, with little difference between men and women.[9]

Many running injuries occur in the lower extremity and low back.[9] More specifically, the tibia, ankle, and foot are the most common injury sites.[103] Medial tibial stress syndrome affects between 13.6% and 20% of runners. The repetitive contraction of the tibialis posterior, soleus, and flexor digitorum longus during the landing and propulsion phases of running places excessive stress on the tibia and results in inflammation of the periosteum.[103] Also, vertical ground reaction forces created during the landing phase interfere with the bone's ability to remodel. Females report medial tibial stress syndrome at a higher rate than males.[9] Hypotheses on females' increased rate include smaller stature, muscular strength and tightness differences, and gait differences.

Nonspecific knee pain is also a common complaint of runners. Studies show incidence to range between 12.7% and 29.5% in male and female adult runners. There are many causes of knee pain, but researchers have noted that the patellar tendon, in particular, is exposed to high and repetitive eccentric loads during running. Patellar tendinopathy occurs in 5.5% to 22.7% of runners during training,[104] but adaptation may occur with training and experience.

Overhead Activities

Shoulder injuries are likely in athletes who perform repetitive motion. Sports such as swimming, wrestling, baseball, rowing, basketball, volleyball, and handball require much of the upper extremity. Shoulder injuries are the fifth most common injury among high school athletes.[17] In an epidemiologic study, Bonza et al[104] examined shoulder injury in high school athletes and found an injury rate of 2.27 shoulder injuries/10,000 AEs in 9 high school sports over 2 seasons. The group concluded that shoulder injuries accounted for 8% of all injuries sustained by high school athletes during that time.[104] In an assessment of collegiate club volleyball players, researchers found that 60% of participants reported a history of shoulder problems, and nearly half said that shoulder problems limited function.[105] In elite overhead athletes, shoulder pain was noted in 41.6% of participants at some point during their career.[106] Although high injury rates to the shoulder are documented in football and wrestling, due to the high amount of contact occurring in each sport, baseball, softball, and volleyball have been noted as having high rates of shoulder injury due to the repetitive motions of the shoulder in these sports.[104]

Constant overhead activity may result in time loss from play, lifelong disability, joint instability, or progressive degeneration. Overhead athletes have specific concerns that affect performance beyond activities of daily living. An athlete-specific questionnaire for upper-extremity assessment called the Kerlan-Jobe Orthopaedic Clinic Overhead Athlete Shoulder and Elbow Score reveals the common complaints of overhead athletes, including difficulty warming up, pain, weakness and/or fatigue, instability of the shoulder or elbow, deterioration of team relationships, change of mechanics, loss of velocity and/or power, loss of endurance, loss of control, and hindrance to fulfilling full sport potential.

Overhead sports affect the elbow, as well. The elbow is the second most common site for osteochondritis dissecans compared to the knee and has a similar incidence to the ankle. Young athletes involved in overhead-dominant sports are more likely to develop osteochondritis dissecans of the elbow. Early diagnosis reduces damage and improves outcomes.[107]

Many risk factors for shoulder pain in overhead athletes exist, including gender, body mass index, sport level, and days of practice per week. Overhead athletes should be carefully supervised and educated about prevention techniques for upper-extremity injury. Supervision should be provided for overhead athletes, with particular attention paid to overuse and excessive repetitions of overhead motions. An emphasis on technique, rather than repetitions, should be provided. Proper mechanics are essential to preventing injury, as well, understanding that the body works as a unit and all parts of the kinetic chain should be assessed.

BRINGING IT TOGETHER

Musculoskeletal injury is a primary concern in athletics. Athletic trainers are charged with preventing injuries, and epidemiological data become a key source of data upon which to base an injury prevention and management program. Youth, college, and professional athletes have unique physical and environmental challenges. Various factors, such as gender, age, sport, participation level, and environment, can have a great influence on musculoskeletal injury. Injury data specific to sports, risk factors, and repetitive motions can be helpful to athletic trainers because they prevent and treat injuries.

REVIEW QUESTIONS

1. A certified athletic trainer is newly hired and given the responsibility of caring for a college women's basketball team. What are all of the considerations that he must make when addressing the prevention of musculoskeletal injury of the players on the team? What are some prevention tools and techniques that he might consider implementing? Compare these choices with teams of varying age, gender, and sport.

2. Discuss the influence of age on musculoskeletal injury. Why is age such an important factor to consider? Discuss the physical and environmental factors of age that influence musculoskeletal injury rate.

3. The population of older, active adults is growing. Provide 3 recommendations for older adults participating in recreational sporting activity to prevent musculoskeletal injury.

LEARNING ACTIVITIES

1. Find 3 exercises that are supported by research to be effective in the prevention of ACL injury. Instruct a friend or classmate on the exercise, provide a demonstration, observe, and provide appropriate, constructive feedback on his or her performance. Consider a variety of landing, cutting, and decelerating techniques for your choices of exercise.

2. List 3 essential upper-extremity muscle groups for a throwing athlete. List one strengthening exercise for each group. Demonstrate the exercises to a partner, have him or her complete them, and provide feedback on his or her technique.

REFERENCES

1. Vierimaa M, Erickson K, Côté J. Positive youth development: a measurement framework for sport. *Int J Sport Sci Coach.* 2012;7(3):601-614.
2. National Council of Youth Sports. *Report on Trends and Participation In Organized Youth Sports, 2008.* Stuart, FL: National Council of Youth Sports; 2008.
3. Ni H, Barnes P, Hardy AM. Recreational injury and its relation to socioeconomic status among school aged children in the US. *Inj Prev.* 2002;8(1):60-65.

4. DiFiori JP, Benjamin HJ, Brenner JS, et al. Overuse injuries and burnout in youth sports: a position statement from the American Medical Society for Sports Medicine. *Br J Sports Med.* 2014;48(4):287-288.

5. Comstock RD, Collins CL, Currie DW. National High School Sports-Related Injury Surveillance Study. http://www.ucdenver.edu/academics/colleges/PublicHealth/research/ResearchProjects/piper/projects/RIO/Documents/2012-13.pdf. Accessed April 7, 2014.

6. Ogden JA. Injury to the growth mechanisms of the immature skeleton. *Skeletal Radiol.* 1981;6(4):237-253.

7. Caine D, DiFiori J, Maffulli N. Physeal injuries in children's and youth sports: reasons for concern? *Br J Sports Med.* 2006;40(9):749-760.

8. Bailey DA, Wedge JH, McCulloch RG, Martin AD, Bernhardson SC. Epidemiology of fractures of the distal end of the radius in children as associated with growth. *J Bone Joint Surg Am.* 1989;71(8):1225-1231.

9. Caine DJ, Caine CG, Lindner KJ. *Epidemiology of Sport Injuries.* Champaign, IL: Human Kinetics; 1996:357-377.

10. Fridman L, Fraser-Thomas JL, McFaull SR, Macpherson AK. Epidemiology of sports-related injuries in children and youth presenting to Canadian emergency departments from 2007-2010. *BMC Sports Sci Med Rehabil.* 2013;5(1):30.

11. Radelet MA, Lephart SM, Rubinstein EN, Myers JB. Survey of the injury rate for children in community sports. *Pediatrics.* 2002;110(3):e28.

12. Yard EE, Schroeder MJ, Fields SK, Collins CL, Comstock RD. The epidemiology of United States high school soccer injuries, 2005-2007. *Am J Sports Med.* 2008;36(10):1930-1937.

13. Knowles SB, Marshall SW, Miller T, et al. Cost of injuries from a prospective cohort study of North Carolina high school athletes. *Inj Prev.* 2007;13(6):416-421.

14. Powell JW, Barber-Foss KD. Injury patterns in selected high school sports: a review of the 1995-1997 seasons. *J Athl Train.* 1999;34(3):277-284.

15. Caine D, Caine C, Maffulli N. Incidence and distribution of pediatric sport-related injuries. *Clin J Sport Med.* 2006;16(6):500-513.

16. Messina DF, Farney WC, DeLee JC. The incidence of injury in Texas high school basketball. A prospective study among male and female athletes. *Am J Sports Med.* 1999;27(3):294-299.

17. Powell JW, Barber-Foss KD. Injury patterns in selected high school sports: a review of the 1995-1997 seasons. *J Athl Train.* 1999;34(3):277-284.

18. Emery CA, Meuwisse WH, Hartmann SE. Evaluation of risk factors for injury in adolescent soccer: implementation and validation of an injury surveillance system. *Am J Sports Med.* 2005;33(12):1882-1891.

19. Caine D, Knutzen K, Howe W. A three-year epidemiological study of injuries affecting young female gymnasts. *Phys Ther Sport.* 2003;4:10-23.

20. Caine D, Cochrane B, Caine C, Zemper E. An epidemiological investigation of injuries affecting young competitive female gymnasts. *Am J Sports Med.* 1989;17(6):811-820.

21. Warren MP. The effects of exercise on pubertal progression and reproductive function in girls. *J Clin Endocrinol Metab.* 1980;51(5):1150-1157.

22. Drinkwater BL, Bruemner B, Chesnut CH III. Menstrual history as a determinant of current bone density in young athletes. *JAMA.* 1990;263(4):545-548.

23. Small E. Chronic musculoskeletal pain in young athletes. *Pediatr Clin North Am.* 2002;49(3):655-662.

24. Brenner JS; American Academy of Pediatrics Council on Sports Medicine and Fitness. Overuse injuries, overtraining, and burnout in child and adolescent athletes. *Pediatrics.* 2007;119(6):1242-1245.

25. Wieberg S. Study: college athletes are full-time workers. USA Today. January 13, 2008. http://usatoday30.usatoday.com/sports/college/2008-01-12-athletes-full-time-work-study_N.htm. Accessed November 15, 2015.

26. Hootman JM, Dick R, Agel J. Epidemiology of collegiate injuries for 15 sports: summary and recommendations for injury prevention initiatives. *J Athl Train.* 2007;42(2):311-319.

27. Ristolainen L, Heinonen A, Waller B, Kujala UM, Kettunen JA. Gender differences in sport injury risk and types of injuries: a retrospective twelve-month study on cross-country skiers, swimmers, long-distance runners and soccer players. *J Sports Sci Med.* 2009;8(3):443-451.

28. Albright JP, Powell JW, Martindale A, et al. Injury patterns in big ten conference football. *Am J Sports Med.* 2004;32(6):1394-1404.

29. Dick R, Putukian M, Agel J, Evans TA, Marshall SW. Descriptive epidemiology of collegiate women's soccer injuries: National Collegiate Athletic Association Injury Surveillance System, 1988-1989 through 2002-2003. *J Athl Train.* 2007;42(2):278-285.

30. Yang J, Tibbetts AS, Covassin T, Cheng G, Nayar S, Heiden E. Epidemiology of overuse and acute injuries among competitive collegiate athletes. *J Athl Train.* 2012;47(2):198-204.

31. McHardy AJ, Pollard HP, Luo K. Golf-related lower back injuries: an epidemiological survey. *J Chiropr Med.* 2007;6(1):20-26.

32. Smoljanovi T, Bojani I, Hannafin JA, Hren D, Delimar D, Pecina M. Traumatic and overuse injuries among international elite junior rowers. *Am J Sports Med.* 2009;37(6):1193-1199.

33. Hale R. Factors important to women engaged in vigorous physical activity. In: Strauss R, ed. *Sports Medicine.* 1st ed. Philadelphia: WB Saunders; 1984:250-269.

34. Cureton KJ, Collins MA, Hill DW, McElhannon FM Jr. Muscle hypertrophy in men and women. *Med Sci Sports Exerc.* 1988;20(4):338-344.
35. Malina RM. Body composition in athletes: assessment and estimated fatness. *Clin Sport Med.* 2007;26(1):37-68.
36. Sallis RE, Jones K, Sunshine S, Smith G, Simon L. Comparing sports injuries in men and women. *Int J Sports Med.* 2001;22(6):420-423.
37. Ireland ML, Ott SM. Special concerns of the female athlete. *Clin J Sports Med.* 2004;23(2):281-298.
38. Dick R, Sauers EL, Agel J, et al. Descriptive epidemiology of collegiate men's baseball injuries: National Collegiate Athletic Association Injury Surveillance System, 1988-1989 through 2003-2004. *J Athl Train.* 2007;42(2):183-193.
39. Li X, Zhou H, Williams P, et al. The epidemiology of single season musculoskeletal injuries in professional baseball. *Orthop Rev (Pavia).* 2013;5(1):e3.
40. Posner M, Cameron KL, Wolf JM, Belmont PJ Jr, Owens BD. Epidemiology of Major League Baseball injuries. *Am J Sports Med.* 2011;39(8):1676-1680.
41. Conte S, Requa R, Garrick JG. Disability days in major league baseball. *Am J Sports Med.* 2001;29(4):431-436.
42. Feeley BT, Kennelly S, Barnes RP, et al. Epidemiology of National Football League training camp injuries from 1998 to 2007. *Am J Sports Med.* 2008;36(8):1597-1603.
43. Kelly BT, Barnes RP, Powell JW, Warren RF. Shoulder injuries to quarterbacks in the National Football League. *Am J Sports Med.* 2004;32(2):328-331.
44. Horn S, Gregory P, Guskiewicz KM. Self-reported anabolic-androgenic steroids use and musculoskeletal injuries: findings from the center for the study of retired athletes health survey of retired NFL players. *Am J Phys Med Rehabil.* 2009;88(3):192-200.
45. Belson K, Pilon M. Concern raised over painkiller's use in sports. The New York Times. Published April 13, 2012. http://www.nytimes.com/2012/04/14/sports/wide-use-of-painkiller-toradol-before-games-raises-concerns.html?pagewanted=alland_r=0. Accessed October 9, 2015.
46. Parekh SG, Wray WH III, Brimmo O, Sennett BJ, Wapner KL. Epidemiology and outcomes of Achilles tendon ruptures in the National Football League. *Foot Ankle Spec.* 2009;2(6):283-286.
47. Williams JH, Akogyrem E, Williams JR. A meta-analysis of soccer injuries on artificial turf and natural grass. *J Sports Med.* 2013;(2013):1-6.
48. Powell J, Schootman M. A multivariate risk analysis of selected playing surfaces in the National Football League: 1980 to 1989. An epidemiologic study of knee injuries. *Am J Sports Med.* 1992;20(6):686-694.
49. Drakos MC, Domb B, Starkey C, Callahan L, Allen AA. Injury in the National Basketball Association: a 17-year overview. *Sports Health.* 2010;2(4):284-290.
50. Yeh PC, Starkey C, Lombardo S, Vitti G, Kharrazi FD. Epidemiology of isolated meniscal injury and its effect on performance in athletes from the National Basketball Association. *Am J Sports Med.* 2012;40(3):589-594.
51. Deitch JR, Starkey C, Walters SL, Moseley JB. Injury risk in professional basketball players: a comparison of Women's National Basketball Association and National Basketball Association athletes. *Am J Sports Med.* 2006;34(7):1077-1083.
52. Ekstrand J, Hägglund M, Waldén M. Epidemiology of muscle injuries in professional football (soccer). *Am J Sports Med.* 2011;39(6):1226-1232.
53. Ekstrand J, Hägglund M, Waldén M. Injury incidence and injury patterns in professional football: the UEFA injury study. *Br J Sports Med.* 2011;45(7):553-558.
54. Giza E, Mithöfer K, Farrell L, Zarins B, Gill T. Injuries in women's professional soccer. *Br J Sports Med.* 2005;39(4):212-216.
55. Kaeding CC, Whitehead R. Musculoskeletal injuries in adolescents. *Prim Care.* 1998;25(1):211-223.
56. Bright RW, Burstein AH, Elmore SM. Epiphyseal-plate cartilage. A biomechanical and histological analysis of failure modes. *J Bone Joint Surg.* 1974;56(4):688-703.
57a. Metaxas TI, Mandroukas A, Vamvakoudis E, Kotoglou K, Ekblom B, Mandroukas K. Muscle fiber characteristics, satellite cells and soccer performance in young athletes. *J Sports Sci Med.* 2014;13(3):493-501.
57b. Sullivan JA, Cross RH, Grana WA, Garcia-Moral CA. Evaluation of injuries in youth soccer. *Am J Sports Med.* 1980. 8(5):325-327.
58. Fridman L, Fraser-Thomas JL, McFaull SR, Macpherson AK. Epidemiology of sports-related injuries in children and youth presenting to Canadian emergency departments from 2007-2010. *BMC Sports Sci Med Rehabil.* 2013;5(1):30.
59. Public Health Agency of Canada. Investing in child and youth injury prevention in sports and recreation. Fact Sheet. 2011. http://www.phac-aspc.gc.ca/inj-bles/2012_1011-fs-fi-eng.php. Accessed November 17, 2015.
60. Clayton RA, Court-Brown CM. The epidemiology of musculoskeletal tendinous and ligamentous injuries. *Injury.* 2008;39(12):1338-1344.
61. Volpi E, Nazemi R, Fujita S. Muscle tissue changes with aging. *Curr Opin Clin Nutr Metab Care.* 2004;7(4):405-410.
62. Lehman RC. Shoulder pain in the competitive tennis player. *Clin J Sports Med.* 1988;7(2):309-327.
63. Aagaard P, Suetta C, Caserotti P, Magnusson SP, Kjaer M. Role of the nervous system in sarcopenia and muscle atrophy with aging: strength training as a countermeasure. *Scand J Med Sci Sports.* 2010;20:49-64.

64. Matheson GO, Macintyre JG, Taunton JE, Clement DB, Lloyd-Smith R. Musculoskeletal injuries associated with physical activity in older adults. *Med Sci Sports Exerc.* 1989;21(4):379-385.

65. Stevens JA, Corso PS, Finkelstein EA, Miller TR. The costs of fatal and non-fatal falls among older adults. *Inj Prev.* 2006;12(5):290-295.

66. Kallinen M, Markku A. Aging, physical activity and sports injuries. An overview of common injuries in the elderly. *Sports Med.* 1995;20(1):41-52.

67. Abrams GD, Renstrom PA, Safran MR. Epidemiology of musculoskeletal injury in the tennis player. *Br J Sports Med.* 2012;46(7):492-498.

68. Hootman JM, Macera CA, Ainsworth BE, Martin M, Addy CL, Blair SN. Association among physical activity level, cardiorespiratory fitness, and risk of musculoskeletal injury. *Am J Epidemiol.* 2001;154(3):251-258.

69. Granan LP, Inacio MC, Maletis GB, Funahashi TT, Engebretsen L. Sport-specific injury pattern recorded during anterior cruciate ligament reconstruction. *Am J Sports Med.* 2013;41(12):2814-2818.

70. Renstrom P, Ljungqvist A, Arendt E, et al. Non-contact ACL injuries in female athletes: an International Olympic Committee current concepts statement. *Br J Sports Med.* 2014;42(6):394-412.

71. Dowling AV, Corazza S, Chaudhari AM, Andriacchi TP. Shoe-surface friction influences movement strategies during a sidestep cutting task: implications for anterior cruciate ligament injury risk. *Am J Sports Med.* 2010;38(3):478-485.

72. Dowling AV, Andriacchi TP. Role of shoe-surface interaction and noncontact ACL injuries. In: Noyes FR, Barber-Westin S, eds. *ACL Injuries in the Female Athlete.* 1st ed. Berlin, Germany: Springer-Verlag; 2012:85-86.

73. Orchard J, Seward H, McGivern J, Hood S. Rainfall, evaporation, and the risk of non-contact anterior cruciate ligament injury in the Australian Football League. *Med J Aust.* 1999;170(7):304-306.

74. Orchard J, Seward H, McGivern J, Hood S. Intrinsic and extrinsic risk factors for anterior cruciate ligament injury in Australian footballers. *Am J Sports Med.* 2001;29(2):196-200.

75. Malina RM, Morano PJ, Barron M, Miller SJ, Cumming SP, Kontos AP. Incidence and player risk factors for injury in youth football. *Clin J Sport Med.* 2006;16(3):214-222.

76. Moses B, Orchard J, Orchard J. Systematic review: annual incidence of ACL injury and surgery in various populations. *Res Sports Med.* 2012;20(3-4):157-179.

77. Dick R, Agel J, Marshall SW. National collegiate athletic association surveillance system commentaries: introduction and methods. *J Athl Train.* 2007;42(2):173-182.

78. Agel J, Ransone J, Dick R, Oppliger R, Marshall SW. Descriptive epidemiology of collegiate men's wrestling injuries: National Collegiate Athletic Association Injury Surveillance System, 1988-1989 through 2003-2004. *J Athl Train.* 2007;42(2):303-310.

79. Rechel JA, Yard EE, Comstock RD. An epidemiologic comparison of high school sports injuries sustained in practice and competition. *J Athl Train.* 2008;43(2):197-204.

80. Griffin LY, Albohm MJ, Arendt EA, et al. Understanding and preventing noncontact anterior cruciate ligament injuries: a review of the Hunt Valley II meeting, January 2005. *Am J Sports Med.* 2006;34(9):1512-1532.

81. Rizzo M, Holler SB, Bassett FH III. Comparison of males' and females' ratios of anterior-cruciate-ligament width to femoral-intercondylar-notch width: a cadaveric study. *Am J Orthop (Belle Mead NJ).* 2001;30(8):660-664.

82. Sutton KM, Bullock JM. Anterior cruciate ligament rupture: differences between males and females. *J Am Acad Orthop Surg.* 2013;21(1):41-50.

83. Chandrashekar N, Mansouri H, Slauterbeck J, Hashemi J. Sex-based differences in the tensile properties of the human anterior cruciate ligament. *J Biomech.* 2006;39(16):2943-2950.

84. Stijak L, Herzog RF, Schai P. Is there an influence of the tibial slope of the lateral condyle on the ACL lesion? a case-control study. *Knee Surg Sport Traumatol Arthrosc.* 2008;16(2):112-117.

85. McDonald KM, Schultz E, Albin L, et al. *Care Coordination Measures Atlas.* Rockville, MD: Agency for Healthcare Research and Quality; 2010.

86. Shultz SJ, Schmitz RJ, Nguyen AD, et al. ACL Research Retreat V: an update on ACL injury risk and prevention, March 25-27, 2010, Greensboro, NC. *J Athl Train.* 2010;45(5):499-508.

87. Ruedl G, Ploner P, Linortner I, et al. Interaction of potential intrinsic and extrinsic risk factors in ACL injured recreational female skiers. *Int J Sports Med.* 2011;32(8):618-622.

88. Kumar GS, Klein R. Effectiveness of case management strategies in reducing emergency department visits in frequent user patient populations: a systematic review. *J Emerg Med.* 2013;44(3):717-729.

89. Malinzak RA, Colby SM, Kirkendall DT, Yu B, Garrett WE. A comparison of knee joint motion patterns between men and women in selected athletic tasks. *Clin Biomech (Bristol, Avon).* 2001;16(5):438-445.

90. Bonci CM. Assessment and evaluation of predisposing factors to anterior cruciate ligament injury. *J Athl Train.* 1999;34(2):155-164.

91. Myer G, Ford KR, Khoury J, Succop P, Hewett TE. Development and validation of a clinic-based prediction tool to identify female athletes at high risk for anterior cruciate ligament injury. *Am J Sports Med.* 2012;38(10):2025-2033.

92. Knapik JJ, Bauman CL, Jones BH, Harris JM, Vaughan L. Preseason strength and flexibility imbalances associated with athletic injuries in female collegiate athletes. *Am J Sports Med.* 1991;19(1):76-81.

93. Stevenson JH, Beattie CS, Schwartz JB, Busconi BD. Assessing the effectiveness of neuromuscular training programs in reducing the incidence of anterior cruciate ligament injuries in female athletes: a systematic review. *Am J Sports Med.* 2015;43(2):482-490.

94. Ettlinger CF, Johnson RJ, Shealy JE. A method to help reduce the risk of serious knee sprains incurred in alpine skiing. *Am J Sports Med.* 1995;23(5):531-537.

95. Tashjian RZ. Epidemiology, natural history, and indications for treatment of rotator cuff tears. *Clin Sports Med.* 2012;31(4):589-604.

96. Itoi E, Tabata S. Rotator cuff tears in the adolescent. *Orthopedics.* 1993;16(1):78-81.

97. Yamaguchi K, Ditsios K, Middleton WD, Hildebolt CF, Galatz LM, Teefey SA. The demographic and morphological features of rotator cuff disease. A comparison of asymptomatic and symptomatic shoulders. *J Bone Joint Surg Am.* 2006;88(8):1699-1704.

98. Minagawa H, Itoi E. Clinical relevance of the rotator cuff in the shoulder with pain and dysfunction [in Japanese]. *Kansetsugeka.* 2006;25:923-929.

99. Sipes R. The incidence of shoulder injury among collegiate overhead athletes. *J Intercoll Sport.* 2009;2(2):260-268.

100. Reinold MM, Gill TJ. Current concepts in the evaluation and treatment of the shoulder in overhead-throwing athletes, part 1: physical characteristics and clinical examination. *Sports Health.* 2010;2(1):39-50.

101. Prokopy MP, Ingersoll CD, Nordenschild E, Katch FI, Gaesser GA, Weltman A. Closed-kinetic chain upper-body training improves throwing performance of NCAA Division I softball players. *J Strength Cond Res.* 2008;22(6):1790-1798.

102. Reinold MM, Gill TJ, Wilk KE, Andrews JR. Current concepts in the evaluation and treatment of the shoulder in overhead throwing athletes, part 2: injury prevention and treatment. *Sports Health.* 2010;2(2):101-115.

103. Lopes AD, Hespanhol Júnior LC, Yeung SS, Costa LO. What are the main running-related musculoskeletal injuries? A systematic review. *Sports Med.* 2012;42(10):891-905.

104. Bonza JE, Fields SK, Yard EE, Dawn Comstock R. Shoulder injuries among United States high school athletes during the 2005-2006 and 2006-2007 school years. *J Athl Train.* 2009;44(1):76-83.

105. Reeser JC, Joy EA, Porucznik CA, Berg RL, Colliver EB, Willick SE. Risk factors for volleyball-related shoulder pain and dysfunction. *PM R.* 2010;2(1):27-36.

106. Mohseni-Bandpei M, Keshavarz R, Minoonejhad H, Mohsenifar H, Shakeri H. Shoulder pain in Iranian elite athletes: the prevalence and risk factors. *J Manipulative Physiol Ther.* 2012;35(7):541-548.

107. Nissen CW. Osteochondritis dissecans of the elbow. *Clin Sports Med.* 2014;33(2):251-265.

108. Agel J, Dompier TP, Dick R, Marshall SW. Descriptive epidemiology of collegiate men's ice hockey injuries: National Collegiate Athletic Association Injury Surveillance System, 1988-1989 through 2003-2004. *J Athl Train.* 2007;42(2):241-248.

109. Dick R, Lincoln AE, Agel J, Carter EA, Marshall SW, Hinton RY. Descriptive epidemiology of collegiate women's lacrosse injuries: National Collegiate Athletic Association Injury Surveillance System, 1988-1989 through 2003-2004. *J Athl Train.* 2007;42(2):262-269.

110. Agel J, Palmieri-Smith RM, Dick R, Wojtys EM, Marshall SW. Descriptive epidemiology of collegiate women's volleyball injuries: National Collegiate Athletic Association Injury Surveillance System, 1988-1989 through 2003-2004. *J Athl Train.* 2007;42(2):295-302.

111. Boden BP, Lin W, Young M, Mueller FO. Catastrophic injuries in wrestlers. *Am J Sports Med.* 2002;30(6):791-795.

Mental Health

Melanie Adams, PhD, CSCS, AT-Ret

CHAPTER OBJECTIVES

- Increase awareness of mental health as part of patient-centered health care.
- Identify signs and symptoms associated with depression, anxiety, substance abuse, and eating disorders.
- Consider the role of an athletic trainer in a comprehensive medical team that educates, recognizes, and refers athletes with psychological concerns.
- Understand how physical activity contributes to positive mental health.

INTRODUCTION

Mental health is more than the absence of a psychological concern, such as clinical depression, an eating disorder, or substance abuse. It is a state of well-being that enables people to deal with the normal stresses of life and realize their potential personally and professionally.[1] Regular physical activity promotes physical and mental health. Longitudinal cohort studies are evidence that regular exercise lessens the risk of depression, reduces stress and anxiety, and improves quality of life. The mechanisms by which physical activity affects mental health are less well understood than those discussed in Chapter 2, but it is clear that meeting the American College of Sports Medicine guideline for physical activity (at least 150 minutes/week of moderate physical activity) is as important for the brain as it is for the heart. Emotions are not separate from physiology. Feelings of stress, anger, worry, and disappointment are linked to the release of hormones and neurotransmitters that change how cells repair and replicate throughout the body.[2,3]

Participation in sports is believed to have a positive effect on the social, physical, and emotional development of young people, and dedication to one's sport is positively viewed in

Adams M, Swiger W.
Epidemiology for Athletic Trainers: Integrating Evidence-Based Practice (pp 167-203).
© 2016 Taylor & Francis Group.

our culture. Athletes, however, are not immune to psychological concerns; in some ways, sports participation exposes them to greater risks. Athletes experience stress related to time demands; performance expectations; and their relationships with parents, coaches, and teammates. Health care professionals working with athletes should be knowledgeable about mental health concerns and provide effective referrals for athletes when appropriate, according to a consensus statement developed jointly by the National Athletic Trainers' Association (NATA) and National Collegiate Athletic Association (NCAA) in 2013. This chapter reviews prevalence data of several mental health conditions in general and athletic populations and describes the risk factors, signs, and symptoms. The goal of patient-centered care is to meet the needs of the individual, which are not limited to physical injuries.

Classification of Psychological Concerns

Mental health professionals use guidelines from the American Psychiatric Association (APA) to determine the type and severity of a psychological concern. The *Diagnostic and Statistical Manual* (DSM) outlines the criteria for 16 categories of mental health concerns. This chapter reviews the 4 categories mostly like to affect athletes, including mood disorders, anxiety disorders, substance abuse, and eating disorders.

The terminology used in psychology can be confusing to lay people. *Clinical* refers to a condition that meets the DSM criteria, meaning that this is a confirmed diagnosis of a condition. A psychological concern is *subclinical* if it does not meet DSM guidelines but still presents a disruption to a patient's life. Particularly in research on depression, there is a difference between measuring symptoms and actual diagnosis of depression. Having one or more symptoms of a mental health concern does not mean that an individual can be diagnosed with such. In fact, a condition is clinically significant only if it interferes significantly with being productive in work or school and enjoyment of daily activities. Most psychological symptoms fall on a continuum in terms of severity and duration. The DSM uses the terms *mild, moderate,* or *severe* to indicate severity and in partial remission, in full remission, or prior history to describe the stage of the concern. One notable deviation from this is the term *major,* which is used to distinguish clinical depression from the less-intense chronic form.

The occurrence of mental health conditions is measured in prevalence rather than incidence. Unlike athletic injuries, which are usually short periods of disability, psychological concerns are long lasting and prone to reoccurrence. This makes the combination of newly diagnosed and ongoing cases a more accurate picture of how many people are living with a particular condition. The typical age of onset for psychological concerns ranges from adolescence to early adulthood,[4] making high school and college important years for recognition and treatment. Fewer than half of those with a mental health concern will receive treatment. Athletes seek help for psychological concerns at a lower rate, despite evidence that the prevalence is the same in athletes compared to the general population.[5] Several factors contribute to athletes underusing mental health services. One is that the sport culture values toughness. Athletes fear the perception that an emotionally based concern is a sign of weakness or think they are immune to mental health issues because of their toughness.[5] Another factor is a lack of suspicion for psychological concerns by medical staff because of bias toward physical ailments or the belief in athlete toughness.[6,7]

Mental Health Professionals

Only trained and licensed mental health professionals should evaluate and treat psychological concerns. The role of athletic trainers and team physicians is to recognize the need for a mental health referral and to facilitate that referral. Five professions provide mental health services. A psychiatrist is a licensed physician with a specialty in psychiatry and/or neurology. They diagnose disorders, prescribe medication, and may provide cognitive-behavioral therapies. Psychologists

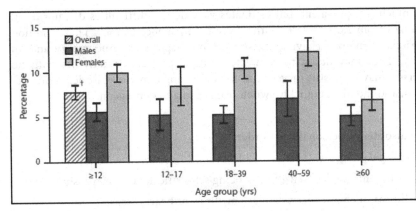

Figure 9-1. Annual prevalence of depression, 2011. (Reprinted with permission from the Centers for Disease Control and Prevention. QuickStats: prevalence of current depression among persons aged ≥12 years, by age group and sex — united states, national health and nutrition examination survey, 2007–2010. *MMWR.* 2012;60(51):1747.)

have a doctoral degree in psychology and can evaluate and treat emotional and behavioral conditions but do not prescribe medications. Clinical psychologists, in particular, use talk therapy to improve coping or change problem behaviors. Depending on their level of education (bachelor's to doctorate) and the state in which they work, psychiatric nurses or nurse practitioners provides many of the same services as a psychiatrist or psychologist. Licensed social workers with master's degrees assess mental health concerns and provide cognitive therapy in various settings. Lastly, licensed professional counselors hold a master's degree in psychology or counseling and can assess mental health concerns and provide therapy.

Prevalence in the General Population

Mental health data come from the following 3 types of reporting: self-report of symptoms or diagnosis, physician/psychologist diagnosis, or in-patient treatment records. Each method underestimates the true number of people living with a mental health concern. Many people hide or deny their psychological concerns, even on anonymous surveys, and do not seek help. This makes epidemiology and the use of mental health studies challenging. Increases and decreases in rates of disorders may be influenced by public awareness, improved detection, or access to treatment rather than actual changes in the number of people with the condition.[8]

According to the US Substance Abuse and Mental Health Services Administration's (SAMHSA) report, 43.7 million adults (18.6% of Americans ages 18 and older) reported experiencing a mental illness in 2012. Young people (aged 12 to 17 years) have a higher rate of mental health disorders, with 20% to 25% meeting diagnostic criteria.[4] Conservatively, that would mean that approximately 20% of the athletes with whom sports injury specialists work are dealing with a psychological concern. Athletes can be successful despite the diagnosis, and sports may have a positive effect on their mental health.[6]

Mood Disorders

Mood-related concerns include major depressive episodes; chronic depression, termed *dysthymia*; and bipolar disorder. Depression is more than feeling sad. Key symptoms of depression include extreme fatigue, sense of hopelessness, loss of enjoyment in pastimes, problems concentrating or making decisions, insomnia, and thoughts of suicide.[7] These are long lasting (≥ 2 weeks). Depression also frequently reoccurs. Lifetime prevalence has been reported to be 16.5%,[9] although the annual rate is 6.9% (Figure 9-1). It is twice as likely to affect women as men. Dysthymia is a less intense form that is prolonged (≥2 years) and often presents with other psychological concerns, such as anxiety or substance abuse. The APA states that the onset of depression typically happens between the ages of 20 and 30 years.

Bipolar disorder is much less prevalent, but estimates vary due to difficulties diagnosing it. Lifetime prevalence ranges from 2.6% to 7.8%, with an annual incidence of 1%.[10] This condition is recognizable by periods of manic behavior, when a person displays extreme energy and an exaggerated personality. They may desire to complete multiple projects or activities with no need for sleep. The person may be hostile or very fun loving during a manic episode. Periods of depression are also seen, and mood can quickly switch from mania to depression.

Risk Factors

- History of anxiety disorder or personality disorder
- Abuse of alcohol or illegal drugs
- Personality traits, such as having low self-esteem, being self-critical, or being pessimistic
- Serious or chronic illness, such as cancer, diabetes mellitus, or heart disease
- Traumatic or stressful events
- Family history of depression, bipolar disorder, alcoholism, or suicide

Anxiety Disorders

Feeling anxious, nervous, or worried in specific situations is a normal human experience. People living with anxiety disorders have more intense physical reactions to stressful stimuli and develop maladaptive coping strategies to ease their worries and fears. According to Merikangas et al,[4] 31% of teenagers meet the criteria for an anxiety-related condition. Psychological concerns classified as anxiety related include social phobias, panic attacks, generalized anxiety disorder (GAD), obsessive compulsive disorder (OCD), social anxiety disorder, and posttraumatic stress disorder (PTSD). Unlike situational anxiety, which everyone experiences, anxiety disorders significantly interfere with normal living. They are chronic (≥ months) and pervasive. A person may go to great lengths to avoid situations that are anxiety producing, as in a phobia, or use repetitive behaviors to cope as with OCD. The annual prevalence for all anxiety disorders combined for US adults is 18.1%.[9] As with depression, women are more at risk than men for anxiety. Social anxiety has the highest prevalence in adults (6.8%)[9] and children/adolescents (5.5%).[4] For adults, PTSD (3.5%), general anxiety (3%), and panic attacks (2.7%) are the next most common concerns.[9] In children and adolescents, they are PTSD (4%) and panic attacks (2.3%).[4]

Risk Factors

- Female
- Traumatic or stressful events
- Stress (significant life event or daily worry)
- Personality traits, such as low self-esteem, being self-critical, or being pessimistic
- Other mental health disorders
- Family history of anxiety disorder
- Abuse of alcohol or illegal drugs

Substance Abuse

The APA 2013 guidelines for substance abuse include recurrent use that fits one or more of the following qualifications: use in hazardous situations such as while driving; results in failure to meet major obligations, such as work- or school-related deadlines; recurring legal problems due to use, such as arrests or fines; or use that is continued despite ongoing social conflicts, such as arguments or fights.

Alcohol is the most commonly abused substance in the United States. The SAMHSA survey found that 23% of those surveyed (N = 68,309) age 12 years or older reported one episode of binge

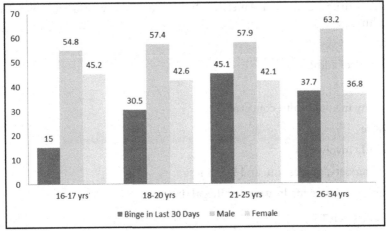

Figure 9-2. Percentage of the population that binge drank by age and gender, 2012. (Adapted from SAMHSA 2012. http://media.samhsa.gov/data/NSDUH/2012SummNatFindDetTables/NationalFindings/NSDUHresults2012.pdf.)

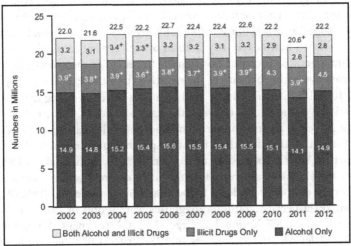

Figure 9-3. Substance abuse or dependence, 2002 to 2012. (Adapted from SAMHSA 2012. http://media.samhsa.gov/data/NSDUH/2012SummNatFindDetTables/NationalFindings/NSDUHresults2012.pdf.)

drinking in the past 30 days. Binge drinking is defined as 5 or more drinks on one occasion in the past 30 days. Heavy drinking is when there are 5 or more binge drinking episodes in the past 30 days. An estimated 6.5% of the population is heavy drinkers. The numbers of people binging or drinking heavily peaks between ages 21 and 25 years. Alcohol abuse is more common in men than in women (Figure 9-2).[11]

Other frequently abused drugs are marijuana, painkillers, cocaine, stimulants, tranquilizers, and hallucinogens. Almost 24% of those surveyed in the SAMHSA reported using an illicit drug in the past month. An illicit drug is one that is illegal to obtain or, in the case of prescription medications, is used outside of medical need. Rates of alcohol and illicit drug abuse or dependency (an increased tolerance and focus on obtaining substance) in the United States have remained fairly constant over the past 10 years at 22% (Figure 9-3). The SAMHSA report found small differences between race/ethnic groups in percentage of the population that is dependent or abusing alcohol or drugs, except for American Indians and Native Alaskans who have twice the rate of other ethnicities.

Risk Factors

- Family history of addiction
- Male
- History of any mental health concern
- Peer pressure
- Lack of family involvement
- Presence of anxiety, depression, and loneliness
- Use of highly addictive medications or illegal drugs

Eating Disorders

The APA has recently revised its diagnostic criteria for eating disorders. The changes were necessary because too many cases were categorized as eating disorders not otherwise specified (EDNOS) and did not accurately reflect how many people were struggling with anorexia nervosa, bulimia nervosa, or binge eating. Prior to revision, EDNOS was the most commonly diagnosed eating disorder. The updated DSM reduced some criteria for anorexia nervosa and bulimia nervosa and created a new category, called *binge eating*. The EDNOS category remained but is much less used than before. Table 9-1 outlines the key features of each type of eating disorder. Binge eating is distinct from bulimia because there are no attempts to get rid of the excess calories. Binge eating is also different from overeating because of the negative emotions experienced by the binge eater.

An estimated 10 million females and 1 million males have an eating disorder in the United States.[12] Nearly all are young people between the ages 12 and 26 years, with 86% reporting an onset prior to age 20 years. Depression frequently accompanies eating disorders. The mortality rates are higher for eating disorders than for other psychological concerns.[13] The prevalence of any eating disorder in Americans aged 13 to 18 years is 2.7%, with females (3.8%) being 3 times more likely than males (1.3%)[4] to self-report. Binge eating disorder is more common than anorexia and bulimia. A survey of college students found that 3% of female and 0.4% of males had been diagnosed with anorexia nervosa. Bulimia diagnoses were found in 2% of women and 0.2% of the men according to the 2007 National College Health Assessment. Napolitano and Himes[14] reported that 8.4% of female undergraduates met the criteria of binge eating disorder. Adults report a lifetime prevalence of 0.9% for anorexia nervosa, 0.6% for bulimia nervosa, and 2.8% for binge eating. Smink et al[8] found that anorexia nervosa has the highest mortality rate of all mental health conditions. Suicide occurs in 5.1/1000 cases of anorexia nervosa, and health complications from obesity combined with depression are thought to contribute to the 3.3/1000 deaths in those with EDNOS.[15]

Several studies have found that college athletes have higher rates of eating disorders than nonathletic peers[16-18] and that athletic females in particular have the greatest risk.[7] Factors related to the prevalence of eating disorders in sport along with suggestions for screening and return to play are discussed later in this chapter.

Risk Factors

- Female
- Age (preadolescent through early 20s)
- Family history of eating disorder
- Presence of mental health concern, such as depression, anxiety, or OCD
- Recent history of successful dieting

TABLE 9-1
KEY FEATURES OF EATING DISORDERS

ANOREXIA NERVOSA	BULIMIA NERVOSA	BINGE EATING DISORDER	EDNOS

• Fear of gaining weight
  ◦ Despite thin appearance
• Denial of hunger
  ◦ Rarely eats in public
• Preoccupation with food
  ◦ Counting calories
  ◦ Rituals for eating
• Extreme limits to portions
• Irritable
• Negative body image
  ◦ Talk of being overweight
• Socially withdrawn
• Flat emotions
• Complains of stomach pain
• Cold even in warm weather
  ◦ Wears bulky clothing
  ◦ Develops fine hairs on skin
• Arrhythmia and hypotension
	• Secret eating
	  ◦ Loss of control
	• Compensatory behavior after eating
	  ◦ 1 to 2 times/week
	• Spends longer than normal times in bathroom during or after meals
	• Preoccupied with weight and body shape
	• Low self-esteem
	• Normal to overweight
	• Frequently diets/fasts
	• Poor oral health
	  ◦ Frequent cavities
	  ◦ Sores, swollen gums
	• Arrhythmia
		• Secret eating
		  ◦ Large volumes
		  ◦ Eating quickly
		• No compensatory behavior
		• Feelings of guilt or depression over binge
		  ◦ Distress once a week for 3 months
		• May be normal, overweight, or obese
			• Prior to 2013
			• Similar to binge eating disorder food-related behaviors that do not met the criteria of the 3 prior conditions
			• Extreme dieting
			• Compensatory behaviors
			• Distorted body image
			• Unreasonable limits on food type or amount

TABLE 9-2
BEHAVIORS OF CONCERN FROM THE
NATA-NCAA CONSENSUS STATEMENT

- Changes in eating or sleeping habits
- Change in emotion: loss or mood swings
- Problems concentrating or focusing
- Withdrawn and uninterested
- Complaints of fatigue, illness, or injury
- Irritable or easily angered
- Complaints of gastrointestinal problems or frequent headaches
- Excessive worry or anxiety
- Drug and or alcohol abuse
- Gambling
- Fighting or legal issues
- Talk about death, dying, or going away
- Unexplained wounds (self-harm)
- Lying or lack of responsibility

Adapted from Bonci CM, Bonci LJ, Granger LR, et al. National Athletic Trainers' Association position statement: preventing, detecting, and managing disordered eating in athletes. *J Athl Train*. 2008;43(1):80-108.

- Life transitions, including moving, going to college, relationship break up
- Career or avocations, such as sports, acting, dancing, and modeling

STRESS, ANXIETY, AND DEPRESSION IN ATHLETES

Research on athletes' mental health is limited to small cross-sectional studies and case reports. Rather than being immune from psychological concerns, athletes may experience more stress than nonathletes and be predisposed to anxiety, depression, and substance abuse.[5] Athletes must meet expectations from coaches, teammates, loved ones, and fans. Student-athletes are especially stressed. At all levels, they report feeling overtaxed physically and mentally by school, training, travel, competition, and injury.[19] That type of constant overload can trigger psychological concerns. Most athletes will experience and cope with these stressors in healthy ways, but sports medicine professionals need to recognize signs and symptoms of declining mental health and provide proper referral. Table 9-2 provides a list of behaviors to watch for in student-athletes. The next section explains the impact of stress on health and is followed by a review of the types of anxiety commonly experienced by athletes and the comorbidities associated with depression.

The Stress Response

The autonomic nervous system is responsible for the cascade of hormones that create a rapid physiologic response to stress. The purpose of the stress response is to mobilize energy and prepare

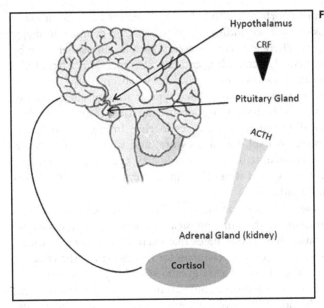

Figure 9-4. The stress response.

the body for intense physical activity ("fight or flight"). The increase in heart rate, blood pressure, breathing, circulating glucose, and mental alertness are meant to assist in winning the physical battle between you and your stressor. Unfortunately, most stress cannot be handled by hitting it or running away from it. People encounter daily stressors that are not physical threats but that create internal pressure, such as an argument or a deadline. Even a loud, hot, or crowded physical environment can spur on the stress response.

In the initial stage, the amygdala alerts the hypothalamus, and the hypothalamus activates the adrenal glands, which secrete epinephrine and norepinephrine. This step typically occurs before a person is even aware of the stressor. If this initial surge is not enough, the hypothalamus, pituitary gland, and adrenal glands, referred to as the HPA axis, keep the symptomatic nervous system turned up by releasing corticotrophin-releasing factor (CRF). CRF acts on the pituitary gland to secrete adrenocorticotropic hormone (ACTH), which then tells the adrenal gland to release cortisol into the blood stream (Figure 9-4). Cortisol is a steroid, specifically a glucocorticoid. It helps to increase glucose levels in the blood and is anti-inflammatory in the short term.

If the stressful situation is not resolved, the HPA axis continues to fuel the stress response at a lower intensity. This means that the body and brain are in a heightened physiologic state with higher-than-normal levels of circulating CRF, ACTH, and cortisol. Humans keep the HPA axis engaged by worrying or replaying stressful events in their minds.[3] Prolonged activation of the HPA axis is believed to suppress immune function, damage hippocampal neurons, and lead to dysregulation of the HPA axis. Cortisol levels are monitored by the hippocampus, hypothalamus, and pituitary gland; once a high enough level has been reached, the flow of CRF and ACTH stops. Chronic stress makes the HPA less sensitive to cortisol and lengthens the time needed to return to homeostasis. Cortisol inhibits lymphocyte function and can slow wound healing. Chronically elevated levels wear out the glucocorticoid receptors on cytokines so that inflammation is no longer held in check.[20]

Psychoneuroimmunology is the study of interconnections between the brain (neurology and neurochemistry), the mind (thoughts and emotions), and the processes of the immune and endocrine systems. Stress is so related to health that it is listed as a risk factor for cardiovascular diseases[21] and type 2 diabetes mellitus[22] and is a key component in the etiology of anxiety, depression, substance abuse, and eating disorders.[22,23] Epidemiology studies have found a history of depression to increase the risk of Alzheimer's disease.[24] The 2 are linked by neuron damage from chronic stress. Reducing stress is an important health behavior. Stressors come from many sources and range from small daily hassles, such as finding a parking spot on campus, to major life events, such as recovering from surgery. There are acute stressors, such as almost being hit by a car, and chronic stressors, such as continuously demanding courses. Stressors do not have to be negative. Even positive events, such as going on vacation or starting a new job, create the increased need for energy and focus that the stress response provides. Each type of stressor contributes to the allostatic load. Measuring the allostatic load is challenging because the stress response involves multiple body systems, including the cardiovascular, nervous, endocrine, immune, and limbic systems. Some biomarkers include salivary cortisol, blood pressure, and waist circumference. Questionnaires also attempt to quantify the volume of stress people are experiencing. Learning Activity number 2 asks you to measure your current stress through surveys on major life events and the balance between daily hassles and uplifts.

Physical activity plays an important role in reducing the effects of stress on the body. Exercise is a specific type of stress that produces many of the same physical and hormonal events as the stress response. The cross-stressor adaptation hypothesis states that exercise is a way of training the body to deal with the response.[25] A more specific mechanism for this benefit is the effect of fitness on the cortisol feedback loop. Regular exercisers have a greater sensitivity to cortisol at the hippocampus and hypothalamus so that the stress response shuts off more quickly.[26] Human and animal studies have shown a moderate reduction in signs of a stress response (increased heart rate, blood pressure, epinephrine levels) with acute bouts of exercise and chronic exercise training.[27] Animal studies have provided a neurochemical link between stress, physical activity, depression, and dementia. A consequence of increased stress hormones is a reduction in neurogenesis (new neuron growth). Rodents that are given access to running wheels had more capillaries, dendrites, new neurons, and better survival of new neurons than did the control animals.[26,28] The ability of the brain cells to regenerate and adapt is called *neuroplasticity* and is associated with improved mood, less anxiety, less depression, and reduced cognitive decline.[29] Recall from the discussion of Alzheimer's disease in Chapter 1 that brain scans showed a loss of tissue. Similar findings can be seen in those who have major depressive disorder.

Anxiety

Thoughts and emotions play a large part in the stress response, as well. The amygdala, hippocampus, and hypothalamus (Figure 9-5) are key structures of the limbic system, the seat of emotions in the brain. Concerns about important or difficult situations produce mini-stress responses. The body is preparing to meet a challenge, such as taking an examination or performing for an audience, and increases to heart rate, blood pressure, and mental alertness are helpful. We recognize these as symptoms of the specific situation and refer to them as nerves or butterflies. For most people, the sensation of being nervous dissipates quickly once the task begins. Someone with an anxiety-related psychological concern can have severe physical responses, such as dizziness, perfuse sweating, hyperventilation, and heart palpitations.[7] They do not get relief from symptoms by engaging in the task and may avoid anxiety-producing situations to prevent the overwhelming panic or fear they experience.

GAD and social anxiety are thought to be more common among athletes than social phobias or OCD,[5,30] although few studies have been conducted. Generalized anxiety is excessive worry over multiple facets of life. Sleep disruption, irritability, and muscle tension are symptoms. High levels of trait anxiety are present, and the people often view potential problems or errors as catastrophes.[7] A study of national-level athletes in France found that 6% of the sample met the diagnostic criteria for GAD. The highest rates were seen in women (39%) and athletes in aesthetic sports (17%).[30] Social anxiety has some similarities, especially in sleep disturbance, but the anxiety is specific to social situations when the person feels as though he or she is being judged. A survey of 398 college students, including 105 student-athletes, found that signs of social anxiety were

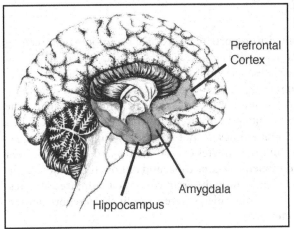

Figure 9-5. Hippocampus, amygdala, and prefrontal cortex.

SIDE BAR 9-1

State anxiety: Feelings of anxiety (nervousness, rapid heartbeat) that are specific to a situation (eg, a test); the anxiety is temporary and relieved when the threat is removed.

Trait anxiety: A more stable condition of high reactivity to stressful situations; someone with high trait anxiety experiences more frequent state anxiety. Trait anxiety is viewed as a personality characteristic.

---

more common among female athletes than all others (males and nonathletes), although clinical diagnosis levels were not different.[31]

Performance anxiety is related to GAD and social anxiety. Athletes who are extremely nervous over their performance display characteristics of GAD or social anxiety.[5,7] Those with high trait anxiety apply the same pressure-filled expectations to sport as they do to other areas of their life.[32] Those with more state anxiety are overly conscious of how others are evaluating their performance. Sport psychology has devoted much research to performance anxiety and measuring state and trait anxiety (Side Bar 9-1).[33,34]

Powell[32] estimated that 2% of the adult population suffers from debilitating performance anxiety, including college and elite athletes. Comorbidities are also present in one-third of those with performance anxiety, including GAD, social anxiety disorder, depression, and eating disorders. Higher levels of performance anxiety have been noted in female college athletes with symptoms of eating disorders.[18] Normal anxiety is temporary and manageable, meaning that it does not interfere with work, school, and social obligations. Anxiety lasting more than 6 months that interferes with daily activities should be referred, especially if the athlete tries to avoid the stressful circumstance or has constant dread of the situation.[5]

Risk Factors in Athletes

- Unrealistic performance expectations
- Recent injury, especially season or career ending
- Personality traits, such as low self-esteem, being self-critical, or being very competitive
- Individual sports in which mistakes are viewed by many (eg, diving, gymnastics, and wrestling)

Depression

Studies of depression in athletes are limited to reports of depressive symptoms or screening surveys rather than actual diagnosis of major depressive episodes or dysthymia. Yang et al[35] stated that 21% of a Division I university's student-athletes had symptoms of depression. Although greater than the 8.7% seen in adults,[36] it is similar to rates of other college students.[7,31] Women were more likely than men to report symptoms, regardless of athletic status, and freshmen appeared to be at the greatest risk for feelings of depression.[35] Injury and retirement from sport have been cited as triggers for depression in athletes,[6] but recent studies do not completely support this theory. Appaneal et al[37] tracked depression scores in injured athletes over 3 months and compared them to noninjured controls. Symptoms decreased moderately over time, and although the injured had higher scores at weeks 1 and 4, they were not significantly different from the noninjured athletes. Weigand et al[38] found that current Division I student-athletes were more likely to report signs of depression (16.8%) than former student-athletes (8%).

There is evidence that sport is protective against depression and suicide. According to Armstrong and Oomen-Early,[39] student-athletes have less risk for depression and suicide because of their higher self-esteem, greater sense of social connection, and regular exercise. Studies of high school athletes show inverse relationships between sports participation and depression and suicidal thoughts.[4] There are multiple personal, social, and biological factors interacting here. Exercise and sport participation are associated with higher self-esteem and better stress management. Social support is related to self-esteem and fewer feelings of hopelessness and loneliness. Miller and Hoffman[42] looked more closely at how one's self-identity related to depression and attempted suicide. College students who identified as athletes (focused on academic, athletic performance and teamwork) were less likely to attempt suicide and reported less depression, whereas those who identified as jocks (heavy focus on risk taking and individualism) had nearly twice the incidence of suicide attempts despite only small differences in depression.

Risk Factors

- Female
- Recent injury, especially season or career ending
- Overtraining
- Family history of depression

Comorbidities

Depression is associated with substance abuse, insomnia, and overtraining. The temporal sequence of these comorbidities is not clear. Researchers are working to understand if they are maladaptive coping mechanisms or if they contribute in part to the development of depression. For example, alcohol and drugs may be a way to self-medicate, or substance abuse may change neurotransmitters and hormones in the brain, making depression more likely.[43]

Substance Abuse

According to the 2012 SAMHSA report, adults and adolescents are more likely to abuse substances if they also experience depression. Figure 9-6 shows that 20.8% of adults who reported an episode of major depression were also substance dependent or abused substances within the past year. Only 7.9% of those reporting depression did not report abusing substances. An estimated 3.3 million adults had depression and substance abuse or dependency. Figure 9-7 illustrates the overlap in between major depression and substance abuse in youths. Youth who experienced a major depressive episode were more than 3 times as likely to have abused alcohol or drugs in the past year compared to youth without depression (16% to 5.1%).

The stress response is the neurological link between depression and substance abuse or dependency. CRF is thought to be a pathogen for depression. Reduced neurogenesis occurs during

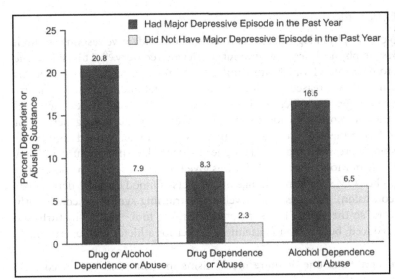

Figure 9-6. Substance abuse and dependency among adults with major depression. (SAMHSA, 2012)

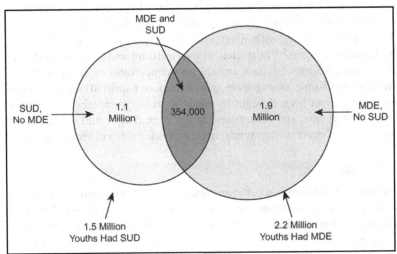

Figure 9-7. Youth depression and substance abuse/dependency. Abbreviations: MDE: major depressive episode; SUD: substance use disorder. (SAMHSA, 2012.)

periods of stress, and loss of brain plasticity is another factor in the etiology of depression.[44] Alcohol or drug use creates a different type of neuroplasticity in which structural and biochemical changes at nerve synapses make sensation seeking more ingrained.[45]

Insomnia

Changes in sleep patterns are a well-known sign of depression. Ninety percent of patients with depression complain of insomnia.[46] There is evidence that insomnia is a risk factor for depression, and its existence prior to the onset of depression has been documented in youth and young and older adults.[47] A longitudinal study of adults who were depression free at baseline found that the incidence of depression 4 years later increased linearly with the number of sleep issues that were reported and measured objectively. The relative risk of depression was 3.23 for participants that had 3 or more symptoms of insomnia.[48] This may be a contributing factor in college students because lack of sleep is an often-reported health concern. Brand et al[49] concluded that athletes have less insomnia than nonathletes and that volume of exercise predicted sleep quality.

Overtraining Syndrome

Overtraining is a neurological, physiological, and psychological maladaptive response to high volumes or high intensities of physical activity without sufficient recovery.[50] This syndrome has many signs and symptoms, some of which are similar to depression. Signs and symptoms of overtraining syndrome include decreased physical performance, fatigue, malaise, difficulty sleeping, depressed mood, changes in appetite, decreased ability to concentrate, increased irritability or anxiety, and lower motivation for sport.[50] Changes to mood during periods of overtraining have been well documented. College swimmers, for example, showed significant increases in feelings of tension, depression, anger, and fatigue during peak training volumes.[51,52] A questionnaire called the Profile of Mood States (POMS) was given to athletes prior to and during periods of intense training. The POMS measures change in 6 aspects of mood (tension, depression, anger, vigor, fatigue, and confusion). Athletes who develop overtraining syndrome consistently have higher scores than peers, so the POMS is a suggested screening tool.[53] Mood disturbance improves when training is reduced, but return to baseline is slower for athletes with overtraining syndrome.

Overtraining and depression share one or more mechanisms in their etiologies. According to Raglin and Kenttä,[53] 80% of athletes with overtraining syndrome have clinically significant depression. Changes in serotonin and cortisol are thought to impact the hypothalamus' regulation of neurotransmitters and growth factors,[50] resulting in physiologic and neurologic fatigue.

There is a tendency to diagnose athletes with overtraining and prescribe rest rather than consider depression as the broader concern.[5,6] Suspicion of overtraining and depression should be particularly high for endurance athletes because annual prevalence rates range from 7% to 21%.[53] Research on overtraining syndrome among team sport and power sport athletes is almost nonexistent, but anaerobic training has been thought to create a greater sympathetic response, leading to insomnia, increased heart rate, and restlessness rather than fatigue and depression.[50] Similar to depression, prior history of overtraining syndrome leaves one more vulnerable to future episodes.[53]

Concussion and Depression

Recent studies have examined the relationship between concussion and symptoms or diagnosis of depression. Long- and short-term associations have been documented, but the studies used self-report of concussions, depression, or both. Guskiewicz et al[54] first reported that former National Football League players with a history of 3 or more concussions were 3 times as likely to report a diagnosis of depression and that those with 1 to 2 concussions had 1.5 times the risk as those reporting no concussions. A longitudinal follow-up study 9 years later found a similar dose-response relationship, with relative risk starting at 2.3 for 1 to 2 concussions and increasing to 5.8 for 10 or more concussions.[55] A greater prevalence of depression in those with at least one previous concussion has been found in adolescents (ages 12 to 17 years).[56] Symptoms of depression and changes in mood are evident 2 to 14 days after a concussive blow,[57] but temporally, it is not clear if the depression symptoms result from concussions. Covassin et al[58] reported that athletes with higher depression scores had lower ImPACT scores and more concussion symptoms in a baseline assessment than athletes reporting less depression. These symptoms are more than the athlete feeling "down" because of his or her limited status. Studies using functional magnetic resonance imaging[59] and neurocognitive tests[57] have found a significant relationship between depression scores and changes in brain function. Also, depression symptoms are highly associated with postconcussive syndrome and may be a contributing factor for athletes whose concussion symptoms do not resolve normally.[60]

One hypothesis is that neuron loss is sped up by brain lesions caused by the metabolic insult of a concussion and increases in neurotransmitters over time wear down receptors, resulting in cell death.[61] In young, healthy athletes, neurogenesis is likely, and the symptoms of depression are temporary. However, the long-term effects of repeated concussive and subconcussive blows are just beginning to be explored. Mood and behavior disturbances years after participation in collision and contact sports may be a sign of significant structural changes in the brain.

Initially, evidence of brain damage in athletes came from boxers who took repeated blows to head. The term *punch drunk* was first used in the 1920s to describe the tremors, staggered gait, and speech difficulties seen in retired boxers. An autopsy study of a professional football player in 2005[62] opened researchers to the possibility that head trauma in other sports could permanently damage the brain. Chronic traumatic encephalopathy (CTE) is a progressive degeneration of brain tissue that affects cognition, behavior, and mood. It first presents with bouts of depression, aggression, and difficulties with memory and concentration and progresses to Parkinson-like tremors and speech and movement issues.[63] Similar to Alzheimer's disease, neurofibrillary tangles and tau proteins develop, and brain mass decreases. However, the location and pattern of these changes is distinctly different. More dense, irregular patches of tau proteins are found superficially in the frontal and temporal cortices, and atrophy is seen in the cerebral hemispheres rather than the overall decrease found in patients with Alzheimer's disease.[64] Also, less than half of CTE brains have beta amyloid plaques. Symptoms are thought to increase in number and severity with the length of playing career, number of concussion, and their severity.[63] Stern et al[64] suggested that CTE develops years after concussion symptoms have resolved and is not the continuation of postconcussion syndrome but is a separate pathology. The exact frequency and severity of the head trauma needed to start the CTE is not known but likely includes concussive and subconcussive intensities.[63,64]

SUBSTANCE ABUSE AND RISKY HEALTH BEHAVIORS IN ATHLETES

Athletes are often portrayed as models of physical strength, endurance, and health by the media. The belief that participation in sport is a natural deterrent to harmful lifestyle choices has been refuted by data showing rates of use and abuse of alcohol,[65] ergogenic substances (stimulants, steroids, nutritional supplements),[66,67] smokeless tobacco,[67,68] unplanned sex,[69] and driving while intoxicated[65] are higher among high school[68] and college student-athletes[70] than their nonathletic peers. But, athletes are less likely to smoke tobacco[68] or marijuana and use illicit drugs (methamphetamine, cocaine, ecstasy) than nonathletes.[67,71] The culture of sport may explain in part why drug use and risk taking is more prevalent in this population. Greater physical competence coupled with youthfulness lead to a strong sense of invincibility, and health risks are interpreted less seriously.[69] The work-hard, play-hard mentality may be integrated into the athletic identity.[72] Social and financial links between alcohol and sports are culturally accepted, with constant advertising during events, focus on tailgate parties, and use of alcohol to celebrate or console wins and losses. Higher rates of use among athletes also increases the social norms for drinking and drug use.[73] Athletes may also be more prone to sensation seeking, place more emphasis on the use of substances to enhance enjoyment,[70] and perceive that there is a greater expectation and acceptance of use than nonathletes.

Patterns of use are important to consider. Alcohol use may increase the risks of trying other drugs[74] and is associated with risky health behaviors and negative consequences.[75] The development and enforcement of alcohol and drug policies requires that coaches and medical staff present clear messages about expectations and consequences. A sample of policies and prevention programs is reviewed later in the chapter.

Risk Factors

- Male
- White
- Member of Greek organization
- Strongly identifies with jock image
- Family history of substance abuse
- For ergogenic substances: unrealistic performance expectations

Alcohol

Several authors have reported that a greater percentage of athletes use alcohol than their nonathletic peers and that there is a higher prevalence of binge drinking among athletes.[70,71,76] An accurate rate of alcohol use is difficult to find due to the use of self-report data, different time frames for reporting, and varied sample sizes. The most recent NCAA study in 2009 found that 83% of male and female athletes consumed alcohol in the past 12 months. However, in a systematic review in 2006, Martens et al[70] estimated the prevalence among college athletes as 80% to 87%, with 80% to 84% of nonathletes using in the past year. The NCAA report showed an increase from 2005, when 77% of student-athletes reported use. These variations suggest that social desirability and, possibly, fear of repercussions may be impacting the data, despite assurances that all responses were anonymous.

The NCAA study and those reviewed by Martens et al[70] contained large samples (N ≈ 12,000 to 51,000) but are not comparable to other large national surveys, such as the National College Health Assessment and the National Survey on Drug Use and Health, because of the different reporting time frames. The NCAA study used a 12-month time period, whereas 3 key studies[72,77,78] in the Martens et al[70] review asked for alcohol use in the past 2 weeks. The national SAMHSA and College Health surveys used past 30 days or past month for reporting and found that 60% to 65% college students are current users. Smaller studies using the 1-month time frame provide better evidence of a difference between college athletes and nonathletes. A study at a Division I institution (N = 893) found that 85% of male athletes and 77% of female athletes drank within the past month.[67] Stronger associations between sports participation and use of alcohol can be seen in middle and high school students. A large national cohort study (N = 45,000) found that eighth graders who played competitive sports were more likely to report using alcohol in the past month than nonathletes.[79]

Differences between athletes and nonathletes are seen in rates of binge drinking. Team sports participation was strongly related to binge drinking in high school students compared to those playing individual sports or exercising.[79] In a large study by Nelson and Wechsler,[77] college athletes were 42% more likely than nonathletes to engage in binge drinking in the past 2 weeks. Male athletes had the largest gap in prevalence (58% to 49%) compared to nonathletic males, but female athletes also had a significantly higher rate of binge drinking than nonathletic females (48% to 40%). A similar pattern was seen by Yusko et al,[67] who reported that male athletic binge drinkers (71%) significantly outnumbered male nonathletes (59%) and all females (48%). Time of year or in-/off-season differences may impact reporting because there were no differences when participants were asked about use over 12 months. Student-athletes were more likely to report using alcohol to excess when drinking and drinking for the purpose of becoming intoxicated than nonathletes.[77] Data also show a concentrated pattern of use on Fridays and Saturdays for athletes, particularly males.[80]

Risk factors for binge drinking among all college students are being male, White, and a member of a Greek organization.[70] The deeper one's involvement in athletics, the higher the risk for excessive use. Team leaders reported the highest number of drinks per week compared to team members and nonathletes.[72] They also drank more per week than leaders in other campus organizations. Students with high school and college sports experience were more likely to binge drink than high school athletes and those with no scholastic sports experience. According to Hildebrand et al,[4] those with at least high school sports experience drank at nearly twice the rate as nonathletes. This finding is supported by others,[73,76] who found that identifying as an athlete and the belief that alcohol consumption was part of being an athlete were predictive of binge drinking.[76] There is less prevalence of binge drinking among Blacks and other minority athletes, and although female athletes drank more than their nonathlete peers, their rates of binge drinking are lower than nonathlete males.[73,76]

Differences in alcohol use between scholarship and nonscholarship athletes and between sports have been found. According to the NCAA, slightly more Division III athletes (85.3%) report using alcohol than Division I athletes (81.7%). Men's ice hockey and lacrosse had the highest prevalence with 95%, followed by golf (90%) and baseball (88%). For women, field hockey (94.2%), golf (89.9%), and softball (88%) were the sports with the most users. Men's and women's track athletes had the lowest prevalence at 69.8% and 68.8%, respectively.

The reasons behind the greater prevalence of drinking in athletes has been well studied but without definitive results. Motives for alcohol use include social enhancement, positive reinforcement from peers, and coping with stress. In addition, exaggerated perceptions exist among student-athletes as to what normal drinking is.[80] Martens et al[81] found that using alcohol as a coping mechanism was more strongly related to experiencing negative consequences (ie, fights, team punishments, legal problems, and unplanned sex) than it was to binge drinking or alcohol use. Athletic trainers should have a heightened concern for students who express needing alcohol to cope with stress.

Tobacco and Marijuana

The negative effect of smoking on athletic performance, particularly for aerobic athletes, likely explains the lower prevalence of cigarette and marijuana use. The inflammatory response to smoke reduces respiratory function, thus lowering cardiac output. Comparisons between athletes and nonathletes are complicated by the time intervals used to collect self-report data. The SAMHSA and College Health surveys show that between 14% and 21% of full-time students smoked cigarettes in the past 30 days. Meanwhile, the NCAA reported an annual prevalence of 15.5% among athletes. Almost 23% of college athletes used marijuana in the past year compared to the monthly rate of 18.3% in all college students. The use of smokeless tobacco products (dip, snuff, chew) is greater in athletes than nonathletes. Male athletes, in particular, are more likely to use smokeless tobacco products than their peers. Yusko et al[67] found that 32% of male college athletes had used smokeless tobacco in the past year compared to 6% of nonathletic males and 3.8% of female athletes. The NCAA study reports a slightly lower usage of 27% in males and 2.7% in females for the banned substance. Roughly 50% of college ice hockey athletes, baseball players, and wrestlers reported using. In terms of race, Black athletes have the lowest prevalence (4.7%), whereas Native Americans (24.5%) and Whites (20%) have the highest numbers of users. Studies of smokeless tobacco use in high school athletes are limited. A review by Diehl et al[68] estimated that 26% of high school athletes had used smokeless tobacco at some point in their life.

Marijuana use among athletes is high considering the consequences to eligibility.[82] The potential scholarship loss may account for lower rates of use in Divisions I and II. Twenty-eight percent of Division III athletes reported using marijuana in 2009 compared to 17% (D1) and 21% (D2). Males were more likely use marijuana in the past year than females.[67] According to the NCAA, few racial and sport differences were found among marijuana users. Prevalence was highest among men's lacrosse (48.5%) and women's field hockey (35.7%) players. Few studies are specific to marijuana use in high school athletes. Terry-McElrath et al[79] estimated that as many as 56% of high school

TABLE 9-3 ERGOGENIC DRUG USE BY NCAA STUDENT-ATHLETES IN 2009						
		BY DIVISION			BY GENDER	
	Overall	I	II	III	Male	Female
Amphetamines	3.7%	3.7%	3.2%	4.1%	4%	3.3%
Anabolic steroids	.4%	.4%	.4%	.5%	.5%	.2%
Ephedrine	.9%	1.1%	.9%	.9%	.9%	.9%

students have tried marijuana but that athletic participation lowers the risk of use. Reasons for use and risk factors appear to be similar for athletes and nonathletes. Buckman et al[82] found that ratings of social enhancement and sensation seeking were higher in college athlete users. Prior history of cigarette smoking was consistently reported by athletes and nonathletes. Odds ratios for cigarette smoking were 7.15 for men and 3.63 for women.

Ergogenic Substances

Substances that could improve physical performance or aid in the recovery from exercise are known as ergogenic. These include anabolic-androgenic steroids, growth and insulin hormones, blood transfusions, stimulants (amphetamines, ephedrine), and nutritional supplements (creatine, amino acids, and vitamins) that claim muscle development or energy production. Not all ergogenic aids are completely banned by sport. Caffeine, for example, is permitted below a threshold even though performance benefits are gained at lower levels.[83] Many substances that are purported to enhance performance lack scientific evidence, such as injections of vitamin B. What was once thought only to be a problem at the highest level of sport (professionals and olympians) has trickled down to high school and youth levels. A study of Minnesota middle and high school students found that 5.2% of males and 3.3% of females report use of steroids at some point in their lives.[84] Athletes are at a higher risk for using ergogenic aids than the general population due to the competitive environment. What has surprised researchers in the past decade are the numbers of recreational and fitness participants that use. Yusko et al[67] reported that 3.9% of nonathletic college males took a known banned ergogenic substance in the past year. Use among females not involved in sports is also high. Elliot et al[85] saw a significantly higher percentage of steroid use among nonathletes (62%) compared to team sport participants (38%) in a large sample of female high schools students.

The most recent NCAA study found that approximately 5% of athletes had taken a banned ergogenic aid in the past year. Amphetamines were the most widely used substance, with 3.7% reporting use. Only 0.4% of athletes admitted to using steroids, and 0.9% reported taking ephedrine. These rates are down from 2005 when 4.2% used amphetamines and 1.1% reported taking steroids. Division III athletes reported slightly higher use of amphetamines and steroids than Division I and II athletes (Table 9-3). More males used amphetamines and steroids than females, but use of ephedrine was the same for both genders (see Table 9-3). Athletes from the Pacific Islands were twice as likely to report amphetamine (8.2%) and ephedrine (2.3%) use as Whites, and athletes of Asian descent reported the highest prevalence of steroid use at 1%. Men's sports with the highest use of amphetamines were lacrosse (12.2%) and ice hockey (6.9%). Steroid use had decreased from 2.4% among football players in 2005 to 0.8% in 2009. Baseball and wrestling athletes also reported less use, decreasing from 2.1% to 0.6% and 0%. Targeted interventions, such as drug education and testing programs, may account for the improvement. Currently, men's lacrosse has the highest rate of steroid use at 1.5%. Among women's teams, lacrosse athletes report the greatest prevalence of amphetamines (9.7%), followed by field hockey (5.9%) and softball (5.2%). Steroid use ranged from 0% in field hockey and golf to 0.4% in swimming.

Long-term effects of these substances have not been well documented, and knowledge of how they might affect young people over time is particularly lacking. Potential consequences of steroid use include dyslipidemia, cardiomyopathy, thrombosis, acne, baldness, depression, and some cancers.[86] The risk of cardiac arrest and heatstroke is increased in athletes abusing stimulants.[87] Products that contain multiple stimulants, or stacks, are widely available on the Internet. Because they are sold as nutritional supplements, manufacturers do not have to follow federal guidelines for label or quality assurance. Young, healthy athletes often rationalize their use as normal for their sport and assume that because the products are openly sold that they are safe.

Risky Health Behaviors

Athletes are often make headlines because of poor choices they made, usually under the influence of alcohol or other drugs. Although the public expresses disappointment with the athlete, the culture of sport encourages athletes to take more risks and normalizes the behavior. According to Martens et al,[70] 46% of college athletes have regretted actions they took while intoxicated compared with 33% of nonathletes. In addition, more athletes report interactions (arrests, citations, warnings) with police while drinking than nonathletes. The higher prevalence of alcohol use and abuse by athletes compared to their nonathletic peers puts them at higher risks for behaviors associated with alcohol use, such as use of other drugs,[74] driving under the influence,[65] and unprotected sex.[69] Also, injuries that are sport-related[70] and from falls and physical altercations occur more often[80] in athletes who are using alcohol or drugs.

Users of illicit drugs and banned substances also abuse alcohol, leading to the hypothesis that alcohol is a gateway drug.[74] Alcohol use in the early teenage years is a risk factor for marijuana, heroin, and cocaine use.[88] Studies of athletes add support to the gateway concept. Marijuana use is linked to binge drinking in college athletes and nonathletes.[4] Athletes who report using steroids were also heavy users of alcohol, marijuana, and tobacco compared to nonsteroid users.[85,90]

Thirty-one percent of motor vehicle deaths are due to accidents involving an alcohol-impaired driver.[91] Combine that statistic with the fact that motor vehicle crashes are the leading cause of death for Americans aged 14 to 24 years, and you can understand why driving while impaired (DWI) prevention programs target 15 to 30 year olds. Twenty-nine percent of college students reported DWI in the past year,[92] whereas 13% of 11th graders had driven under the influence and 24% had ridden with a driver who was impaired in the past 30 days.[93] Risk factors for DWI include being male,[94] intoxication before age 19,[94] and prior experience riding with an intoxicated driver.[95] Studies of athletes and impaired driving are limited. Hildebrand et al[65] asked high school and college athletes if they never, sometimes, or weekly engaged in DWI. A staggering 49% and 62.9% said they sometimes drove after drinking, respectively, and 8.8% and 9.9% of participants had driven impaired in the past week. A significantly higher proportion of nonathletes (50.6%) reported never DWI vs 42.2% and 27.2% of high school and college athletes. Only 6.6% of nonathletes had driven impaired in the past week. Nelson and Wechsler[77] also found that college athletes were more likely to drive after drinking than their peers but by a smaller margin.

Unprotected sex and having multiple sexual partners are risk factors for sexually transmitted infections (STIs). STIs are spread through direct contact with genitals, semen, or vaginal secretions and include herpes, chlamydia, gonorrhea, human papillomavirus, syphilis, and HIV. The Centers for Disease Control and Prevention estimates that 110 million Americans have a new or ongoing STI. Half of all new infections occur in young people aged 15 to 24 years.[96] Unprotected sex and multiple partners are related to alcohol use, especially episodes of heavy drinking. A meta-analysis by Rehm et al[97] found that intentions to have unsafe sex increased linearly with blood alcohol levels. No differences were seen between men and women in this study, but studies of student-athletes have reported gender differences. Overall, college male athletes reported riskier sexual behavior than female athletes. However, when binge drinking is involved, women are more than twice as likely to engage in unprotected or casual sex (odds ratio [OR] = 2.8) as men (OR = 1.37).[98] As seen with DWI, precollege experiences with alcohol and sex may be key risk factors. Hingson et al[99] found that college students who reported being drunk before age 13 were twice as likely as those who 19 years or older to have unplanned or unprotected sex. Specifically in male athletes, a history of binge drinking and sex while intoxicated in high school had been associated with more sexual partners and a greater likelihood of engaging in unprotected sex in college.[100]

Prevention Programs

Athletic trainers are often called on to participate in substance abuse education and policy making at high school and college levels. Guidelines for these programs come from governing bodies, such as the NCAA, state high school athletic associations, or boards of education. Typically, a combination of drug testing and educational elements is aimed at preventing the use of recreational drugs and ergogenic aids. Unfortunately, few studies have examined the effectiveness of drug testing, prevention programs, or both.

The purpose of drug testing amateur athletes, according to the International Olympic Committee and the NCAA, is to protect the health of athletes and the ethics and fairness of the sport. Athletes have largely accepted the culture of drug testing. The most recent NCAA survey found that 58.8% of participants agreed that the NCAA should conduct drug tests. Since 2006 when the New Jersey State Interscholastic Athletic Association became the first to conduct regular drug tests, high school athletes are increasingly screened for alcohol, marijuana, and ergogenic drugs. Terry-McElrath et al[101] reported that 11% of a nationally represented sample of high school students attend schools that randomly drug test athletes.

Two quality studies have examined the effectiveness of drug testing programs on deterring substance use. The first conducted by Goldberg et al[102] compared the past month's and past year's usage of alcohol, marijuana, cocaine, amphetamines, opiates, barbiturates, lysergic acid diethylamide, and anabolic-androgenic steroids between athletes enrolled at high schools with drug testing programs (N = 653) and athletes who attended high schools without testing programs (N = 743). Student-athletes self-reported drug use and attitudes about drug use 5 times over 2 years. Results were mixed. No difference in the past month's use of any substances was found. However, there was a significant reduction in past year's use for alcohol and illicit drugs in the students at the drug testing schools. Steroid use was unchanged by the drug testing program.[102] A longer prospective study of high school students (N = 173,000) determined the OR for past month's use of marijuana and any other drug under specific drug testing protocols (no testing, random, or for-cause) and among specific groups (athletes, general students, and nonathletic extracurricular activities). Alcohol and steroids were not included in this study. Random drug testing for general students and targeted groups, such as athletes, lowered the risk of marijuana use (OR = 0.85, all students; 0.76, athletes) but was associated with a slightly higher risk of other illicit drugs (OR = 1.11, all students; OR = 1.19, athletes).[101] Athletes also have mixed feelings on the efficacy of drug testing to prevent abuse. Only 22% of college athletes strongly agreed that drug testing by the NCAA was a deterrent to substance use, and fear of drug testing was cited by a small percentage of athletes as the main reason for not using (0.6% for alcohol, 4% for steroids, 2.6% for ephedrine, and 10% for marijuana).

Substance abuse educational programs take multiple forms, and programs often combine strategies for behavior change and negative consequences. The NCAA requires that student-athletes be informed about banned substances and the penalties for a negative drug test. Approximately 90% of Division I and 60% of Division II and III schools provide more in-depth educational programs. The content of these programs varies greatly. Most use some mix of the following: basic knowledge of drugs and consequences, adjusting perceptions of social norms, alternative decision making, expectations for prosocial behavior, stress management, and development of self-esteem.[103] Few schools collect outcome data, and because content and participation shifts from year to year, it is difficult to evaluate the effectiveness of these programs. One method that is supported by research is the use of social norming to reduce alcohol abuse. Athletes, in particular, overestimate how much and how many of their peers are drinking. Perkins and Craig[104] found that an ongoing media campaign of social norming reduced athlete misperceptions about alcohol consumption, self-reported alcohol use, and consequences from heavy drinking to about 30% in a sample of Division III athletes.

Two programs that target ergogenic aids in high school athletes also have reported positive results. The Athletes Training and Learning to Avoid Steroids (ATLAS) and Athletes Targeting Healthy Exercise and Nutrition Alternatives (ATHENA) interventions promote improved sports performance through healthy training, sound nutrition, and avoidance of alcohol and drugs. The intervention is conducted with individual teams and stresses interaction between teammates as they examine peer norms and decision making. A large study of ATLAS participants found that risk factors for use (belief of harm and ability to turn down drugs) and reported use (alcohol, marijuana, steroids, and nutritional supplements) were lower than controls immediately after and 1 year later.[105] Results from a study of ATHENA participants showed similar positive outcomes for refraining from stimulants, body image, use of seatbelts, refusal skills, and intentions to use diet pills or vomit for weight loss.[105]

Although the evidence is lacking, drug testing and drug education programs are commonplace in high school and college athletic departments. Policies regarding banned substances, including alcohol for minors, testing and sanctions, should be in writing and given to students each year. Coaches and athletic staff must also be knowledgeable about the policy, identify students who are at risk, and participate in educational programs.

EATING DISORDERS IN ATHLETES

Athletes' bodies are displayed and focused on intently in sport. Their physical attributes are critiqued and measured because characteristics such as height, weight, and lean body mass are integral to success. Some sports require tight-fitting or revealing uniforms, which may increase the attention paid to their physique. Despite these pressures, high school and college athletes are less likely to report symptoms of eating disorders than nonathletes.[17,106] Eating disorders are particularly challenging to identify and treat. Athletic trainers are in a position to notice signs of disordered eating. Types of eating disorders, their risk factors, and prevalence are discussed here. In 2008, NATA recommended that guidelines for referring athletes with eating and body image concerns should be in place just as other medical referrals are.

The latest DSM provides criteria for the following 3 types of eating disorders: binge eating disorder, anorexia nervosa, and bulimia nervosa. Binge eating disorder is characterized by recurring episodes of high-volume eating and experiencing negative feelings of self-disgust, guilt, and embarrassment. Often, the binges occur in private and are not initiated by hunger. This is not overeating, but a regular pattern of consumption (1 time/week for 3 months) and loss of control. The key features of anorexia nervosa include a fear of becoming fat and a distorted sense of body image leading the person to lose weight. The clinical diagnosis is weight based and occurs when someone weighs less than 85% of their expected weight based on height.[10] Bulimia nervosa is described as frequent bouts of binge eating followed by vomiting or other methods to reduce weight gain, such as laxatives or excessive exercise. The diagnostic criteria for bulimia nervosa is binge and purge behaviors occurring once a week over 3 months. Eating disorders develop over time. Individuals often begin with healthy weight loss that increases to deeper restrictive or purging behaviors. Focus on food and weight intensifies. Fear of weight gain, feelings of guilt, and loss of control manifest until the person reaches the criteria for an eating disorder.[16] The Disordered Eating Continuum illustrates this progression (Figure 9-8).

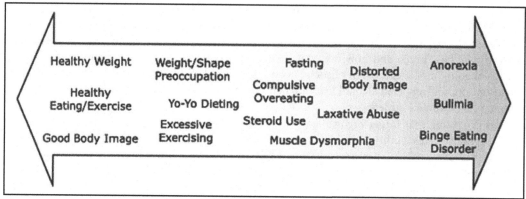

Figure 9-8. Disordered eating continuum.

Prevalence

As with other psychological concerns, finding exact numbers of athletes who live with eating disorders is difficult due to the multiple ways in which eating disorders are measured. There are data for self-reported symptoms and prior diagnosis of eating disorders, but few studies used actual medical records. Too often, researchers use different self-report questionnaires, including unvalidated ones, making comparisons between studies difficult. In addition, the new DSM standards for anorexia nervosa and bulimia nervosa are less stringent than before, meaning that higher rates of both conditions should be expected. The addition of binge eating disorder will also impact epidemiology data. It is not clear yet if the prevalence of binge eating is similar to that of EDNOS or if there will be cases that do not fit any of the 3 categories. Most of the prominent literature on eating disorders in athletes was published prior to 2013 and will have to be updated to match new clinical standards. The data presented here predate the newer standards. The discussion here begins with the overall lifetime prevalence, then considers college and high school students, and finally athletes.

Nationwide, the lifetime prevalence of anorexia nervosa in the United States is 0.9% for women, 0.3% for males,[11] and 0.3% for adolescent males and females.[107] Lifetime prevalence of bulimia nervosa has been reported to range between 0.9% and 1.5% in women and between 0.1% and 0.5% among men.[11] Bulimia nervosa appears to be more prevalent among Latinos (2%) and Blacks (1.3%) than non-Latino Whites (0.5%).[108] Among adolescents, lifetime prevalence was 1.3% for girls and 0.5% for boys.[107] The prevalence of EDNOS was higher in all age groups. Adult women had a lifetime prevalence of 3.5%. Male prevalence was 2% in the same study. Of adolescents, 2.3% of females and 0.8% of males reported a history of EDNOS.[11] Hudson et al[11] projected the lifetime prevalence of binge eating disorder from these EDNOS data and reported an increase between 0.1% and 3.6% for women and 2.1% for men.[11]

Prevalence data for the most at-risk age group (14 to 25 year olds) is usually collected as point-prevalence, meaning that the conditions are current (within 1 to 6 months). As with the national data, EDNOS or subclinical behaviors, such as vomiting and laxative use, were more common than actual diagnoses of eating disorders in college-aged adults. The College Health Assessment for 2007 found that 3% of females and 0.4% of males reported current anorexia nervosa. Bulimia nervosa was less common, with 2% of women and 0.2% of men reporting it. But, 4% and 1%, respectively, had used some compensatory behavior in the past 30 days. In a study on adolescents, Allen et al[109] followed participants aged 14 to 20 years to assess the prevalence of eating disorders using the new DSM standards and to track changes in the prevalence over time. At each age, the percentage affected was higher for females than males (Table 9-4). Bulimia nervosa was the most common type of eating disorder among females, regardless of age. Males also had the highest rates

TABLE 9-4
PREVALENCE OF EATING DISORDER SYMPTOMS BY AGE[109]

Eating Disorder	MALE			FEMALE		
	14 yrs	17 yrs	20 yrs	14 yrs	17 yrs	20 yrs
Anorexia nervosa	0%	0%	0%	.3%	1.4%	.6%
Bulimia nervosa	.4%	.7%	1.6%	2.7%	8.7%	7.9%
Binge eating disorder	0%	1.2%	.7%	1.8%	1.4%	4.15
Any	1.2%	2.6%	2.9%	8.5%	15.2%	15.2%

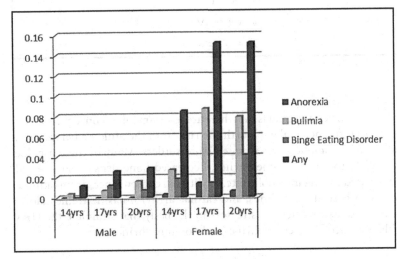

Figure 9-9. Change in eating disorder symptoms from 14 to 20 years of age. (Adapted from Allen KL, Byrne SM, Oddy WH, Crosby RD. DSM–IV–TR and DSM-5 eating disorders in adolescents: prevalence, stability, and psychosocial correlates in a population-based sample of male and female adolescents. *J Abnorm Psychol.* 2013;122[3]:720-732.)

of bulimia nervosa at ages 14 and 20, but at age, 17 binge eating disorder was the most prevalent. The rates of any eating disorder doubled between ages 14 and 17 and remained stable at age 20 (Figure 9-9).

Considerable research has compared the rates of eating disorders between athletes and nonathletes. Some found that athletes are more at risk than nonathletes,[18,110] and others concluded that there is no difference between the groups[17,106] or that nonathletes had greater symptoms.[111] The term *disordered eating* is often used when studying athletic populations. Disordered eating refers to a behavior pattern that is below the criteria for an eating disorder and represents a subclinical level of the disease. DiPasquale and Petrie[17] reported that athletes may experience disordered eating more than nonathletes. The risk is greater for females, especially those in aesthetic sports (gymnastics, cheerleading, diving) and those participating in track, cross-country, swimming, or ballet.[112]

Melin et al[113] estimated that 18% to 45% of female athletes and 0% to 28% of male athletes suffer from disordered eating or an eating disorder. The prevalence of eating disorders increases with the level of competition. At the olympic and professional level, as many as 20% of female athletes and 8% of male athletes are thought to have a diagnosable eating disorder compared with 9% and 0.5% of nonathletes, respectively.[114] Among US college athletes, the reported prevalence of diagnosable eating disorders ranges from 2% to 5.7% in women[115] and 0% to 1% in men.[116] Subclinical levels are found in 18.3% to 25.5% of female athletes and 16.6% to 19.2% of male athletes. Binge eating accounts for a large percentage of the disordered eating, with 6.2% to 16.2% of college female athletes and 4.8% to 12.6% of male college athletes reporting binges.[117,118]

TABLE 9-5
POTENTIAL HEALTH CONSEQUENCES OF EATING DISORDERS

• Dehydration	• Constipation
• Osteopenia, osteoporosis	• Abdominal pain
• Menstrual dysfunction in women	• Ruptures of esophageal or gastric lining
• Decreased testosterone in men	
• Delayed puberty	• Muscle cramps
• Bradycardia	• Tooth decay
• Hypotension	• Short stature
• Arrhythmia	• Obesity
	• Depression

Potential Health Consequences

One reason eating disorders are difficult to treat is that there are few immediate consequences.[113] In addition, improvements in performance make it worth the risk from the athlete's perspective. Table 9-5 lists the potential medical complications from eating disorders. Many of these are due to chronically low energy availability, such as amenorrhea, decreased bone density, suppressed hormone production, and decreased resting metabolic rate. Additional consequences from bulimia nervisa include dehydration, acid-base abnormalities, and cardiac arrhythmias. Extreme calorie restriction, repeated vomiting, and laxative use are stressors to the body that stimulate the HPA axis and increases the circulation of cortisol, epinephrine, and norepinephrine.[113]

Risk Factors

Eating disorder research is lacking in long-term prospective studies, which are key to establishing risk factors. Most research relies on scores from eating attitudes and behavior surveys to determine clinical and subclinical levels of eating disorders. The true incidence of eating disorders is not often measured. The available evidence suggests that eating disorders have multiple associations. Personal characteristics, such as perfectionism, may be predisposing, whereas others factors, such as competitive pressure or injury, may act as triggers or perpetuate the behavior.[119,120] Female athletes are more at risk than male athletes, and the risk is higher in some sports than others. Also, eating disorders are more prevalent at higher levels of competition.[110,114] Table 9-6 summarizes the risk factors currently being studied by researchers.

Schaal et al[30] reported that endurance sports and aesthetic sports had the highest prevalence of eating disorders for women, whereas sports with weight classes have the greatest risk for male athletes.[30] However, this distinction may not apply to adolescents, for whom few sport-specific differences have been reported.[121] The gender difference is more than just sport related. Eating disorders manifest differently in men and women. Anorexia nervosa is much less common in males than females. Male athletes suffering from eating disorders are striving to gain muscle mass and may view themselves as undersized even when they are not.[16] This is known as muscle dysmorphia. Female athletes have a drive for thinness and view themselves as overweight even when they are underweight (Side Bar 9-2).[17]

Aspects of an athlete's personality may place them at a higher risk for an eating disorder. Predisposing factors, such as a high achievement orientation, obsessive compulsive traits, body dissatisfaction, and perfectionism, have been proposed links to disordered eating. The combination

TABLE 9-6
POSSIBLE EATING DISORDER RISK FACTORS FOR ATHLETES

- Body dissatisfaction
- Parental or coach influence
- Perfectionism
- Performance anxiety
- Type of uniform
- Belief that thinness increases performance
- Sports with weight classes

- History of dieting
- History of abuse or trauma
- Exercise addiction
- Aesthetic sport
- Endurance sport
- Peer pressure
- Early specialization

SIDE BAR 9-2

ENDURANCE SPORTS	AESTHETIC SPORTS	WEIGHT CLASS SPORTS
• Cycling	• Ballet/dance	• Boxing
• Crew	• Diving	• Judo/martial arts
• Triathlon	• Equestrian	• Olympic lifting
• Swimming	• Gymnastics	• Power lifting
• XC running	• Cheerleading	• Wrestling
• XC skiing	• Figure skating	

of perfectionism and body dissatisfaction has been associated with symptoms of eating disorders in adolescent females. The evidence in athletes is limited, but some cross-sectional studies have shown moderate to strong associations between perfectionism and body dissatisfaction[122] and between perfectionism and risk for eating disorders.[123]

The presence of a predisposing factor is not enough to initiate an eating disorder. Often, an event triggers an athlete's experimentation with behaviors such as fasting, vomiting, or laxative use. That event could be a negative comment from a coach, parent, or teammate or perceived pressure to improve performance. Coaches that focus heavily on leanness as a way to increase ability and closely monitor their athletes' weights may push a susceptible athlete toward disordered eating unknowingly.[119] Krentz et al[120] found that desire for leanness to improve performance was predictive of disordered eating in youth participating in gymnastics, figure skating, diving, and ballet. Injury may be another contributing factor. Athletes who have long recovery periods may gain weight or lose muscle mass while away from training. The desire to make a quick return to sport could spur an athlete to use unhealthy dieting or purging behaviors.

The sport itself may perpetuate disordered eating. Sports that are judged in part based on the physique of the athlete or are meant to be visually pleasing can be categorized as aesthetic sports. Body size and proportion may be important in the skills of the sport, such as in gymnastics where the ability to generate rotational force increases with smaller frames and greater muscle mass. Krentz and Warschburger[124] found that adolescents in aesthetic sports had more symptoms of disordered eating than age-matched adolescents who played ball sports. Other sports in which athletes compete in weight classes are also concerning. Wresting and weight lifting emphasize power in the smallest body possible to gain a competitive advantage. Eating disorders in male athletes are most likely to occur in the sports of wrestling, crew, and track.[30,106] Recent changes to weigh-in rules in wrestling appeared to decrease the practice of weight cutting in NCAA Division I athletes.[125]

Early specialization in aesthetic or weight class sports may leave young athletes at a disadvantage if they grow out of the physical characteristics key to those sports.[114,119] Efforts to resist puberty-induced growth spurts may lead an athlete to restrictive dieting. Intense training is known to slow the onset of puberty in females. Puberty marks a critical change in how adolescents view their bodies. Postpubescent females had greater body dissatisfaction and restricted between-meal eating than those who were prepubescent, and postpubescent males reported more desire to increase muscle and lose weight than prepubescent males.[126] The potential loss of a sport they have been involved with from an early age is an additional threat during an important stage of physical and emotional growth.

Higher levels of competition are thought to increase the prevalence of eating disorders. However, direct comparisons between high school, college, and elite athletes are lacking. There is evidence that adolescents and adults who compete at elite levels in Norway (regional or national teams) have higher rates of eating disorders than their nonathlete peers.[110,114] Prevalence among elite adolescents was reported as 7% vs 2.3% of adolescent nonathletes.[110] Sundgot-Borgen and Torstveit[114] found even great rates of eating disorders in the adult elites (13.5%) with a slightly higher prevalence in nonathletes (4.6%). A comparison of risk factors between elite and nonelite adolescent athletes found that elite females had significantly higher risk than nonelite females, but no differences existed between male athletes.[4] Several studies of specific sports show high rates of eating disorders among elite athletes in the United States, but these did not compare prevalence directly to other levels of participation.[123,128]

Screening and Referral

All concerns, comments, or observations regarding an athlete's diet or weight must be taken seriously. Athletes with eating disorders rarely self-report, but their behavior and anxiety about food and weight are likely to be noticed by coaches and teammates who notify the athletic trainer. Athletic trainers play key roles in preventing, identifying, and referring those with eating disorders.

Several questionnaires are used in research and by clinical psychologists to assess someone's risk for disordered eating, including surveys specifically for athletes (Table 9-7). Unfortunately, most are copyrighted and are not widely available. The Female Athletic Screening Test is one of few free surveys. The 2008 NATA position statement cautioned against using questionnaires as the primary tool to identify at-risk athletes. Screening for eating disorders should be incorporated into the preparticipation examination and include an assessment of body composition and changes in weight, history of injuries, review of menstrual cycles in women, and questions about food intake, dieting, and use of laxatives or other purging behaviors. A less than optimal medical history combined with reports or observed behaviors are signals to intervene.

A well-defined protocol should be established and reviewed by the medical team (team physician, athletic trainers, mental health professional, and dietician). The initial step in the referral process is to meet individually with the athlete and explain the concerns and any physical results that are indicative. Confidentiality is essential to building the trust of the athlete who will be defensive. The athlete should then follow-up with a physician or mental health professional with training in eating disorders. If an eating disorder is confirmed, a course of treatment will be prescribed by the specialist. This may range from weekly meetings with a counselor and continued sports participation or an inpatient treatment program with limits on physical activity. Athletic trainers must stay within their scope of practice and not take on the role of counselor. They may provide support and help the athlete advocate for themselves during the referral and treatment process.

TABLE 9-7	
EATING DISORDER SCREENING SURVEYS FROM THE NATA POSITION STATEMENT	
Survey of Eating Disorders among Athletes	33 items to identify abnormal eating behaviors and underlying factors, such as belief that thinness is required for sport
Athletic Milieu Direct Questionnaire	19 items to identify eating disorders and disordered eating, validated in a study of Division I female athletes
Female Athlete Screening Tool	33 items that examine atypical exercise and eating behaviors http://www.watainc.org/uploads/pdfs/Annual%20 Meeting/2013_Annual_Meeting/Foos%20-%20Female%20 Athlete%20Screening%20Tool.pdf
College Health Related Information Survey	32 items groups into 4 areas: mental health problems, eating problems, risk behaviors, and performance pressure; appropriate for both genders
Physiologic Screening Test	4 self-report items combined with 4 physiologic measures; based on the presence of changes to physical health rather than eating behaviors www.acsmstore.org/ProductDetails. asp?ProductCode=9781606790694
Health, Weight, Dieting, and Menstrual History Questionnaire	53 items divided into 4 categories: general health, body weight, dieting behaviors, and body image

Education programs for coaches and athletes can improve awareness of disordered eating in sport. The NCAA advises that all schools provide information on the risks factors and potential consequences of eating disorders, but programs are not mandatory. Prevention programs for youth and high school athletes may be more effective because the onset of disordered eating typically begins prior to college.[129] The ATHENA program, a female-specific intervention, has shown improvements in body satisfaction, nutrition, and dieting or use of purging behaviors.[130]

Return to Play

The decision to continue sports during treatment and return to play after treatment rests with the team or personal physician as outlined by the 2008 NATA position statement. No specific guideline exists, and the physician must consider the recommendations of the mental health professional and dietician along with any test results (cardiac, endocrine, bone density, body composition) and physical examination. The central questions to answer are, "When has an athlete recovered?" and "Is participation safe prior to recovery?"[16] Recovery can be evaluated physically, as in maintaining a healthy body weight, or emotionally, such as a realistic estimation of body size. Conditions may be placed on the athlete in order to return to play (eg, continued counseling or regular weight assessments). Eating disorders are pervasive, meaning they affect many aspects of a person's life. Those suffering with eating disorders can be good at hiding their disease, and relapse is common. Any stipulations or supervision of an athlete with an eating disorder must be carefully considered so as not create further hiding of behaviors.

MENTAL HEALTH BENEFITS OF PHYSICAL ACTIVITY

In 1996, the Surgeon General's Report on Physical Activity and Health stated that physical activity may have a role in reducing depression and anxiety, improving overall well-being, and preventing chronic disease. This announcement spurred research into the mental health benefits related to physical activity. Four aspects of mental health (mood, stress, cognition, and quality of life) now have cross-sectional and longitudinal data to support a positive relationship between physical activity and better outcomes. The limitations of this research are that physical activity is almost always self-reported, as are depressive symptoms, stress, and quality of life. Interventions have also been promising, especially in delaying cognitive decline.[131] The impact of physical activity on the HPA axis and neurogenesis is likely the mechanism for improved mood, lower risk of depression, less stress reactivity, and improved cognition. Other factors have also been reported and explain, in part, why physical activity is protective. These include social interaction, increased self-confidence, distraction, and learning of new skills.[132,133]

Changes in mood were noted as early as 1980 with aerobic exercise. The term *runner's high* referred to the positive feelings reported by people who regularly completed vigorous exercise sessions. It was hypothesized that an increase in circulating endorphins was responsible for improving mood and reducing stress.[134] At the time, elevated mood was seen as an acute effect and that any lessening of risk of depression would be due to consistent bouts of endorphin release from exercise. Depression screenings in longitudinal cohort studies consistently showed that lower risk of depression was associated with volumes and intensities of physical activity that were lower than the original running studies.[135,136] This led researchers to consider another mechanism beside vigorous exercise. It appeared that even slower-paced walking was beneficial. More recent longitudinal cohort studies have shown lower incidences of depression in young adults who participated in physical activity during adolescence.[135] The protective effect seems to fade over time. Studies of middle-age and older adults found that physical activity within the last few years was most beneficial,[137,138] but any volume and intensity was an improvement over inactivity. The results of physical activity interventions on patients with clinical depression have been mixed. Studies with no control or placebo group generally show improved symptoms,[139] as do those with supervised programs.[140] However, at-home individual programs were less successful because depression reduces the motivation for physical activity.[141,142]

Laboratory experiments with mice provided the first evidence that physical activity reduced the stress response. Mice who used a running wheel daily had lower levels of cortisol in the blood after a stressful event than mice who were confined,[143] and in studies of chronic stress, the exercising mice were more resilient and maintained neurogenesis, whereas nonexercisers lost brain volume.[144,145] Observational studies in humans found similar results. Levels of cortisol and self-reported stress levels are lower in people who are more physically active.[146,147] This is not to say that exercisers do not experience stress. They are still susceptible to deadlines, traffic, and major life events. But, the HPA axis shuts off sooner, decreasing the levels of cortisol, CRF, and ACTH. Chronically elevated levels of these hormones slow neurogenesis and negatively impact the immune system, especially as people age.[148] The stress response deduces one's ability to resist infection, fight inflammation, and reproduce healthy cells.[2] Studies have even linked stress to athletic injury.[149] Sport-related and life stress may lead to greater susceptibility to injury due to a narrowing of attention. During stress, the mind can focus sharply on individual tasks but has difficulty shifting attention or maintaining a broader view of our surroundings.[150] For example, a basketball player with narrowed perception may be so focused on completing his or her blocking assignment that he or she is unaware of a turnover and collides with another player. This is known as the stress-injury model. Stress can harm the recovery from injury, as well. Cortisol amplifies the inflammatory process so that more mast cells, leukocytes, and neutrophils are present, potentially prolonging the acute injury phase.[151]

The cognitive benefits of physical activity have been seen in studies of children, middle-aged adults, and older adults.[152-154] Diagnosis of dementia or scores from memory and problem-solving tests have been used to show that individuals who are physically activity have less dementia, including Alzheimer's disease,[153,155] and better cognitive function[152,156] than those who are inactive. The effect appears to be strongest in those who are most at risk for dementia. Interventions in older adults and those with the e4 allele show that regular physical activity can decrease the rate of cognitive decline[157] and help people maintain their independence longer.[158] Results are also promising for children who increase their physical activity from zero to 40 minutes/day.[159] The improved brain function is likely due to a combination of mechanisms, including neurogenesis. Also thought to contribute is the increased cerebral blood flow and growth factors, such as brain-derived neurotropic factor[154] seen with acute physical activity.

Quality of life refers to someone's overall sense well-being and satisfaction with life. It takes into account people's positive and negative perceptions of their physical, mental, and emotional health; relationships; employment; and living conditions. Detailed surveys are used to measure the multiple components included in this broad concept. A higher quality of life is a sign that someone feels good about his or her self, is productive, and is coping well with life's stressors. People who are more physically active report a higher quality of life,[160,161] and quality of life can be increased by physical activity.[162] Older adults and individuals living with chronic illnesses also benefit from greater levels of physical activity.[161] The relationship between sports participation and quality of life is inconsistent. Some research suggests that current and former student-athletes may have lower health-related quality of life than their nonathletic peers[163,164] and that the presence of sport-related injuries may negatively impact athletes' quality of life.[165]

Similar Mechanisms

The lack of neurogenesis links depression and dementia to the stress response. The effect of cortisol on the regeneration of brain cells seems to contribute to maintaining the neurochemistry needed for positive affect and the synaptic connections for memory and cognition. Modern life is full of stressors, and many Americans, including students, complain about high levels of stress in their lives. Although one can recognize the immediate effects of the stress response (increased heart rate, blood pressure, insomnia), most people do not understand how significantly health can be impacted by chronic stress. Physical activity can reduce the harm done by cortisol by training the HPA axis to quickly turn off the hormone cycle.[26] Reports of depression and CTE after repeated concussions lead to questions of possible similarities in the mechanisms. How are the HPA axis and neurogenesis affected by concussion? Research, particularly epidemiological studies, are needed to determine the relationship between concussions and depression and CTE and, eventually, on neurogenesis postconcussion.

BRINGING IT TOGETHER

- Athlete rates of anxiety and depression are similar to those in the general population. Athletes may be at higher risk for substance abuse. Rates of eating disorders are higher in aesthetic and weight class sports, although the overall rate of eating disorders is similar to nonathletic populations. Athletes are less likely to seek help for psychological concerns due to the stigma associated with mental health conditions.

- Mental health professionals use the DSM to define and grade psychological concerns. Not all signs and symptoms rise to the level of a clinical diagnosis. Subclinical concerns can have a negative impact on one's life as well.

- Depression is fairly common among young adults. In addition to depressed mood, key symptoms include extreme fatigue, sense of hopelessness, problems concentrating or making decisions, insomnia, and thoughts of suicide. Depression frequently reoccurs.

- Anxiety-related concerns include social phobias, panic attacks, GAD, OCD, social anxiety disorder, and PTSD. Approximately one-third of adolescents experience anxiety. The stress response is initiated and maintained by anxiety-producing situations and worry over possible reoccurrences.

- Alcohol is the most commonly abused substance in the United States. Abuse is defined as recurrent use and as one or more of the following: use in hazardous situations; failure to meet major obligations, such as work or school-related deadlines; legal problems; or social conflicts. The cultural aspects of sport appear to contribute to a higher prevalence of alcohol use and abuse by athletes at all levels. Binge drinking is associated with several risky health behaviors.

- The 3 classifications of eating disorders include anorexia nervosa, bulimia nervosa, and binge eating disorder. The lifetime prevalence of eating disorder is low, but it is significantly greater during adolescence. Females are more likely than males to suffer from eating-related behaviors.

- Key risk factors in athletes include the following:

  o Depression: Age between early and mid-20s, overtraining, substance abuse, history of insomnia, and, possibly, history of concussion

  o Binge drinking: More males than females, White, member of Greek organization, team leader, lower level of competition for college athletes (Division III > Division I)

  o Eating disorders: More females than males, aesthetic or weight class sports, ages 12 to 17 years, body dissatisfaction, perfectionism, and higher levels of competition

- Stress has a profound impact on health. Neurotransmitters and hormones released during the stress response affect heart rate, blood pressure, neurogenesis, and the inflammatory process. Researched has linked stress to depression, cognitive decline, and sport-related injury.

- Athletic trainers should be knowledgeable of risk factors and signs of depression, anxiety, substance abuse, and eating disorders. A protocol for mental health referrals should be established ahead of any identified need. Athletic trainers must understand their role in the treatment of athletes with psychological concerns and never attempt to counsel an athlete.

- Physical activity protects again depression, cognitive decline, and stress. The leading hypothesis for these benefits is that physical activity makes the hypothalamus more sensitive to cortisol and quickens the negative feedback loop. This, along with increased cerebral blood flow and levels of brain-derived neurotropic factor, improve neurogenesis.

LEARNING ACTIVITIES

1. Take the Daily Hassles and Uplifts and Major Life Events. What stress reduction strategies, including physical activity would you be willing to try to reduce your scores? Copies of the surveys can be found at https://students.asu.edu/files/StressChecklist.pdf and http://bama.ua.edu/~sprentic/large101%20Hassles-Uplifts%20Scale.pdf.

2. Develop a handout to educate coaches on their role in preventing and recognizing eating disorders. The toolkit from the National Eating Disorders Association is a good resource (www.nationaleatingdisorders.org/sites/default/files/Toolkits/CoachandTrainerToolkit.pdf).

3. Select a complementary and alternative health practice, such as message therapy, reflexology, yoga, mediation, reiki, or Ayurveda. Search the Internet for information on it's theory, philosophy, and practices. What benefit would this practice be to an athlete in recovery from an injury and why?

REFERENCES

1. World Health Organization. Mental health: strengthening our response. http://www.who.int/mediacentre/factsheets/fs220/en/. Updated August 2014. Accessed November 29, 2014.
2. Pert CB. The wisdom of the receptors: neuropeptides, the emotions, and bodymind. *Adv Mind Body Med.* 2002;18(1):30-35.
3. Brosschot JF, Gerin W, Thayer JF. The perseverative cognition hypothesis: a review of worry, prolonged stress-related physiological activation, and health. *J Psychosom Res.* 2006;60(2):113-124.
4. Merikangas KR, He JP, Burstein M, et al. Lifetime prevalence of mental disorders in U.S. adolescents: results from the National Comorbidity Study--Adolescent Supplement (NCS-A). *J Am Acad Child Adolesc Psychiatry.* 2010;49(10):980-989.
5. Esfandiari A, Broshek DK, Freeman JR. Psychiatric and neuropsychologic issues in sports medicine. *Clin Sports Med.* 2011;30(3):611-627.
6. Reardon CL, Factor RM. Sport psychiatry: a systematic review of diagnosis and medical treatment of mental illness in athletes. *Sports Med.* 2010;40(11):961-980.
7. Kamm RL. Diagnosing emotional disorders in athletes: a sport psychiatrist's perspective. *J Clin Sport Psychol.* 2008;2(2):178-201.
8. Smink FR, Van Hoeken D, Hoek H. Epidemiology of eating disorders: incidence, prevalence and mortality rates. *Curr Psychiatry Rep.* 2012;14(4):406-414.
9. Kessler RC, Chiu WT, Demler O, Merikangas KR, Walters EE. Prevalence, severity, and comorbidity of twelve-month DSM-IV disorders in the National Comorbidity Survey Replication. *Arch Gen Psychiatry.* 2005;62(6):617-627.
10. Sadock BJ, Sadock VA. *Kaplan and Sadock's Synopsis of Psychiatry: Behavioral Sciences/Clinical Psychiatry.* 10th ed. Philadelphia, PA: Lippincott Williams and Wilkins; 2007.
11. Substance Abuse and Mental Health Services Administration. 2012 report. http://media.samhsa.gov/data/NSDUH/2012SummNatFindDetTables/NationalFindings/NSDUHresults2012.pdf. Accessed December 2, 2015.
12. Breeden L, Marchesani A. Eating disorders 101. *School Counselor.* 2013;(Winter):13-14.
13. Crow SJ, Peterson CB, Swanson SA, et al. Increased mortality in bulimia nervosa and other eating disorders. *Am J Psychiatry.* 2009;166(12):1342-1346.
14. Napolitano MA, Himes S. Race, weight, and correlates of binge eating in female college students. *Eat Behav.* 2011;12(1):29-36.
15. Arcelus J, Mitchell AJ, Wales J, Nielsen S. Mortality rates in patients with anorexia nervosa and other eating disorders. A meta-analysis of 36 studies. *Arch Gen Psychiatry.* 2011;68(7):724-731.
16. Bratland-Sanda S, Sundgot-Borgen J. Eating disorders in athletes: overview of prevalence, risk factors and recommendations for prevention and treatment. *Eur J Sport Sci.* 2013;13(5):499-508.
17. DiPasquale LD, Petrie TA. Prevalence of disordered eating: a comparison of male and female collegiate athletes and nonathletes. *J Clin Sport Psychol.* 2013;7(3):186-197.
18. Holm-Denoma JM, Scaringi V, Gordon KH, Van Orden KA, Joiner TE Jr. Eating disorder symptoms among undergraduate varsity athletes, club athletes, independent exercisers, and nonexcercisers. *Int J Eat Disord.* 2009;42(1):47-53.
19. Wilson G, Pritchard M. Comparing sources of stress in college student athletes and non-athletes. *Athl Insight.* 2005;7(1):1-8.
20. Yeager MP, Pioli PA, Guyre PM. Cortisol exerts bi-phasic regulation of inflammation in humans. *Dose Response.* 2011;9(3):332-347.
21. Steptoe A, Kivimäki M. Stress and cardiovascular disease. *Nat Rev Cardiol.* 2012;9(6):360-370.
22. Pouwer F, Kupper N, Adriaanse MC. Does emotional stress cause type 2 diabetes mellitus? A review from the European Depression in Diabetes (EDID) Research Consortium. *Discov Med.* 2010;9(45):112-118.
23. Ehlert U, Gaab J, Heinrichs M. Psychoneuroendocrinological contributions to the etiology of depression, post-traumatic stress disorder, and stress-related bodily disorders: the role of the hypothalamus–pituitary–adrenal axis. *Biol Psychol.* 2001;57(1-3):141-152.
24. Aznar S, Knudsen GM. Depression and Alzheimer's disease: is stress the initiating factor in a common neuropathological cascade? *J Alzheimers Dis.* 2011;23(2):177-193.

25. Sothmann MS. Cross-stressor adaptation hypothesis. In: Acevedo EO, Ekkekakis P, eds. *Psychobiology of Physical Activity*. Champaign, IL: Human Kinetics; 2006:149-160.

26. Stranahan AM, Lee K, Mattson MP. Central mechanisms of HPA axis regulation by voluntary exercise. *Neuromolecular Med*. 2008;10(2):118-127.

27. Ramirez E, Wipfli B. Exercise and stress reactivity in humans and animals: two meta-analyses. *Int J Exerc Sci*. 2012;5(4):144-156.

28. Swain RA, Harris AB, Wiener EC, et al. Prolonged exercise induces angiogenesis and increases cerebral blood volume in primary motor cortex of the rat. *Neuroscience*. 2003;117(4):1037-1046.

29. Swain RA, Berggren KL, Kerr AL, Patel A, Peplinski C, Sikorski AM. On aerobic exercise and behavioral and neural plasticity. *Brain Sci*. 2012;2(4):709-744.

30. Schaal K, Tafflet M, Nassif H, et al. Psychological balance in high level athletes: gender-based differences and sport-specific patterns. *PLoS One*. 2011;6(5):e19007.

31. Storch EA, Storch JB, Killiany EM, Roberti JW. Self-reported psychopathology in athletes: a comparison of intercollegiate student-athletes and non-athletes. *J Sport Behav*. 2005;28(1):86-98.

32. Powell DH. Treating individuals with debilitating performance anxiety: an introduction. *J Clin Psychol*. 2004;60(8):801-808.

33. Kleine D. Anxiety and sport performance: a meta-analysis. *Anxiety Research*. 1990;2(2):113-131.

34. Woodman T, Hardy L. The relative impact of cognitive anxiety and self-confidence upon sport performance: a meta-analysis. *J Sports Sci*. 2003;21(6):443-457.

35. Yang J, Peek-Asa C, Corlette JD, Cheng G, Foster DT, Albright J. Prevalence of and risk factors associated with symptoms of depression in competitive collegiate student athletes. *Clin J Sport Med*. 2007;17(6):481-487.

36. Strine TW, Mokdad AH, Balluz LS, et al. Depression and anxiety in the United States: findings from the 2006 Behavioral Risk Factor Surveillance System. *Psychiatr Serv*. 2008;59(12):1383-1390.

37. Appaneal RN, Levine BR, Perna FM, Roh JL. Measuring postinjury depression among male and female competitive athletes. *J Sport Exerc Psychol*. 2009;31(1):60-76.

38. Weigand S, Cohen J, Merenstein D. Susceptibility for depression in current and retired student athletes. *Sports Health*. 2013;5(3):263-266.

39. Armstrong S, Oomen-Early J. Social connectedness, self-esteem, and depression symptomatology among collegiate athletes versus nonathletes. *J Am Coll Health*. 2009;57(5):521-526.

40. Sabo D, Miller KE, Melnick MJ, Farrell MP, Barnes GM. High school athletic participation and adolescent suicide: a nationwide US study. *Int Rev Sociol Sport*. 2005;40(1):5-23.

41. Taliaferro LA, Rienzo BA, Pigg RM Jr, Miller MD, Dodd VJ. Associations between physical activity and reduced rates of hopelessness, depression, and suicidal behavior among college students. *J Am Coll Health*. 2009;57(4):427-436.

42. Miller KE, Hoffman JH. Mental well-being and sport-related identities in college students. *Sociol Sport J*. 2009;26(2):335-356.

43. Brady KT, Sinha R. Co-occurring mental and substance use disorders: the neurobiological effects of chronic stress. *Am J Psychiatry*. 2005;162(8):1483-1493.

44. Masi G, Brovedani P. The hippocampus, neurotrophic factors and depression possible implications for the pharmacotherapy of depression. *CNS Drugs*. 2011;25(11):913-931.

45. Niehaus JL, Cruz-Bermudez ND, Kauer JA. Plasticity of addiction: a mesolimbic dopamine short-circuit? *Am J Addict*. 2009;18(4):259-271.

46. Tsuno N, Besset A, Ritchie K. Sleep and depression. *J Clin Psychiatry*. 2005;66(10):1254-1269.

47. Baglioni C, Battagliese G, Feige B, et al. Insomnia as a predictor of depression: a meta-analytic evaluation of longitudinal epidemiological studies. *J Affect Disord*. 2011;135(1-3):10-19.

48. Cukrowicz KC, Otamendi A, Pinto JV, Bernert RA, Krakow B, Joiner TE Jr. The impact of insomnia and sleep disturbances on depression and suicidality. *Dreaming*. 2006;16(1):1-10.

49. Brand S, Gerber M, Beck J, Hatzinger M, Pühse U, Holsboer-Trachsler E. Exercising, sleep-EEG patterns, and psychological functioning are related among adolescents. *World J Biol Psychiatry*. 2010;11(2):129-140.

50. Armstrong LE, VanHeest JL. The unknown mechanism of the overtraining syndrome: clues from depression and psychoneuroimmunology. *Sports Med*. 2002;32(3):185-209.

51. O'Connor PJ, Morgan WP, Raglin JS, Barksdale CM, Kalin NH. Mood state and salivary cortisol levels following overtraining in female swimmers. *Psychoneuroendocrinology*. 1989;14(4):303-310.

52. Raglin JS, Morgan WP, O'Connor PJ. Changes in mood states during training in female and male college swimmers. *Int J Sports Med*. 1991;12(06):585-589.

53. Raglin JS, Kenttä G. A psychological approach toward understanding and preventing overtraining syndrome. In: Echemendía RJ, Moorman Ct, eds. *Praeger Handbook of Sports Medicine and Athlete Health: Psychological Perspectives*. Santa Barbara, CA: Praeger Publishing; 2010:64-76.

54. Guskiewicz KM, Marshall SW, Bailes J, et al. Association between recurrent concussion and late-life cognitive impairment in retired professional football players. *Neurosurgery*. 2005;57(4):719-726.

55. Kerr ZY, Marshall SW, Harding HP Jr, Guskiewicz KM. Nine-year risk of depression diagnosis increases with increasing self-reported concussions in retired professional football players. *Am J Sports Med.* 2012;40(10):2206-2212.

56. Chrisman SP, Richardson LP. Prevalence of diagnosed depression in adolescents with history of concussion. *J Adolesc Health.* 2014;54(5):582-586.

57. Kontos AP, Covassin T, Elbin RJ, Parker T. Depression and neurocognitive performance after concussion among male and female high school and collegiate athletes. *Arch Phys Med Rehabil.* 2012;93(10):1751-1756.

58. Covassin T, Elbin RJ III, Larson E, Kontos AP. Sex and age differences in depression and baseline sport-related concussion neurocognitive performance and symptoms. *Clin J Sport Med.* 2012;22(2):98-104.

59. Chen JK, Johnston KM, Petrides M, Ptito A. Neural substrates of symptoms of depression following concussion in male athletes with persisting postconcussion symptoms. *Arch Gen Psychiatry.* 2008;65(1):81-89.

60. Hou R, Moss-Morris R, Peveler R, Mogg K, Bradley BP, Belli A. When a minor head injury results in enduring symptoms: a prospective investigation of risk factors for postconcussional syndrome after mild traumatic brain injury. *J Neurol Neurosurg Psychiatry.* 2012;83(2):217-223.

61. Vaidya VA, Terwilliger RM, Duman RS. Role of 5-HT2A receptors in the stress-induced down-regulation of brain-derived neurotrophic factor expression in rat hippocampus. *Neurosci Lett.* 1999;262(1):1-4.

62. Omalu BI, DeKosky ST, Minster RL, Kamboh MI, Hamilton RL, Wecht CH. Chronic traumatic encephalopathy in a National Football League player. *Neurosurgery.* 2005;57(1):128-134.

63. McKee AC, Cantu RC, Nowinski CJ, et al. Chronic traumatic encephalopathy in athletes: progressive tauopathy after repetitive head injury. *J Neuropathol Exp Neurol.* 2009;68(7):709-735.

64. Stern RA, Riley DO, Daneshvar DH, Nowinski CJ, Cantu RC, McKee AC. Long-term consequences of repetitive brain trauma: chronic traumatic encephalopathy. *PM R.* 2011;3(10 suppl 2):S460-S467.

65. Hildebrand KM, Johnson DJ, Bogle K. Comparison of patterns of alcohol use between high school and college athletes and non-athletes. *Coll Stud J.* 2001;35(3):358-365.

66. Humphreys BR, Ruseski JE. Socio-economic determinants of adolescent use of performance enhancing drugs: evidence from the YRBSS. *J Socio Econ.* 2011;40(2):208-216.

67. Yusko DA, Buckman JF, White HR, Pandina RJ. Alcohol, tobacco, illicit drugs, and performance enhancers: a comparison of use by college student athletes and nonathletes. *J Am Coll Health.* 2008;57(3):281-290.

68. Diehl K, Thiel A, Zipfel S, Mayer J, Litaker DG, Schneider S. How healthy is the behavior of young athletes? A systematic literature review and meta-analyses. *J Sports Sci Med.* 2012;11(2):201-220.

69. Wetherill RR, Fromme K. Alcohol use, sexual activity, and perceived risk in high school athletes and non-athletes. *J Adolesc Health.* 2007;41(3):294-301.

70. Martens MP, Dams-O'Connor K, Beck NC. A systematic review of college student-athlete drinking: prevalence rates, sport-related factors, and interventions. *J Subst Abuse Treat.* 2006;31(3):305-316.

71. Lisha NE, Sussman S. Relationship of high school and college sports participation with alcohol, tobacco, and illicit drug use: a review. *Addict Behav.* 2010;35(5):399-407.

72. Leichliter JS, Meilman PW, Presley CA, Cashin JR. Alcohol use and related consequences among students with varying levels of involvement in college. *J Am Coll Health.* 1998;46(6):257-262.

73. Ford JA. Alcohol use among college students: a comparison of athletes and nonathletes. *Subst Use Misuse.* 2007;42(9):1367-1377.

74. Kirby T, Barry AE. Alcohol as a gateway drug: a study of US 12th graders. *J Sch Health.* 2012;82(8):371-379.

75. Nelson TF, Xuan Z, Lee H, Weitzman ER, Wechsler H. Persistence of heavy drinking and ensuing consequences at heavy drinking colleges. *J Stud Alcohol Drugs.* 2009;70(5):726-734.

76. Green K, Nelson TF, Hartmann D. Binge drinking and sports participation in college: patterns among athletes and former athletes. *Int Rev Sociol Sport.* 2014;49(3-4):417-434.

77. Nelson TF, Wechsler H. Alcohol and college athletes. *Med Sci Sports Exerc.* 2001;33(1):43-47.

78. Wechsler H, Dowdall GW, Maenner G, Gledhill-Hoyt J, Lee H. Changes in binge drinking and related problems among American college students between 1993 and 1997. Results of the Harvard School of Public Health College Alcohol Study. *J Am Coll Health.* 1998;47(2):57-68.

79. Terry-McElrath YM, O'Malley PM, Johnston LD. Exercise and substance use among American youth, 1991-2009. *Am J Prev Med.* 2011;40(5):530-540.

80. Yusko DA, Buckman JF, White HR, Pandina RJ. Risk for excessive alcohol use and drinking-related problems in college student athletes. *Addict Behav.* 2008;33(12):1546-1556.

81. Martens MP, Pedersen ER, Smith AE, Stewart SH, O'Brien K. Predictors of alcohol-related outcomes in college athletes: the roles of trait urgency and drinking motives. *Addict Behav.* 2011;36(5):456-464.

82. Buckman JF, Yusko DA, Farris SG, White HR, Pandina RJ. Risk of marijuana use in male and female college student athletes and nonathletes. *J Stud Alcohol Drugs.* 2011;72(4):586-591.

83. Desbrow B, Biddulph C, Devlin B, Grant GD, Anoopkumar-Dukie S, Leveritt MD. The effects of different doses of caffeine on endurance cycling time trial performance. *J Sports Sci.* 2012;30(2):115-120.

84. Vertalino M, Eisenberg ME, Story M, Neumark-Sztainer D. Participation in weight-related sports is associated with higher use of unhealthful weight-control behaviors and steroid use. *J Am Diet Assoc.* 2007;107(3):434-440.

85. Elliot DL, Cheong J, Moe EL, Goldberg L. Cross-sectional study of female students reporting anabolic steroid use. *Arch Pediatr Adolesc Med.* 2007;161(6):572-577.

86. Ciapponi TM, Fahey TD. Health risks of anabolic steroids: update 2003. *Medicina Sportiva.* 2003;7(2):E41-E47.

87. Avois L, Robinson N, Saudon C, Baume N, Mangin P, Saugy M. Central nervous system stimulants and sport practice. *Br J Sports Med.* 2006;40(suppl 1):i16-i20.

88. Barnes GM, Welte JW, Hoffman JH. Relationship of alcohol use to delinquency and illicit drug use in adolescent: gender, age, and racial/ethnic differences. *J Drug Issues.* 2002;32(1):153-178.

89. Wechsler H, Davenport AE, Dowdall GW, Grossman SJ, Zanakos SI. Binge drinking, tobacco, and illicit drug use and involvement in college athletics. A survey of students at 140 American colleges. *J Am Coll Health.* 1997;45(5):195-200.

90. Buckman JF, Farris SG, Yusko DA. A national study of substance use behaviors among NCAA male athletes who use banned performance enhancing substances. *Drug Alcohol Depend.* 2013;131(1-2):50-55.

91. National Highway Traffic and Safety Administration. Alcohol-Impaired Driving. Washington, DC: National Highway Traffic and Safety Administration; 2012.

92. Hingson RW, Zha W, Weitzman ER. Magnitude of and trends in alcohol-related mortality and morbidity among U.S. college students ages 18-24, 1998-2005. *J Stud Alcohol Drugs* Suppl. 2009(16):12-20.

93. Li K, Simons-Morton BG, Hingson R. Impaired-driving prevalence among US high school students: associations with substance use and risky driving behaviors. *Am J Public Health.* 2013;103(11):e71-e77.

94. Wechsler H, Lee JE, Nelson TF, Lee H. Drinking and driving among college students: the influence of alcohol-control policies. *Am J Prev Med.* 2003;25(3):212-218.

95. Li K, Simons-Morton BG, Vaca FE, Hingson R. Association between riding with an impaired driver and driving while impaired. *Pediatrics.* 2014;133(4):620-626.

96. Centers for Disease Control and Prevention. Sexually Transmitted Disease Surveillance 2012. Atlanta, GA: Centers for Disease Control and Prevention, US Dept of Health and Human Services; 2013.

97. Rehm J, Shield KD, Joharchi N, Shuper PA. Alcohol consumption and the intention to engage in unprotected sex: systematic review and meta-analysis of experimental studies. *Addiction.* 2012;107(1):51-59.

98. Huang JH, Jacobs DF, Derevensky JL. Sexual risk-taking behaviors, gambling, and heavy drinking among U.S. college athletes. *Arch Sex Behav.* 2010;39(3):706-713.

99. Hingson R, Heeren T, Winter MR, Wechsler H. Early age of first drunkenness as a factor in college students' unplanned and unprotected sex attributable to drinking. *Pediatrics.* 2003;111(1):34-41.

100. Olmstead SB, Roberson PN, Pasley K, Fincham FD. Hooking up and risk behaviors among first semester college men: what is the role of precollege experience? *J Sex Res.* 2014;52(2):186-198.

101. Terry-McElrath YM, O'Malley PM, Johnston LD. Middle and high school drug testing and student illicit drug use: a national study 1998-2011. *J Adolesc Health.* 2013;52(6):707-715.

102. Goldberg L, Elliot DL, MacKinnon DP, et al. Outcomes of a prospective trial of student-athlete drug testing: the Student Athlete Testing Using Random Notification (SATURN) study. *J Adolesc Health.* 2007;41(5):421-429.

103. Pandina RJ, Johnson VL, Lagos LM, White HR, Maher CA. Substance use among high school athletes: implications for prevention interventions. *J Appl Sch Psych.* 2005;21(2):115-143.

104. Perkins HW, Craig DW. A successful social norms campaign to reduce alcohol misuse among college student-athletes. *J Stud Alcohol.* 2006;67(6):880-889.

105. Goldberg L, Elliot DL, Maher CA. Preventing substance use among high school athletes: the ATLAS and ATHENA Programs. *J Appl Sch Psych.* 2005;21(1):63-87.

106. Reinking MF, Alexander LE. Prevalence of disordered-eating behaviors in undergraduate female collegiate athletes and nonathletes. *J Athl Train.* 2005;40(1):47-51.

107. Swanson SA, Crow SJ, Le Grange D, Swendsen J, Merikangas KR. Prevalence and correlates of eating disorders in adolescents. Results from the national comorbidity survey replication adolescent supplement. *Arch Gen Psychiatry.* 2011;68(7):714-723.

108. Marques L, Alegria M, Becker AE, et al. Comparative prevalence, correlates of impairment, and service utilization for eating disorders across US ethnic groups: implications for reducing ethnic disparities in health care access for eating disorders. *Int J Eat Disord.* 2011;44(5):412-420.

109. Allen KL, Byrne SM, Oddy WH, Crosby RD. DSM-IV-TR and DSM-5 eating disorders in adolescents: prevalence, stability, and psychosocial correlates in a population-based sample of male and female adolescents. *J Abnorm Psychol.* 2013;122(3):720-732.

110. Martinsen M, Sundgot-Borgen J. Higher prevalence of eating disorders among adolescent elite athletes than controls. *Med Sci Sports Exerc.* 2013;45(6):1188-1197.

111. Hausenblas HA, McNally KD. Eating disorder prevalence and symptoms for track and field athletes and non-athletes. *J Appl Sport Psychol.* 2004;16(3):274-286.

112. Hausenblas HA, Carron AV. Eating disorder indices and athletes: an integration. *J Sport Exerc Psychol.* 1999;21(3):230-258.

113. Melin A, Torstveit MK, Burke L, Marks S, Sundgot-Borgen J. Disordered eating and eating disorders in aquatic sports. *Int J Sport Nutr Exerc Metab.* 2014;24(4):450-459.

114. Sundgot-Borgen J, Torstveit MK. Prevalence of eating disorders in elite athletes is higher than in the general population. *Clin J Sport Med.* 2004;14(1):25-32.

115. Greenleaf C, Petrie TA, Carter J, Reel JJ. Female collegiate athletes: prevalence of eating disorders and disordered eating behaviors. *J Am Coll Health.* 2009;57(5):489-495.

116. Petrie TA, Greenleaf C, Reel J, Carter J. Prevalence of eating disorders and disordered eating behaviors among male collegiate athletes. *Psychol Men Masc.* 2008;9(4):267-277.

117. Carter JE, Rudd NA. Disordered eating assessment for college student athletes. *Women in Sport and Physical Activity Journal.* 2005;14:62-71.

118. Johnson C, Powers PS, Dick R. Athletes and eating disorders: the National Collegiate Athletic Association study. *Int J Eat Disord.* 1999;26(2):179-188.

119. Currie A. Sport and eating disorders - understanding and managing the risks. *Asian J Sports Med.* 2010;1(2):63-68.

120. Krentz EM, Warschburger P. A longitudinal investigation of sports-related risk factors for disordered eating in aesthetic sports. *Scand J Med Sci Sports.* 2013;23(3):303-310.

121. Martinsen M, Bratland-Sanda S, Eriksson AK, Sundgot-Borgen J. Dieting to win or to be thin? A study of dieting and disordered eating among adolescent elite athletes and non-athlete controls. *Br J Sports Med.* 2010;44(1):70-76.

122. Krane V, Stiles-Shipley JA, Waldron J, Michalenok J. Relationships among body satisfaction, social physique anxiety, and eating behaviors in female athletes and exercisers. *J Sport Behav.* 2001;24(3):247-264.

123. Voelker DK, Gould D, Reel JJ. Prevalence and correlates of disordered eating in female figure skaters. *Psychol Sport Exerc.* 2014;15(6):696-704.

124. Krentz EM, Warschburger P. Sports-related correlates of disordered eating: a comparison between aesthetic and ballgame sports. *Int J Sport Psychol.* 2011;42(6):548-564.

125. Oppliger RA, Utter AC, Scott JR, Dick RW, Klossner D. NCAA rule change improves weight loss among national championship wrestlers. *Med Sci Sports Exerc.* 2006;38(5):963-970.

126. O'Dea JA, Abraham S. Onset of disordered eating attitudes and behaviors in early adolescence: interplay of pubertal status, gender, weight, and age. *Adolescence.* 1999;34(136):671-679.

127. Francisco R, Narciso I, Alarcão M. Individual and relational risk factors for the development of eating disorders in adolescent aesthetic athletes and general adolescents. *Eat Weight Disord.* 2013;18(4):403-411.

128. Gapin JI, Kearns B. Assessing prevalence of eating disorders and eating disorder symptoms among lightweight and open weight collegiate rowers. *J Clin Sport Psychol.* 2013;7(3):198-214.

129. Hildebrandt TB. A review of eating disorders in athletes: recommendations for secondary school prevention and intervention programs. *J Appl Sch Psych.* 2005;21(2):145-167.

130. Elliot DL, Goldberg L, Moe EL, et al. Long-term outcomes of the ATHENA (Athletes Targeting Healthy Exercise and Nutrition Alternatives) Program for female high school athletes. *J Alcohol Drug Edu.* 2008;52(2):73-92.

131. Forbes D, Forbes S, Morgan DG, Markle-Reid M, Wood J, Culum I. Exercise programs for people with dementia. *Cochrane Database Syst Rev.* 2013(12):CD006489.

132. Netz Y. Physical activity and three dimensions of psychological functioning in advanced age: cognition, affect, and self-perception. In: Tenenbaum G, Eklund RC, eds. *Handbook of Sport Psychology.* 3rd ed. Hoboken, NJ: John Wiley and Sons; 2007:492-508.

133. Wankel LM. The importance of enjoyment to adherence and psychological benefits from physical activity. *Int J Sport Psychol.* 1993;24(2):151-169.

134. Carr DB, Bullen BA, Skrinar GS, et al. Physical conditioning facilitates the exercise-induced secretion of beta-endorphin and beta-lipotropin in women. *N Engl J Med.* 1981;305(10):560-563.

135. Colman I, Zeng Y, McMartin SE, et al. Protective factors against depression during the transition from adolescence to adulthood: findings from a national Canadian cohort. *Prev Med.* 2014;65:28-32.

136. Stavrakakis N, Roest AM, Verhulst F, Ormel J, de Jonge P, Oldehinkel AJ. Physical activity and onset of depression in adolescents: a prospective study in the general population cohort TRAILS. *J Psychiatr Res.* 2013;47(10):1304-1308.

137. Pinto Pereira SM, Geoffroy MC, Power C. Depressive symptoms and physical activity during 3 decades in adult life: bidirectional associations in a prospective cohort study. *JAMA Psychiatry.* 2014;71(12):1373-1380.

138. Griffiths A, Kouvonen A, Pentti J, et al. Association of physical activity with future mental health in older, mid-life and younger women. *Eur J Public Health.* 2014;24(5):813-818.

139. Josefsson T, Lindwall M, Archer T. Physical exercise intervention in depressive disorders: meta-analysis and systematic review. *Scand J Med Sci Sports.* 2014;24(2):259-272.

140. Patel A, Keogh JW, Kolt GS, Schofield GM. The long-term effects of a primary care physical activity intervention on mental health in low-active, community-dwelling older adults. *Aging Ment Health.* 2013;17(6):766-772.

141. Pfaff JJ, Alfonso H, Newton RU, Sim M, Flicker L, Almeida OP. ACTIVEDEP: a randomised, controlled trial of a home-based exercise intervention to alleviate depression in middle-aged and older adults. *Br J Sports Med.* 2014;48(3):226-232.

142. Clegg A, Barber S, Young J, Iliffe S, Forster A. The Home-based Older People's Exercise (HOPE) trial: a pilot randomised controlled trial of a home-based exercise intervention for older people with frailty. *Age Ageing.* 2014;43(5):687-695.

143. Kannangara TS, Lucero MJ, Gil-Mohapel J, et al. Running reduces stress and enhances cell genesis in aged mice. *Neurobiol Aging.* 2011;32(12):2279-2286.

144. van Praag H. Exercise, neurogenesis, and learning in rodents. In: Acevedo EO, Ekkekakis P, eds. *Psychobiology of Physical Activity.* Champaign, IL: Human Kinetics; 2006:61-73.

145. Colcombe SJ, Erickson KI, Scalf PE, et al. Aerobic exercise training increases brain volume in aging humans. *J Gerontol A Biol Sci Med Sci.* 2006;61(11):1166-1170.

146. George ES, Jorm L, Kolt GS, Bambrick H, Lujic S. Physical activity and psychological distress in older men: findings from the New South Wales 45 and up study. *J Aging Phys Act.* 2012;20(3):300-316.

147. Traustadóttir T, Bosch PR, Matt KS. The HPA axis response to stress in women: effects of aging and fitness. *Psychoneuroendocrinology.* 2005;30(4):392-402.

148. McEwen BS. Sex, stress and the hippocampus: allostasis, allostatic load and the aging process. *Neurobiol Aging.* 2002;23(5):921-939.

149. Johnson U, Ivarsson A. Psychological predictors of sport injuries among junior soccer players. *Scand J Med Sci Sports.* 2011;21(1):129-136.

150. Williams JM, Tonymon P, Anderson MB. The effects of stressors and coping resources on anxiety and peripheral narrowing. *J Appl Sport Psychol.* 1991;3(2):126-141.

151. Toumi H, Best TM. The inflammatory response: friend or enemy for muscle injury? *Br J Sports Med.* 2003;37(4):284-286.

152. Dregan A, Gulliford MC. Leisure-time physical activity over the life course and cognitive functioning in late mid-adult years: a cohort-based investigation. *Psychol Med.* 2013;43(11):2447-2458.

153. Grande G, Vanacore N, Maggiore L, et al. Physical activity reduces the risk of dementia in mild cognitive impairment subjects: a cohort study. *J Alzheimers Dis.* 2014;39(4):833-839.

154. Etnier JL, Labban JD. Physical activity and cognitive function: theoretical bases, mechanisms, and moderators. In: Acevedo EO, ed. *The Oxford Handbook of Exercise Psychology.* 1st ed. New York, NY: Oxford University Press; 2012:76-96.

155. Podewils LJ, Guallar E, Kuller LH, et al. Physical activity, APOE genotype, and dementia risk: findings from the Cardiovascular Health Cognition Study. *Am J Epidemiol.* 2005;161(7):639-651.

156. Weuve J, Kang JH, Manson JE, Breteler MM, Ware JH, Grodstein F. Physical activity, including walking, and cognitive function in older women. *JAMA.* 2004;292(12):1454-1461.

157. Etnier JL, Caselli RJ, Reiman EM, et al. Cognitive performance in older women relative to ApoE-epsilon4 genotype and aerobic fitness. *Med Sci Sports Exerc.* 2007;39(1):199-207.

158. Vreugdenhil A, Cannell J, Davies A, Razay G. A community-based exercise programme to improve functional ability in people with Alzheimer's disease: a randomized controlled trial. *Scand J Caring Sci.* 2012;26(1):12-19.

159. Schaeffer DJ, Krafft CE, Schwarz NF, et al. An 8-month exercise intervention alters frontotemporal white matter integrity in overweight children. *Psychophysiology.* 2014;51(8):728-733.

160. Klavestrand J, Vingård E. The relationship between physical activity and health-related quality of life: a systematic review of current evidence. *Scand J Med Sci Sports.* 2009;19(3):300-312.

161. Bertheussen GF, Romundstad PR, Landmark T, Kaasa S, Dale O, Helbostad JL. Associations between physical activity and physical and mental health--a HUNT 3 study. *Med Sci Sports Exerc.* 2011;43(7):1220-1228.

162. Dale CE, Bowling A, Adamson J, et al. Predictors of patterns of change in health-related quality of life in older women over 7 years: evidence from a prospective cohort study. *Age Ageing.* 2013;42(3):312-318.

163. Simon JE, Docherty CL. Current health-related quality of life is lower in former Division I collegiate athletes than in non-collegiate athletes. *Am J Sports Med.* 2014;42(2):423-429.

164. Snyder AR, Martinez JC, Bay RC, Parsons JT, Sauers EL, Valovich McLeod TC. Health-related quality of life differs between adolescent athletes and adolescent nonathletes. *J Sport Rehabil.* 2010;19(3):237-248.

165. Valovich McLeod TC, Bay RC, Parsons JT, Sauers EL, Snyder AR. Recent injury and health-related quality of life in adolescent athletes. *J Athl Train.* 2009;44(6):603-610.

SUGGESTED READINGS

American College Health Association National College Health Assessment. Reference group data report. http://www.acha-ncha.org/docs/ACHA-NCHA_Reference_Group_Report_Spring2007.pdf. Published Spring 2007.

American Psychiatric Association. DSM. http://www.psychiatry.org/practice/dsm.

Bonci CM, Bonci LJ, Granger LR, et al. National Athletic Trainers' Association position statement: preventing, detecting, and managing disordered eating in athletes. *J Athl Train.* 2008;43(1):80-108.

Harvard Medical School. Understanding the stress response. http://www.health.harvard.edu/newsletters/Harvard_Mental_Health_Letter/2011/March/understanding-the-stress-response. Published March 1, 2011.

Herring SA, Boyajian-O'Neill LA, Coppel DB, et al. Psychological issues related to injury in athletes and the team physician. http://www.concussiontreatment.com/images/Herring_2010_Psychological_issues_related_to_injury_in_athletes_and_the_team_physician.pdf. Published 2006.

Kersey RD, Elliot DL, Goldberg L, et al. National Athletic Trainers' Association's position statement: anabolic-androgenic steroids. *J Athl Train*. 2012;47(5):567-588.

Kessler RC, Berglund PA, Bruce ML, et al. The prevalence and correlates of untreated serious mental illness. *Health Serv Res*. 2001;36(6 pt 1):987-1007.

National Alliance on Mental Illness. Types of mental health professionals. http://www.nami.org/Learn-More/Treatment/Types-of-Mental-Health-Professionals.

National Association of Anorexia Nervosa and Associated Disorders. Eating disorders statistics. http://www.anad.org/get-information/about-eating-disorders/eating-disorders-statistics/.

National Collegiate Athletic Association. NCAA doping, drug education and drug testing task force. http://www.ncaa.org/health-and-safety/policy/ncaa-doping-drug-education-and-drug-testing-task-force. Published 2013.

National Collegiate Athletic Association. NCAA drug education and drug testing survey: preliminary results. http://www.ncaa.org/sites/default/files/15.%20INstitutional%20Drug%20Education%20and%20Testing%20Survey%202011.pdf. Published December 2011.

National Collegiate Athletic Association. National study of substance use trends among NCAA college student-athletes. http://www.ncaapublications.com/productdownloads/SAHS09.pdf. Published January 2012.

Nattiv A, Loucks AB, Manore MM, et al. American College of Sports Medicine position stand. The female athlete triad. *Med Sci Sports Exerc*. 2007;39(10):1867-1882.

Neal TL, Diamond AB, Goldman S, et al. Inter-association recommendations for developing a plan to recognize and refer student-athletes with psychological concerns at the collegiate level: an executive summary of a consensus statement. *J Athl Train*. 2013;48(5):716-720.

US Department of Health and Human Services. 1996 surgeon general's report on physical activity. http://www.cdc.gov/nccdphp/sgr/index.htm.

III

Screening and Prevention of Sport-Related Injury

10

Pre-Activity Screening

Wanda Swiger, EdD, ATC, CES and Melanie Adams, PhD, CSCS, AT-Ret

CHAPTER OBJECTIVES

- Identify the necessary components to include in a pre-participation physical examination (PPE) as recommended by contemporary guidelines (eg, American Heart Association, American Academy of Pediatrics Council on Sports Medicine and Fitness).
- Explain the role of the PPE in identifying conditions that might predispose the athlete to injury or illness.
- Identify and describe the standard tests, test equipment, and testing protocols that are used for measuring fitness, flexibility, muscular strength, power, speed, agility, and endurance.
- Explain the basic concepts and practice of fitness and wellness screening.
- Identify the research steps to establish a screening test as predictor of injury.
- Describe the field tests for dynamic valgus and dynamic stability.

INTRODUCTION

Procedures that identify susceptibility to injury or illness are called *screenings*. Typically, screenings occur prior to sports participation and consist of medical history questionnaires, physical examinations and specialized tests. The goal of screening is to identify athletes that are at higher risk of injury and then lower their risk through education, monitoring of health status, better physical conditioning, and protective equipment or by limiting an athlete's exposure. In order to prevent injury, screening procedures must be valid measures of risk factors. This chapter will describe key elements of well-established screening procedures in sport, specifically focusing on the PPE, the health history questionnaires, the Tanner Maturation Scale, general fitness tests,

Adams M, Swiger W.
Epidemiology for Athletic Trainers: Integrating Evidence-Based Practice (pp 207-239).
© 2016 Taylor & Francis Group.

and some screenings for specific for sport-related injury. The chapter will also review the evidence for newer screening tests such as the Functional Movement Screen™ and Dynamic Valgus testing.

GOALS OF THE PRE-PARTICIPATION PHYSICAL EXAMINATIONS

For decades, physicians have been conducting PPE on athletes prior to competition. Initially, PPEs consisted of the triple H (history, heart, hernia).[1,2] The primary goals of the original PPE was to detect life-threatening conditions, identify ailments that would predispose athletes to injury, and address legal/insurance requirements.[1,2] Initial PPEs had a limited physical examination where a physician determined if the athlete was cleared to participate in sport. In 1992 with the collaboration of 5 medical associations (American Academy of Family Physicians, American Medical Society of Sports Medicine, American Academy of Pediatrics, American Orthopedic Society of Sports Medicine, and American Osteopathic Academy of Sports Medicine), comprehensive guidelines were established in an attempt to improve the process of the PPE. This was the first true attempt to standardize the components and the procedures of the PPE. These medical organizations joined the American College of Sports Medicine (ACSM) in 2010 to publish the 4th edition of the PPE. The PPE-4 monograph provides the most current guidelines for standardized forms and screening tools and include recommendations on timing, setting, and structure of a physical examination specific to athletics.[1,3] In 2014, the National Athletic Trainers' Association (NATA) published a position statement on PPE's. This position statement provides best practices guidelines based on the level of scientific data in medical literature regarding the various components of a PPE and other screening tools commonly used for pre-participation for athletics regardless of age, level of participation, or sport.

At the high school level, all states, require a PPE prior to participation in interscholastic athletics.[1-3] While the National Federation of State High School Associations considers the PPE a pre-requisite for participation, it has not adopted a standardized PPE[3] for all states to use. Some state associations require yearly PPE's, but most require the PPE only at initial entry to the institution. A yearly update to the athlete's history questionnaire is required in most states after the initial PPE.[3,4] Similarly, at the collegiate level, both the National Collegiate Athletic Association (NCAA) and the National Association for Intercollegiate Athletics (NAIA) require a PPE upon entrance to the institution's athletic program and a yearly updated health history questionnaire.

It has been reported that the PPE serves as the only annual medical evaluation for a large percentage of youth.[4] Therefore, many in the medical community have advocated for expanding the role of the PPE. Entities charged with revising guidelines for PPEs (high school associations, medical associations, state health agencies), have their own agendas which has led to a number of secondary objectives. While many support these secondary objectives,[4] others recognize that the PPE should not be the sole component of the health care for these student-athletes. The PPE will be most effective if the goals remain focused on sport participation.

Since 1994, the American Medical Association has contended that each physician performing a PPE for athletic participation should identify those student-athletes who have a medical condition (life threatening or disabling) that may increase their risk for sudden death or injury and ensure additional screening for conditions that may predispose an athlete to injury or illness. The focus was to provide every attempt to not disqualify the athlete from participation,[1-3] and to ensure the health and safety of every athlete. These have remained the primary objectives for the PPE-4. Secondary objectives of the PPE have developed and may include determining general health, establishing a relationship with a health care system, and initiating discussion on health-related topics.[1,3] Secondary objectives in the PPE-4 guidelines[1-3] include the following:

- Classification of the athlete[5]
  - Class 1 = Low risk
  - Class 2 = Some health concerns, moderate risk
  - Class 3 = Significant concerns, significant risk
  - Class 4 = High risk
- Disclosure of defects that may limit participation[1,2]
  - Detection of underlying conditions that require additional testing
    - Medical conditions, such as heart murmur that increases with Valsalva indicative of hypertrophic cardiomyopathy (HCM)
    - Congenital anomalies, like atlanto-axial instability in Down syndrome athletes
  - Detection of previous medical history (PMH) (including previous injuries) that are potential problems for the athlete
    - Musculoskeletal injuries, such as post-operative ACL, tibia fracture, or humeral fracture

Provide provisions for students to compete who have either physiologic or pathologic health conditions that may preclude full approval. The PPE-4 provides several options for clearance.

  - Cleared for all sports without restriction
  - Cleared for all sports without restriction with recommendations for further evaluation or treatment for…
  - Not cleared
    - Pending further evaluation
    - For any sport
    - For certain sports (MD will list appropriate sport based on risk)
- Must provide medical rationale
- Fulfilment of legal and insurance requirements for organized athletic programs
- Evaluation of size and level of maturation of younger athletes
  - Males with delayed growth and physical maturity may be at increased risk of injury in collision sport[2]
  - Peri-pubital females may be at increased risk for chronic injuries[6]
    - Provide an opportunity to counsel youth on health and personal questions
    - Provide an entry point into local sports medicine systems
  - Establish a doctor-patient relationship
  - Establish a database and record keeping system
    - Improvement of fitness and performance
  - Determination of the optimal level of performance
  - Proprioceptive ability, strength, endurance, flexibility, and body composition have been linked to injury risk[6]
  - Fitness components are typically performed by coaches, strength coaches, or athletic trainers[2,3] at an alternative time and location prior to competition.

The PPE-4 Recommended forms for the physical exam, history and participation clearance are available at www.aap.org/en-us/about-the-aap/Committees-Councils-Sections/Council-on-sports-medicine-and-fitness/Pages/PPE.aspx.

EFFECTIVENESS OF THE PRE-PARTICIPATION PHYSICAL EXAMINATIONS AND THE NEED FOR STANDARDIZATION

Lack of standardization of the PPE in the United States has led to studies indicating poor effectiveness.[3,4] Controversy over which components and procedures continues to limit the evaluation of the effectiveness of the PPE.[2] Several studies have attempted to establish a level of standardization in the United States. While all 50 states require a PPE for high school students, there is a lack of consistency across all states in almost all components.[1,4,7,8] In 2005, a study found that 81% of states had adequate PPEs[4] but that 85% of states had PPEs that predated the 1996 AHA guidelines for CV screening.[8] Findings were similar at the collegiate level, where both the NCAA and the NAIA require a PPE upon entrance to the institution, but there is a lack of standardization as to what constitutes a good PPE.[7]

The majority of the literature on the PPE consists of level 5 and 6 evidence, including opinion papers, literature reviews, and case reports from respected authors and sports medicine societies. Only a few studies have attempted to establish evidenced based outcomes for the PPE. In a comprehensive literature search, Wingfield et al[9] identified 310 articles that met the selection criteria, with 25 articles identified as original research directly relating to the PPE. The majority of these examined cardiovascular diseases and screening procedures. The 5 studies that assessed the format or effectiveness of the PPE concluded that it was inadequate. Several studies have concluded that the PPE was not standardized and did not consistently address the AHA recommendations for cardiovascular screening history and physical exams. Additionally, there were a variety of health care professionals that administered the PPE's (some of which did not have adequate training) which may increase the lack of consistency. Carek and Mainous[10] reviewed 176 articles to determine whether the PPE in the literature satisfied the basic requirements for medical screening as required by the United States Preventive Services Task Force (USPSTF) (www.uspreventiveservicestaskforce.org). Both the Wingfield[9] and the Carek and Mainous[10] reviews identify lack of standardization of the PPE as a key issue in the PPE not meeting the standards for a reliable screening tool.

Researchers in Germany, reviewed the medical histories adolescent athletes and found that over 16% needed follow up with musculoskeletal system pathologies, nearly 16% needed follow up with general medical conditions, and only 1% answered questions that indicated follow up for cardiovascular conditions.[11] When compared to clinical examinations, almost 34% of the athletes had suspicious findings for musculoskeletal conditions, almost 10% had general medical conditions,[11] and 3% had cardiovascular issues.[7,11]

ADMINISTRATION OF THE PRE-PARTICIPATION PHYSICAL EXAMINATIONS

The PPE should be completed 4 to 6 weeks prior to participation.[1-3] This allows time for any follow up screenings. Individual or multi-station PPE screening methods are acceptable methods of administration. A licensed physician (MD or DO) is the most appropriate medical professional to direct the PPE.[1,2] The qualification of the health care professional who performs the PPE is based on practitioner availability, clinical expertise, and individual state laws, but the training of MD/DO physicians makes them the best qualified to perform the exam. For adolescent athletes, it is recommended that their primary care physician perform the PPE. However, it has been reported that there are several states that allow non-physician providers (physician assistants, nurse practitioners, and chiropractors) to perform the PPE.[7]

Determining participation is based on information gathered during the PPE and is arguably the most important purpose of the PPE. As a result of the PPE, the physician will take the following actions[2,3]:

- Unconditional clearance (cleared for all sports and levels of participation)
- Cleared with recommendation for follow up (evaluation or treatment)
- Not cleared with clearance status to be determined by further evaluation, treatment or rehabilitation
- Not cleared for any sport or level of competition

There is general agreement in the literature on the rates for athletes qualifying (85% to 97%), qualifying with conditions (3% to 13%), or being disqualified (less than 2 to 3%) for sports participation.[3,10] If the athlete is not cleared for participation, the rationale must be communicated to the individual, parent (if athlete is a minor), medical staff (including AT), and the coaching staff.[2,10] HIPPA and FERPA guidelines must be followed. A conference meeting is preferred and allows the physician to discuss all issues.

Most clearance issues revolve around the physician identifying musculoskeletal system conditions where a follow up therapy and/or treatment is recommended. These orthopedic issues temporarily restrict an athlete from full participation.[2,10] In some cases, medical conditions may require an athlete to be restricted until he or she is fully recovered from an illness (fever), some may require a follow up with his or her primary care MD for medication treatment (asthma), and others may require specific monitoring pre, during, and post exercise (diabetes). Certain medical conditions may restrict an athlete from participating in types of sports.[2] For example, an athlete with Down syndrome that has been diagnosed with atlantoaxial instability is likely restricted from collision sports but may have clearance for contact or non-contact sports. Many athletes qualify and are cleared for participation in sports today that previously would have presented with conditions that were considered disqualifying. For example, an athlete with Marfan syndrome, with its high association to SCD, may be required to submit to regular serial cardiac, ophthalmologic, and musculoskeletal evaluations as well as being required to sign written consent or a legal waiver in order to participate,[2] but may not be restricted.

Recommended Components of the Pre-Participation Physical Examinations

Medical screening tools used to determine clearance for athletic participation include the health history questionnaire and the pre-participation examination. The 12-element cardiovascular screening and the 90-second musculoskeletal screening are 2 components that should be included in the physical (clinical) examination. Policies or legal mandates may require additional screenings to determine athlete readiness and/or maturity (ie, Tanner Maturation Scale).

Health History Questionnaire

A comprehensive medical and family history gives the athlete the ability to disclose any past illness, injuries, or conditions critical to sport participation. Most medical professionals identify the history as the most critical component of an evaluation. A comprehensive medical history is the most sensitive and specific component of the PPE.[1,10] Research supports that a comprehensive history identifies 75% to 92% conditions that can affect athletic participation.[1,10] The Health History Questionnaire contains over 50 questions organized by system,[1] but the validity of Questionnaire recommended in the PPE-4 has not been determined. The PPE-4 recommended example of a Health History Questionnaire can be found at www.aap.org/en-us/about-the-aap/Committees-Councils-Sections/Council-on-sports-medicine-and-fitness/Pages/PPE.aspx.

For minors, it is highly recommended that parents assist their children in completing this form; however, parents and student-athletes may not provide reliable and historical information. This is typical of self-report research data possibly due to inadequate information retrieval. The PPE-4 attempts to limit this by including an educational section for parents and athletes to assist them in understanding the terms, the significance of the questions, and the importance of answering them honestly.[1] Furthermore there appears to be some support for an e-History form. A study completed at Stanford University Athletics, indicated a significant increase in compliance and accuracy with an online history form.[12]

While the history questionnaire probes individual body systems, the history form asks questions specific to the recommendations by the American Heart Association for cardiovascular screening of competitive athletes.[1] Another important component of the history is the section on the musculoskeletal system. Additional recommendations to be highlighted and reviewed include nutritional assessment, heat/hydration-related illness risk factors, and mental health considerations. The PPE-4 also emphasizes menstrual cycle and disordered eating in female athletes. The final portion of the history includes questions regarding the mental health status of the athlete. Any yes answers will require a follow up with the physician to determine follow up assessments and/or referral.

Physical Examination

A general health screening should include vital signs (height, weight, blood pressure, temperature), visual acuity (Snellen Eye Chart), cardiovascular, neurologic, musculoskeletal (orthopedic) and a systematic general medical examination (pulmonary and abdominal screening includes auscultation of the lungs and the abdomen, skin, genitalia for males).[2] Additional recommendations of the general health screening include a review of all medications and supplements used by the athlete. The general health screening is used to determine if any additional testing is required. Laboratory or diagnostic screenings (urinalysis, complete blood count, lipid profiles) are not recommended or required. If the athlete has a history of anemia, hemoglobin and ferritin levels should be measured and the athlete should be advised on treatment. If an athlete presents with diabetes, the athlete should be educated on blood glucose monitoring during sport participation as well as being required to have an annual eye, neurological, and cardiovascular exam, and routinely be evaluated for foot conditions (sensory, motor and reflex). The NCAA requires sickle cell screening if their hemoglobinopathy status is unknown. If an athlete is identified as having sickle cell trait, he or she should be aware of concerns related to hydration, conditioning, and acclimatization. The PPE-4 recommended format is available at; https://www.aap.org/en-us/about-the-aap/Committees-Councils-Sections/Council-on-sports-medicine-and-fitness/Pages/PPE.aspx.

The Musculoskeletal Examination

Because one of the strongest independent predictors of sports injuries is a previous injury,[6,10] including a musculoskeletal component to the PPE is critical.[2] Both the PPE-4 and the NATA position statement recommend the 90-second orthopedic screening examination as one component of the PPE (Table 10-1).

The 90-second assessment simply has the clinician instruct the patient to move their upper limbs, lower limbs, neck, and trunk allowing for basic observation of movement (amount, symmetry, and absence of pain).

A study by Gomez et al[13] found that 91.6% of musculoskeletal conditions were detected by history alone. When comparing an orthopedic examination and the 90-second screening, 14 significant injuries were missed by the detailed orthopedic examination, but were detected by the 90-second screening examination. The results of this study determined the sensitivity

TABLE 10-1
90-SECOND MUSCULOSKELETAL SCREENING EXAMINATION

INSTRUCTION	OBSERVATION
Stand facing examiner	AC joints; general habitus
Look at ceiling, floor, over belt, over shoulders, touch ears to shoulders	Cervical spine motion
Shrug shoulders (resistance)	Upper trapezius strength
Abduct shoulders to 90 degrees; (Resistance at 90 degrees)	Deltoid strength
Perform full external rotation of arm	Shoulder motion
Flex and extend elbows	Elbow motion
Spread fingers, make a fist	Hand, finger motion, strength; deformities
Tighten/relax quadriceps	Symmetry and knee effusion; ankle effusion
Duck walk away/toward examiner	Hip, knee, ankle motion
Stand facing away from examiner	Shoulder symmetry; scoliosis
With knees straight, touch toes	Hip motion, hamstring tightness; functional scoliosis
Raise up on toes; raise up on heels	Calf symmetry, leg strength

of the 90-second screening to be 50.8%, specificity of 97.5%, positive predictive value of 40.9%, and negative predictive value of 98.3%.[13] For asymptomatic athletes with no previous injuries, a 90-second screening musculoskeletal test will detect 90% of significant musculoskeletal injuries.[10] When an athlete indicates a PMH or has current signs and symptoms (pain, limited range of motion, etc) during the general examination, then a site specific examination should be performed.[1,2]

Pre-season, pre-participation screenings may include additional stations to collect other types of musculoskeletal baseline data. Those most commonly performed on athletes evaluate the following:

- Flexibility (ROM versus muscular tightness),

- Muscular strength, weakness or asymmetry (isokinetic or dynamometer testing),

- Levels of joint laxity (ie, Beighton Hypermobility Score [www.shoulderdoc.co.uk/article. asp?article=645] quantifies joint laxity on a 9-point scale, with the higher scores indicating hypermobility)

Junge et al[14] assessed the orthopedic portion of the International Federation of Football Association (FIFA) pre-competition medical assessment (PCMA). Performed by team physicians, the orthopedic examination evaluated the lower extremity using pain complaints for each body segment (Hip/groin/thigh, knee, ankle/lower leg/foot), ROM (hip, ankle/foot), flexibility (hip/ thigh muscles), and stability (lachman's, anterior drawer and other knee laxity assessments, ankle anterior drawer, talar tilt) to identify pre-existing conditions. The results indicate that the feasibility and quality of the PCMA is possible with further instruction on standardizing procedures and responses. The literature does not indicate the length (duration) of the orthopedic portion of the

PCMA. While all these risk factors thought to predispose an athlete to injury, collection of this type of information is extremely time-consuming. Many schools do not have the resources and personnel to collect this type of data. Furthermore, studies have not consistently demonstrated that injuries are prevented by interventions aimed at correcting deficits, such as poor flexibility. Prior injury is a predictor of new or repeat injury and the 90-second musculoskeletal screening adequately identifies these pre-existing conditions. The 90-second Musculoskeletal Screening is a quick and effective tool to identify musculoskeletal conditions.[1,2,10,13] However, research is lacking in regards to the depth needed for an orthopedic examination to be comprehensive.

Cardiovascular Screening

The PPE-4 supports the AHA and includes 12 key elements for pre-participation for competitive athletes.[1-3] This pre-screening incudes a history, knowledge of cardiac conditions in family members, and the presence of a heart murmur designed to identify cardiovascular diseases that designate athletes at risk. The personal history questions focus on symptoms that may be evident during exercise, while the family history questions focus on identifying specific cardiac conditions.[1] Athletes with a past history of heart murmur, family history of premature death, exercise induced chest pain, shortness of breath, or syncope[2,10] should be identified for potential conditions. A positive response to any question should be probed with additional questions to determine the need for follow up. The physical examination for cardiovascular concerns is more specific and detailed compared to the examination of the other body systems.

The cardiovascular examination includes the following (Table 10-2)[1,2,10]:

- Dynamic auscultation of heart murmurs
  - Supine and standing
    - Standing is preferred for recognition of HCM murmur
  - While performing various maneuvers: Valsalva maneuver, deep breath, or squat to stand
- Palpation of radial and femoral pulses
  - Exclude aortic coarctation
- Examination for physical characteristics of Marfan Syndrome
  - Kyphoscoliosis, high arched palate, pectus excavatum, arachnodactyly, arms span greater than height, hyperlaxity, myopia, mitral valve prolapse, aortic insufficiency
- Brachial Artery blood pressure
  - Seated position preferred

The CV screening of the PPE is based on expert opinion and has limited sensitivity and specificity data. It is estimated that it has only 3% to 6% sensitivity. This may be caused by the lack of standardization of PPEs, especially those not incorporating all components of the AHA guidelines and use of examiners who are experienced with cardiac screening.[7] A pilot study,[15] evaluated the inter-observer agreement of the AHA guidelines between physicians. Using cadets at West Point, 3 physicians (2 fellows and 1 cardiologist) evaluated 101 cadets. The referral rate of the 2 fellows was 6% which is consistent with other studies that have shown a 3% to 8% referral rate for questionable findings. However, there was poor agreement amongst the 3 between the when identifying who should be referred. While the study was small and had several limitations, it does raise concerns about consistency between physicians performing the cardiac portion of the PPE. Detection of cardiac murmur of grade III/IV or louder, a diastolic murmur, or a murmur that increases with a Valsalva maneuver should prompt a referral to a cardiologist. Athletes with blood pressure > 135/85 require follow up for repeated BP monitoring.[2,10]

TABLE 10-2	
THE 12-ELEMENT AHA RECOMMENDATIONS FOR PREPARTICIPATION CARDIOVASCULAR SCREENING OF COMPETITIVE ATHLETES	
STEP 1	**PERSONAL HISTORY** • Exertional chest pain/discomfort • Unexplained syncope/near-syncope • Excessive exertional and unexplained dyspnea/fatigue associated with exercise • Prior recognition of a heart murmur • Elevated systemic blood pressure
STEP 2	**FAMILY HISTORY** • Prematuure death (sudden and unexpected, or otherwise) before age 50 due to heart disease in > 1 relative • Disability from heart disease in a close relative < 50 years of age • Specific knowledge of certain conditions in family memebers: hypertrophic or dilated myopathy, long QT syndrome, or other ion channelopathies, Marfan syndrome, or clinically important arrhythmias
STEP 3	**PHYSICAL EXAMINATION** • Heart murmur • Femoral pulses to exclude aortic coarctation • Physical stigmata of Marfan syndrome • Brachial artery blood pressure (sitting position)

Electrocardiogram Screening

In 2005, the European Society of Cardiology published a position statement recommending that electrocardiograms (ECG) be included in the pre-participation cardiac screening for all young athletes in organized sport. This change ignited a debate among US physicians and sports-injury specialists. Should all athletes be tested for HCM or should we continue with physical exams and medical history as the primary pre-participation screening tools? All national team members and the professional male sports teams (NFL, MLB, NBA, NHL) are given baseline ECG tests, but should all youth, high school, and college athletes be required be tested as well?

The key evidence supporting the use of ECG's in pre-participation screening comes from Italy where testing has been conducted since 1982. Corrado et al[16] used longitudinal data from one region to illustrate the incidence of sudden cardiac death (SCD) prior and after the mandated screening. Participants were competitive athletes, ages 12 to 35 years. The relative risk of SCD was 4.19 in the prescreening period (1979 to 1981) and dropped significantly over the next 12 years to 0.87. As striking as this result was, it did not change the guidelines published by the American Heart Association in 2007.

Several reasons why American cardiologists remain opposed to mandatory ECG testing have been pointed out by Este and Link.[17] First is that the incidence of SCD among US athletes remains very low. While incredibly tragic when it does occur, the incidence for high school athletes has

Figure 10-1. ECG tracing.

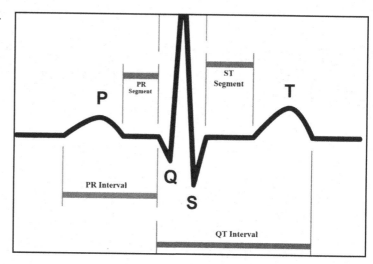

been reported between 1 per 100,000[18] and 1 per 300,000 persons[19] and the NCAA reports 1 per 43,770 athletes.[18] Estimates of relative risk are much lower among US athletes than the Italian cohort report (.44 to 4.19).[20] Second, it is not clear the ECG testing is superior to the current standard of physical exam and medical history. The Corrado et al study did not compare the use of ECG to usual pre-participation screening. According to Este and Link, the incidence rate for SCD is lower among US athletes receiving the standard screening than the Italian participants who were given the additional ECG (1.06 to 1.87 per 100,000).[17] Additionally, a study of Israeli athletes prior to and after their country's ECG legislation showed no benefit.[21] Without replication of positive longitudinal results and no randomized control trails on the effects of ECG on SCD, changing the current guidelines seems premature.

The last 2 reasons cited by opponents of mandatory ECG's are the high rates of false positives and the high cost associated with ECG testing in the United States. The purpose of an ECG is to measure the electrical impulses that initial heart muscle contractions. This can be traced as wave patterns on graph paper (Figure 10-1).

A non-pathological athletic heart can display ECG patterns similar to cardiomyopathy and the 2 can be difficult to distinguish; resulting in a high rate of false positives. The specificity of the ECG to identify abnormalities in athletes varies widely and has been reported to be as low as .64 in children[22] and as high as .89 in adults.[23] This means that somewhere between 4.4% to 9.4% of the ECG tests will result in a permanent disqualification from sports for athletes that are not at risk.[16] The cost of ECG and who bears the burden of that cost is also a major concern. Most European countries have a single payer health care system as opposed to the multiple insurance options used in the United States. With a single payer system there is tight control over the cost of medical procedures and the government sets the rates that it or citizens pay for care. Most American athletes, with the exception of professionals, Olympians, and major college athletes; must use their own insurance to pay for sport-related care. This cost would not be covered by insurance if there is no indication of an abnormality, leaving the individual athlete or the sports organization responsible for the cost. While large universities may be able to support ECG testing through their own medical centers, most will have to pay additional costs to provide this service.

Clearly the debate about required ECG screenings will continue. Future research hopefully will provide evidence to determine the benefits of testing, methods to improve the reliability and validity, and how to best manage the cost of the screening.

TABLE 10-3			
TANNER SEXUAL MATURITY SCALE			
TANNER STAGE	FEMALES		MALES	
	Breasts	*Pubic hair*	*Genitalia*	*Pubic hair*
1	Nipple elevation only	None	Testicles 1 to 2 cm	None
2	Small raised breast bud	Growth along labia, sparse, lightly pigmented	Testicles >2 cm, scrotal enlargement	Sparse, lightly pigmented
3	Breast and areola enlarge with no contour difference	Increases in amount, darkens, starts to curl	Testicles continue to enlarge, penis lengthens	Increases in amount, darkens, starts to curl
4	Further enlargement with areola and nipple projecting to form secondary mound	Resembles adult type, but not spread to medial thighs	Scrotum darkens, widening of glans penis	Resembles adult type, but not spread to medial thighs
5	Adult contour with areola and breast, in same contour, nipple protruding	Spreads to medial thighs, adult distribution	Adult size and morphology	Spreads to medial thighs, adult distribution

Table created using references 25 and 26.

Additional Screenings

Additional screenings may be used to supplement the PPE. It is believed that adolescent growth spurts, age, biologic maturity, and body size are factors predisposing a young athlete to sport injury.[6] Many youth sports group by age or by grade level for competition. Moreover, many of these sport organizations prohibit youth from playing up even if the athlete's skill level and ability warrants. Some high school associations will allow mature and skilled 8th graders to play on high school teams. Maturation, the development of secondary sexual characteristic, occurs during adolescence with individual variation in onset.[24] Therefore, additional assessments can be required to determine physical readiness to protect the health and safety of the athlete.

Tanner Stage of Maturation

The Tanner Stage of Maturation is one tool that has been used to determine biologic maturity (secondary sexual characteristics) (Table 10-3). Physical maturity is part of the process indicating growth plate development.[6] The Tanner Scale is divided into 5 levels of maturity based on the development of a boy's penis and testicles as well as pubic hair. In girls, the Tanner Scale also places the child on 1 of 5 levels based on breast and genital development as well as pubic hair. If females have reached menarche (started menstruating) they are automatically at Tanner 5 and do not have to go through the visual exam.[25,26] The Tanner Scale is often combined with other tests of readiness. For example, in New York State, for those athletes that are at a high level of sport/athletic readiness in grades 7 and 8 and want to compete at the high school level the Tanner Scale is part

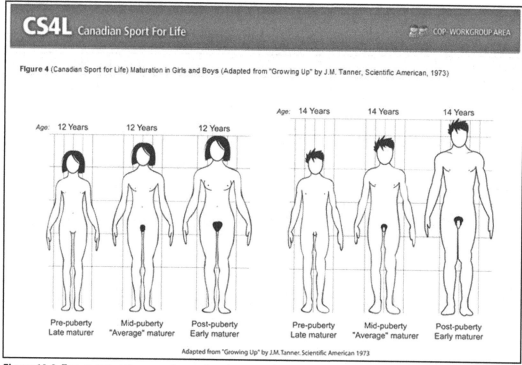

Figure 10-2. Tanner maturation grouping: early to late maturity.

of the Individual Athletic Profile requirement. This profile includes height, weight, developmental rating (the Tanner Stages), athletic performance (Shuttle run, 50-yard dash, 1.5 mile run; standing long jump, stomach curls, and flexed arm hang/pull-ups), and a sport skill assessment by the coach (New York State Board of Education Health Examination Guidelines, www.p12.nysed.gov/sss/documents/SchoolHealthExaminationJune2015Rev9-15.pdf).

Because the Tanner Scale is an intrusive observation by a physician, where the child may feel uncomfortable, there has been increased discussion in the medical community regarding alternative models. The first is self-assessment. Self-assessment is not as reliable as a physician evaluation, however, when coupled with grip strength assessment, the reliability is improved.[25,26] A second alternative is the Pubertal Maturational Observational Scale (POMS), which utilizes parental questionnaires and investigator observations to classify a patient as pre-pubertal (Tanner Stage 1), pubertal (Tanner Stage 2 to 3), or post-pubertal (Tanner Stage 4 to 5) (Figure 10-2). The POMS appears to show reliability in the following indicators: adolescent growth, breast development, menstrual status, axillary and leg hair growth, muscular development, presence of acne, and sweating during physical activity.[27,28]

There has been more research for the Tanner Maturation Scale in males then in females. Unlike females where menarche is the clear transition in maturity, males do not have a clear marker. Standard errors are therefore, greater in boys nearing maturity because of the number of indicators available for assessment.[29] If using the Tanner Scale, timing of maturation with average chronological age is an important component to understand. Median ages for pubic hair transition occur at the following: Stage 1 ~ 11.4, Stage 2 ~ 12.7, Stage 3 ~ 13.5. Furthermore, Monteilh et al[30] determined variables that affected early and later maturers. Beginning at age 8, the shortest boys made the transition to stage 1 and to stage 2 later than the tallest boys at age 8. Besides height, greater weight and BMI at age 8 determined transitions to stage 3. Data for boys older than 14 were not recorded in this study. While 15% of the boys in this study had not reported transitioning to stage 3 by age 14, it was also not reported how many boys had entered stage 4 or 5.

Breast budding is the first sign of puberty in females. There is an additional issue regarding maturational levels with females. Since maturational status is often associated with menarche, associations for females with delayed onset of menarche or dysmenorrhea should be investigated. White girls in the United States now menstruate at an average age of 12.6 years, Black girls at 12.1 years, while Mexican-American girls menstruate at an average age of 12.2 years.[31] A large range for menarche has been reported, between years 8 to 16. However it is widely accepted that intense training and poor nutrition can affect or delay the onset of menarche. Females who have delayed onset are classified as having primary amenorrhea.

Effects of Maturation

Maturation occurs at different rates across gender and within gender. Youth sport and interscholastic sport group competition by age. However, research has supported maturation as a predictor of injury. Furthermore, sexual maturity has some effect on skeletal age, joint laxity, lower extremity power and speed, and grip strength.

Sexual Maturity and Skeletal Age

Most 11 and 12 year old boys are average or on time in terms of skeletal maturation. As boys mature, it has been reported that by age 13, skeletal age and chronological age are close to equal. However, after age 13, there are more boys that have skeletal ages above their chronological age. This is especially true for 15 to 16 year old boys.[29] Early pubertal 10- to 11- and 12- to 13-year-old boys do not differ in skeletal and sexual maturation, but pubertal boys age 14 to 16 are advanced in skeletal maturation height and weight.[29] Advanced skeletal maturity has been associated with greater BMI, muscular strength and power. Malina et al[29] determined that for boys with chronological age of 11 to 16, as skeletal maturity increased, height and weight increased. Ré et al[32] compared boys ages 10 to 16 for height, weight, biological maturity, chronological age, and compared these to performance measures. For all age groups, the higher Tanner Scale (evidence of the secondary sexual characteristics), the taller and heavier the boys were.

Sexual Maturity and Fitness

Ré and colleagues[32] compared boys ages 10 to 16 for height, weight, biological maturity, chronological age, and compared these to performance measures (speed, lower extremity power, aerobic capacity, abdominal strength, hip flexibility, and agility). For all age groups, the only 2 performance measures that were significantly different were lower extremity power and speed. Boys with chronological ages 13 to 16 that were classified in later stages of the Tanner Scale were significantly faster than those with less sexual maturity at the same chronological age. Some research[25] has attempted to link grip strength to the Tanner Scale. Immature boys (Tanner 1 to 3) that were less than 65 inches tall had a grip strength average of less than 25 kg. While mature boys (Tanner 4 and 5) that were taller than 65 inches had grip strength averages above 25 kg. While other studies have attempted to link[26] handgrip and self-assessment instead of a physician evaluation. Boys that rated themselves as a Tanner 3 or less had a grip strength of 24.9 kg and those who rated themselves greater than 3 had grip strength of greater than 24.9 kg. Less than 18% of boys assessed had scores that were in disagreement.

Several studies have reported increased running economy with age and the running economy of females has been reported to be equal or better than boys. However, these previous studies did not take into account sexual maturity and focused more on body mass. Maturation does not appear to affect absolute VO_2 in children age 12 when the data is adjusted for body mass[33] or in relative VO_2max.[34]

Sexual Maturity and Joint Laxity

There have been limited studies that have investigated pubertal status and joint laxity in both male and females. It is common among sport injury specialists to associate increased joint laxity with female athletes. Joint laxity can be assessed in various ways; however, the Beighton Scale

Figure 10-3. Beighton hyper-mobility scale.

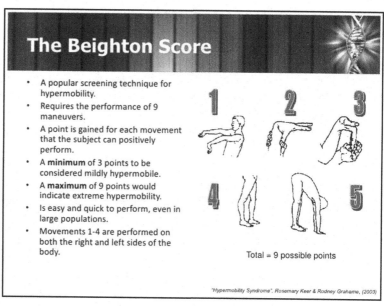

or Beighton-Horan Joint Mobility Index (BHJMI) is commonly used to assess joint laxity in youth[35] (Figure 10-3).

Anterior cruciate ligament (ACL) injury incidence has been reported higher in adolescent females than adolescent males. Prior to puberty there does not appear to be a difference in ACL injury rates. In a study by Quatman et al,[28] there was no joint laxity differences between males and females pre-puberty; however, post puberty, females were significantly more lax than males. Additionally, as females moved through the pubertal stages, they became more lax, while males moved through the pubertal stages and became less lax. While laxity may be a benefit to dancers, gymnasts, and martial arts, it is likely a risk factor in other competitive sports. Several studies have investigated the link between female maturation with increased peak knee abduction angle and post pubertal (post menarche).[24,28,36,37] A number of studies have linked poor dynamic alignment and lower extremity landing to increased risk for injury.[24,28,37,38] Because of these variables, the Tanner Maturation Scale and the BHJMI may be valid measures for assessing school aged children as they move through the levels of puberty.

Linking Tanner Stage to Injury Risk

Age has been linked with an increased injury risk along with grade and age group. It is unclear if this is due to more exposure time or higher level of play. For example, boy's ice hockey has noted increased concussion rate when checking becomes legal and gymnastics has noted increased injury when higher skills are allowed. Body size has been associated with injury risk in various ways. Hockey studies have noted that lighter players are more likely to be injured and Bantam players (13 to 14 y/o, average height = +65 inches; average weight = 134 lbs; average Tanner score 3.86/5) had higher incidence of injury (especially in competition).[39] In American football though, athletes with a high body mass index (BMI) who were considered oversized or obese had an increased risk of injury.[40] However, when age and biologic maturity (skeletal age and sexual maturity) are accounted for, differences are difficult to identify.[39,41-43] While children may have the same chronological age, there may be significant differences in their biologic maturity status. Several studies have attempted to link injury risk with early and late maturing boys as well as linking pre-menstrual and post-menstrual females.

During the period of rapid growth, adolescents appear to be at increased risk for sport related injuries.[43] Rapid growth of the tibia and the femur initiates height increases and raises the center of mass. Increased femur length has been linked to ACL injuries in female skiers and increased center of mass may also be a risk factor.[27] Adolescent growth spurt is associated with rapid growth and peak fracture rates, an increase in epiphyseal fractures in pubescence, and higher injury rates in peri-pubertal females (Tanner stages 2 and 3) compared to other young females (Tanner stages 1, 4, and 5).[6] Another indicator of rapid growth is foot length, this has also been used as a factor in comparing growth to maturation and injury risk.[24] A study by Backous et al[40] found that boys ages 6 to 17 with the highest incidence of injury were tall and weak (measured by grip strength) compared to short and strong. However, sexual maturity was not considered in the study. During maturation, males demonstrate a neuromuscular spurt while females seem to only have a skeletal spurt.[27,36,37,44] Chronological age, skeletal age, and secondary sexual characteristics when used together can provide valuable information to the clinician.

Medical screenings assess the health of the athlete and determine if participation is safe. Sport injury specialists use the health history questionnaire, physical examination, 12-element CV screening, and 90-second musculoskeletal to identify health conditions and pre-existing conditions/injuries that may predispose an athlete to injury or illness. Other screenings (Tanner secondary sexual maturity scales and Beighton Joint Laxity Scale) may assist in determining an adolescent's readiness for increased competition or identify specific predictors of injury. In addition, many clinicians will implement baseline fitness testing.

FITNESS AND DYNAMIC MOVEMENT TESTING

It's common for coaches at all levels to test the fitness components of their athletes prior to the season. The testing serves multiple purposes; to determine a starting point for conditioning programs, assess the effectiveness of off season training, motivate athletes to be compliant with a conditioning program, and possibly predict which athletes will perform well. It has also been assumed that higher levels of fitness decrease one's risk of injury; however, evidence of this is limited. The following section will review widely-used fitness and dynamic movement tests and describe the research supporting or not supporting their use.

Cardiorespiratory Fitness

Maximal oxygen uptake (VO_2max) is the gold standard for measuring cardiorespiratory fitness (CRF). This type of testing requires an athlete to run or bike at increasing intensities until they reach their absolute maximal heart rate and VO_2, which are monitored throughout the test. While very accurate, max testing is expensive and difficult to do with teams. Instead, field tests have been developed that can estimate an athlete's VO_2max from a timed distance of running or level reached. Table 10-4 outlines several of the most frequently used CRF tests.

Tests that require continuous work for at least 8 minutes are considered aerobic. More intense protocols that require sprints are anaerobic. Sports that blend both aerobic and anaerobic metabolic systems such as soccer, basketball, lacrosse, and hockey will either use multiple types of CRF tests or a test that combines both continuous running and sprinting, such as the YoYo test.

Several recent prospective studies have examined the impact of aerobic and anaerobic fitness on injury incidence.[45-49] The different measures used to assess CRF make conclusions about the predictive ability of a test difficult. Aerobic testing may be less useful than anaerobic tests in athletes, but more beneficial in military settings. Poor performance on anaerobic tests such as the 6 minute run and shuttle run increased the risk of injury[46] and the time lost[47] in rugby and Australian-rules football players. The evidence for traditional sports athletes is limited. Frisch et al[45] reported that the shuttle run was not related to the incidence of injury in youth football players. A study of European male soccer players found that poor aerobic conditioning was a risk factor for severe injuries[50] but a study of similar female athletes found no differences

TABLE 10-4		
COMMON FIELD TESTS FOR CARDIORESPIRATORY FITNESS		
NAME	**PROCEDURE**	**SCORING**
Cooper Run	Using a measured distance athletes run as hard as they can for 12 minutes.	The distance reached is correlated to a fitness level based on gender and age (www.exrx.net/Calculators/MinuteRun.html).
1.5 Mile Run	Athletes complete 1.5 miles as fast as possible. Walking is allowed, but lowers score.	Time measured in minutes and seconds is used to determine fitness level for gender and age (www.exrx.net/Calculators/OneAndHalf.html).
YoYo, Multistage, or Beep Test	20 meter distance is marked off and pre-recorded pacing beeps are needed. Athletes start at the 1st cone on the beep and must get to the 2nd cone by the next beep. Each pair of beeps is a stage. The time between beeps shortens with each stage. Recovery time between stages may include jogging and may also decrease as the test continues.	The number of stages completed is used to estimate fitness level based on gender and age (www.brianmac.co.uk/beep.htm).
300 Yard Shuttle Run (anaerobic)	Two cones are set 25 yards apart. Athlete runs the distance back and forth 6 times being sure to touch the marker on each turn.	The time needed to complete 300 yards (6 laps) is recorded. There are no normative data tables to place athletes into fitness levels. Coaches will determine what they believe to be appropriate times for positions.

based on CRF.[51] Grant et al[52] took measures of both aerobic and anaerobic fitness in male college hockey players and found no influence of CRF on injuries. In military and fire recruits, lower baseline scores on the 3 mile run, 3 kilometer run, and max treadmill test were associated with a higher risk of injury.[48,49] Body mass may also play a factor. Studies that assessed BMI and running times found that larger athletes who were fast had an increased injury risk.[46,52] The ability to create force (mass × speed) is another predisposing factor, especially in collision sports.[46] Evidence of cardiorespiratory fitness as a risk factor is lacking. Performance on CRF tests may reflect a readiness for physical training rather than a true risk of injury.

Muscular Tests

Tests that measure neuromuscular elements such as strength, endurance, flexibility, or balance are frequently included in fitness assessments. Muscular strength, endurance, and flexibility are properties that are specific to a muscle or group of muscles that produce a specific movement. Strength is the ability to move a heavy load a limited number of times. Strength tests such as the one repetition max bench press or squat assess the athlete's ability to recruit muscle fibers and maximal force production. Muscular endurance is the ability to contract a muscle over and over and tests the muscle's capacity for work and energy production. Exercises like pull ups, push-ups, or curl ups done to failure are used. Muscle fiber type and history of training will dictate how strong or fatigue resistant a muscle is. Athletes can train to develop both strength and endurance within the same muscles. Muscle flexibility refers to the length of the muscle itself which can be increased with consistent stretching. Muscle shortness is one reason for limited joint ROM. Flexibility is measured as joint ROM. Tests such as the sit and reach and back scratch involve multiple joints. Individual joints can be assessed by goniometry. Balance tests assess the coordination of the muscle actions, kinesthetic awareness, and nerve conduction.[53] Balance can be measured in both static and dynamic conditions. Holding the body stable while standing on one foot is an example of static balance. Maintaining proper alignment while bending forward and lifting the non-stance leg is dynamic balance. The term *dynamic stability* is also used to note a larger contribution of core and trunk muscles needed to perform more challenging movements.

There are numerous tests to assess the muscular strength, endurance, dynamic stability, or flexibility of athletes. Again because so many different tests are used, it is challenging to determine which if any, can be used to predict injury risk. Test results for one muscle group should not be generalized to the whole body. For example, the push up test assesses the muscular endurance of the pectoral and triceps muscles and an athlete may score very poorly on it but very high on maximum repetitions of the leg press. Multiple tests should be conducted if whole body results are desired or coaches may focus on muscular groups and movements that are key to their sport. There is little evidence that general muscular fitness tests are predictive of future injury (Table 10-5).

Some specific measures, uncommon to pre-season assessments, are more sensitive for certain of sport-related injuries. Reviews by Dallinga et al[54] and Murphy et al[55] suggested that tests of dynamic stability, hamstring to quadriceps ratio, ROM, and muscular imbalance at the ankle were clinically useful screenings. The Star Excursion Balance Test (SEBT) may be a particularly good tool for female athletes. Plisky et al[56] found that asymmetries on the anterior reach greater than 4 cm increased the risk of lower extremity injury nearly 3 times. Females with composite reaches <94% of their limb length had 6.5 times the risk of injury as those with better reach scores.[56] Balance and postural sway tests may also be predictive of future ankle injuries. The simple Single Leg Balance (SLB) test was used by Trojian and colleagues[57] to screen high school and college athletes for ankle injury risk. The RR for ankle sprain was 2.54 (95% CI, 1.02 to 6.03) if the SLT was positive.[57] Leetun et al[58] took isometric strength measurements of several trunk muscle groups including hip adductors, abductors, and internal and external rotators in college basketball and track athletes. Only poor hip external rotation was a significant predictor of lower extremity injury. A laboratory study of trunk stability found an increased likelihood of knee injury (OR = 2.14, p = .009) if athletes were unable to resist lateral displacement.[59] Muscular imbalance between the hamstrings and the quadriceps can be measured as a ratio between the 2, known as the H:Q ratio. This test requires an isokinetic dynamometer that is not widely available to most clinicians. Lower ratios indicate quadriceps dominance over the hamstring muscles and has been predictive of ACL injuries in women[60] and in hamstring strains in football.[61] An imbalance of strength or flexibility of the ankle increased the risk of ankle sprains in college-age athletes.[60] Ankle ROM is easily measured with a goniometer yet strength tests are best done with isokinetic equipment. Of the tests reviewed only the SEBT, SLT, and ROM measures are clinically relevant. Because of the lack of field tests to predict injury, clinicians have either developed their own testing programs or adapted laboratory measures. Two examples are the Functional Movement Screen (FMS) (Functional Movement Systems Incorporated) which combines dynamic stability and flexibility and tests of dynamic knee valgus for ACL risk.

Functional Movement Screening

The FMS is a battery of 7 tests that assess one's ability to produce basic multi-joint movements. It was developed by a group of Physical Therapists and Athletic Trainers as a means of evaluating

Table 10-5

Fitness Tests for Muscular Strength, Endurance, and Flexibility

STRENGTH

Name	Equipment	Procedure and Scoring
Grip Strength	Hand Dynamometer	Correctly adjust dynamometer for hand size. Have athlete squeeze slowly and hold for 2 to 3 seconds. Repeat 3 times and take best score (www.topendsports.com/testing/tests/handgrip.htm).
1 Rep Max	Weight Machine, Bench Press, or Squat Rack	Have athlete warm up by selecting a weight they can lift comfortably for 12 to 15 reps. Find the 10 rep max by increasing the weight by 10%. Ask athlete to lift as many times as possible with good form. If they can only complete 10 reps, divide that load by .75. This is their estimated 1 rep max. For every rep above 10 add .025 to the denominator. Divide the 1 rep max load by the athlete's weight to create a strength ratio. Scoring is specific to the lift and not available for all machines, ages or genders (www.sport-fitness-advisor.com/strengthtests.html).
4 Level Abdominal Strength Test	Mat and partner	Athlete will attempt 4 progressively harder forms of a sit up. The quality of the movement is graded from 0 to 4 based on easy of contraction. The 4 sit ups are; knees bent and feet held, knees bent and feet not held, legs straight and feet held, legs straight and feet not held. Only one rep of each form is needed (www.topendsports.com/testing/tests/ab-strength.htm).

ENDURANCE

Name	Equipment	Procedure and Scoring
Partial Curl Up	Mat, Tape, Measuring Tape, Metronome and Stopwatch	Mark a 12 cm distance using 2 pieces of tape. Athlete lays on back with knees bent to 90 degrees positioned so that the tips of their middle finger are touching the top of the first tape line. Set the metronome to 40 bpm. In pace with the tones, the athlete should crunch forward until their fingertips touch the second piece of tape. The athlete should do as many curl ups as possible, but only full reps (fingers touch line) are counted. If athlete cannot hold the slow pace or they reach 75 reps the tests is stopped. Scoring is based on age and gender.

	Males 20 to 29 years	Females 20 to 29 years
Excellent	56 to 75	45 to 70
Good	31 to 55	32 to 44
Average	24 to 30	21 to 31

(continued)

TABLE 10-5 (CONTINUED)		
FITNESS TESTS FOR MUSCULAR STRENGTH, ENDURANCE, AND FLEXIBILITY		
STRENGTH		
Name	*Equipment*	*Procedure and Scoring*
Push-up Test	Mat	Males lift body from toes. Females from knees. Must maintain flat back position throughout. Athletes complete as many reps as possible with good form, without stopping (www.exrx.net/Calculators/PushUps.html).
Bench Press Test	Bench Press Rack and Metronome	Set metronome for 60 bpm. Male athletes lift 80 lbs. Females lift 35 lbs. Keeping pace with the tones, athletes lift bar from chest to full elbow extension as many times as possible without arching their back or touching their chest with the bar (www.exrx.net/Calculators/YBenchPress.html).
FLEXIBILITY		
Name	*Equipment*	*Procedure and Scoring*
Sit and Reach	Sit and Reach Box	Measure each leg separately. Athlete may stretch prior to test. Without shoes, athletes places the sole of one foot on under the platform of the box and bend the opposite knee. Hands should be stacked on each other as the athlete starts with arms overhead and flexes trunk to push the measurement tab forward. Movement should be slow and controlled. Athlete should hold stretched position for 2 to 3 seconds before returning to start. Repeat 3 times on each leg and use the best score for each leg (www.exrx.net/Calculators/SitReach.html).
Back Scratch Test	Measuring Tape or Yard Stick	Ask athlete to touch their hands behind their back. The top arm is in external rotation and the bottom is internally rotated. Measure the distance between the middle fingers or the overlap of the fingertips. Repeat with the other arm on top. Record distances as R/L based on which is the top arm. Scoring is based on touching or not touching fingertips (http://sportsmedicine.about.com/od/fitnessevalandassessment/qt/ShoulderFlex.htm).
Joint Specific ROM	Goniometer	Common joints to measure are the hips, shoulders and ankles.

an athlete's potential athletic performance and risk of injury. The 7 tests are simple movements that require dynamic balance, core stability, and flexibility to accomplish. A full description of the tests can be found in the suggested reading by Cook, Burton, Hoogenboom, and Voight.

Four of the movements assess the right and left sides individually and 3 include a clearing test to check for the presence of pain. Each movement is scored from 0 to 3 and the total of the 7 tests is recorded out of a possible 21 points. Pain with any of the movements results in a score of 0. A score of 3 represents no biomechanical compensations in the movement pattern and no modifications were needed. Compensations are joint actions that assist in accomplishing the movement but are inefficient. For example in order to get the foot over the barrier in the hurdle step test, a patient may externally rotation their hip and bring the foot over the hurdle at an angle rather than straight across. The substitution of the gluteal muscles allows the patient to step over the hurdle but points to a lack of core stability, hip flexor strength, and flexibility in the posterior muscles. Common FMS compensations include side-bending to maintain balance trunk flexion to complete a deep squat and pelvic rotation. Three tests can be modified if a compensatory action is produced on the first try. A score of 2 is given if the patient can complete the movement but uses a compensatory action or can do the movement correctly once it's been modified. A test is graded a 1 if the patient cannot complete the full movement even with a modification or cannot hold the correct starting position without losing balance. The difference between the muscular fitness test described earlier and the FMS is that the quality of the movement pattern is being graded rather than the volume of work.

Assessing Risk of Injury

The FMS assumes that muscular compensations indicate underlying biomechanical inefficiencies (muscular imbalances, limited ranges of motions, lack of core stability) that predispose athletes to injury. A number of longitudinal cohort studies have been conducted to determine if lower scores on the FMS are predictive of sport-related injury. The initial test was conducted by Kiesel and colleagues on 46 professional football players.[62] Screenings were done during pre-season training and injuries resulting in 3 or more weeks of lost time were included. The authors found that those with a score of 14 or lower had a much greater chance of serious injury than those with higher scores (OR = 11.87). The study was repeated in 2013 with a larger sample (N = 238). This time any musculoskeletal injury that resulted in lost time was added to the analysis. The relative risk of injury decreased to 1.8763. An additional finding was that athletes that lacked symmetry (different scores for right and left sides) on one or more tests also had an increased risk of injury (RR = 1.8).[63] A study of female college basketball, soccer and volleyball athletes found a higher risk level for scores ≤14 (OR = 3.85). The risk increased when athletes with repaired ACLs were excluded (OR = 4.58).[64] And, when the shoulder mobility test was removed from the analysis, the relationship between FMS score and lower extremity injuries was very strong (r = .95, p = 0.0003). These studies helped establish 14 as the threshold for increased risk, but that cut point is debatable. Recently, Shojaedin et al[65] saw an increased risk of musculoskeletal injury in soccer, handball, and basketball athletes scoring ≤17 (OR = 4.7). Knapik and colleagues[66] even suggest different cut points for male (≤12) and females (≤15) after studying military academy cadets during their initial training.

Military personnel and firefighters are also frequently used as participants in FMS studies. Injuries during training are costly and result in fewer graduates and increased medical and salary expenses. A study of 108 recruits at a firefighting academy found that those with scores ≤14 were 8 times more likely to be injured over the 16 week training period. And, individual scores of the deep squat and the trunk stability push up were also predictors of future injury.[67] The functional movements of 874 Marines were scored prior to 68 days or 38 days of training. Again, scores ≤14 were associated with higher risks of injury; RR = 1.65 in the longer training group and 1.91 in the shorter training group.[68] O'Connor and colleagues also highlighted the relationship between overall fitness and FMS scores. Only 6.6% of the high-fit Marines had FMS scores ≤14. While 79.8% of the subpar FMS scorers were in the lower fit category.[68] When low FMS scores were combined with slower times on a 3-mile run test the relative risk of injury increased to 4.2.[48]

Studies of athletes have also looked at relationships between other performance and screening tests. Lehr and colleagues[69] strengthened the predictive ability of the FMS by combining scores from the Lower Quarter Y-Balance Test. They divided athletes (N = 63) into high and low risk categories based on an algorithm developed from the 2 tests. The high-risk athletes sustained lower extremity injuries 3 times as often as the low risk group. Correlations between sprint times, leg strength, and power measures and FMS scores are small and non-significant in a group of college golfers.[70] Waist circumference in adults[71] and weight in children[72] were inversely associated with FMS score. Measures of core stability did not correlate well to the 7 FMS movements[73] despite Cook et al's focus on maintaining spinal alignment.

Criticisms of the FMS

Published reviews of the FMS agree that the composite score can distinguish those at higher risks for injury.[74,75] However, concerns about the test's validity, learning effect, cut point, and use as a measure of rehabilitation have been raised. The validity of the FMS is questioned by studies showing that test scores are not well correlated to each other,[76] nor are they strongly related to measures of core stability[73] or static balance.[77] Sensitivity and specificity for the FMS are rather low. The reported sensitivity scores are .45, .54, and .58 with specificities of .71, .74, and .91.[62,64,68] Frost et al[78] points out participants can adjust their movement to better fit the scoring criteria and that changes to the composite score may be from a learning effect rather than from training or functional ability. While several studies do support the use of 14/21 as the cut point for injury risk, some have been critical of the fact that all 7 tests are weighted the same.[75] And there are several studies that support higher[65,79] or lower cut points.[66] Next, functional training programs have not produced scores that are significantly different from traditional weight training programs.[80,81] Lastly, the claim that higher FMS scores relate to better athletic performance has not been substantiated by any research study thus far.[70,73]

Dynamic Valgus Testing

Several authors have suggested that an athlete's risk of ACL injury can be established by looking at knee position and lower leg alignment during jumping and squatting movements.[82-84] Video analysis of non-contact ACL injuries revealed that the knee was often in a valgus position with the hip externally rotated.[85] Further biomechanical analysis of male and female athletes has revealed a number of interesting things; females generally have less knee and hip flexion at landing,[86] their knees and feet are closer together than males at take-off and landing,[87] and in females one or both knees are more likely to pinch inward.[86] Females reach maximal levels of hip adduction, knee flexion, and genu valgus earlier in the declaration phase (landing) than males[88] and changes during puberty have been noted with males decreasing valgus alignments as they mature.[89] As discussed in Chapter 8, women have a significantly greater risk of ACL injury than men, the gender differences seen in biomechanical analysis has lead a number of researchers to propose that a lack of neuromuscular control during jumping, cutting, and stopping maneuvers is a modifiable risk factor for ACL tears.[82-84,87]

Testing for dynamic valgus began with sophisticated video and force analysis equipment in biomechanics labs in the early 2000's, but has become more accessible to coaches and athletic trainers. Several studies have shown screenings using little to no video equipment to be sensitive and reliable.[90,91] Munro points out there are several movement components that make up the position that is commonly referred to as dynamic knee valgus and the degree to which an athlete displays any of these differs. They include hip internal rotation, pelvic drop, hip adduction, tibial external rotation, and mid-foot pronation.[82] Figure 10-4 is a classic example of dynamic knee valgus during landing.

The severity of dynamic knee valgus can be measured as knee separation distance (KSD) and frontal plane projection angle (FPPA) when still video frames are used (Figures 10-5 and 10-6).

Other techniques include counting the number of alignment and balance errors seen, grading scales of mild, moderate and severe, or positive/negative determinations.

Screening Tests

There are several jumping, cutting, and squatting movements in the literature that produce observable dynamic knee valgus in participants. The most commonly used one is the drop vertical

Figure 10-4. Example of dynamic knee valgus on landing.

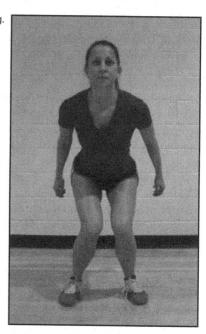

Figure 10-5. Measurement of knee separation distance.

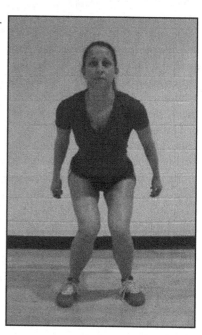

jump (DVJ). An athlete drops or jumps from a 12-inch box, lands, and then performs a vertical jump for maximum height. According to Noyes and colleagues there are 3 positions of interest; pre-land, landing, and take-off.[87] A simple video recorded from the frontal can be reviewed in slow motion. The key sign to look for is the inward movement (adduction) of the knee as the athlete goes from pre-landing (toes just off ground) to the deepest point of knee flexion during the landing and a smaller outward movement of the knee at take-off. All athletes should wear shorts and shoes for testing. Marking bony landmarks (superior iliac crest, mid-patella, mid-tibia, and lateral malleolus) with bright stickers improves the clinician's ability to see changes in the kinetic chain. When scoring the DVJ without computer software, the clinician can grade the severity of

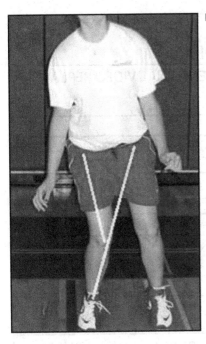

Figure 10-6. Measurement of frontal plane protection angle.

the valgus motion or can grade the test as positive or negative. Single-leg VDJ are equally reliable, but should be conducted after double leg analysis.[82]

Another test developed by Padua et al uses a slightly different jump and is scored by counting the number of misalignments.[92] The landing error scoring system or LESS can be done with or without video recording. The jump for LESS combines a forward motion (Table 10-6).

Instead of coming straight down from a 12-inch box, athletes are instructed to jump out to a distance equal to half their height, and then perform a maximal vertical jump. Higher error scores mean greater dynamic valgus and thus higher risk. If screening without video replay, the athlete should repeat the jump 4 times while the clinician looks for 10 possible errors.[91] If video footage from the front and side are used, then there are 17 possible errors. Errors are weighted as 1 or 2 point mistakes, so that the maximum scores of the tests are 15 and 18, respectively.

A single leg squat will also induce knee valgus in many athletes (Figure 10-7). Ugalde and colleagues found that the single leg squat was equally as effect as 2-D video analysis of DVJ test in high school and middle school athletes.[93] An additional advantage of the single leg squat according to Munro is that it puts the least amount of strain on the ACL and presents the lowest risk of injury.[82]

Algorithms

An algorithm is a mathematical equation that combines multiple factors in order to predict an outcome. Since dynamic knee valgus is made up of several movements and forces acting on the lower extremity, some researchers have sought a way to quantify the various contributions to the misalignment. The equations are individualized for each athlete by using data from biomechanical analysis[94] or more easily attained clinical measures such as BMI, tibial length, knee range of motion, and quadriceps to hamstring strength ratios.[95,96] Studies indicate that these formulas are sensitive enough to predict the amount of shearing force produced during a DVJ called the *knee abduction moment* (KAM). Higher KAMs are thought to a risk factor for ACL tears.[95]

		TABLE 10-6 **LESS SCORING ERRORS**		
	REAL-TIME OBSERVATIONS **MAX = 15**		**2-DIMENSIONAL VIDEO REPLAY** **MAX = 19**	
Trial	*View*		*View*	
1	F	Stance Width too wide or too narrow +1	F	Stance Width too wide +1 Stance Width too narrow +1
1	F	Foot Rotated Internally or Externally +1F	F	Foot Rotated Internally +1 Foot Rotated Externally +1
1	F	Asymmetrical Foot Landing +1	F	Asymmetrical Foot Landing +1
2	F	Maximum Knee Valgus small +1 large +2	F	Knee Valgus Displacement Is toe inline or medial to center of patella +1
2	F	Lateral Trunk Flexion on contact +1	F	Lateral Trunk Flexion at contact +1
3	S	Landing on Heels or Flat-footed +1	S	Landing on Heels or Flat-footed +1
3	S	Knee Flexion after Landing small +2 average +1	S	Knee Flexion after Landing If 45 degrees more than angle at contact +1
4	S	Trunk Flexion after Landing small +2 average +1	S	Trunk Flexion at Contact Lack of trunk flexion, too upright +1
all	S	Joint Displacement from Side View soft landing +0 average absorption +1 stiff landing +2	S	Joint Displacement from Side View soft landing +0 average absorption +1 stiff landing +2
all		Overall Impression excellent +0 average +1 poor +2	F S	Overall Impression excellent +0 average +1 poor +2
			S	Knee Flexion at contact Not at least 30 degrees +1
			S	Hip Flexion at contact If thigh is in line with trunk +1

(continued)

	REAL-TIME OBSERVATIONS MAX = 15		2-DIMENSIONAL VIDEO REPLAY MAX = 19	
TABLE 10-6 (CONTINUED) **LESS SCORING ERRORS**				
Trial	View		View	
			F	Knee Valgus at contact Is mid-foot medial to center of patella +1
			S	Hip Flexion at Max Knee Flexion No increase in Hip Flexion after contact +1
			S	Trunk Flexion at Max Knee Flexion +1 No increase Trunk Flexion after contact

Adapted from Padua DA, Boling MC, DiStefano LJ, Onate JA, Beutler AI, Marshall SW. Reliability of the landing error scoring system-real time, a clinical assessment tool of jump-landing biomechanics. *J Sport Rehabil.* 2011;20:145-156 and Padua DA, Marshall SW, Boling MC, Thigpen CA, Garrett WE, Beutler AI. The Landing Error Scoring System (LESS) is a valid and reliable clinical assessment tool of jump-landing biomechanics: The JUMP-ACL study. *Am J Sport Med.* 2009;37(10):1996-2002.

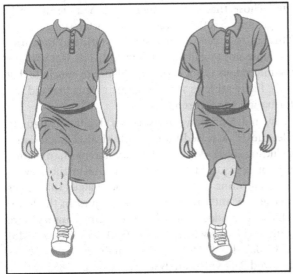

Figure 10-7. Dynamic knee valgus in single leg squat.

Relationship to Athlete Maturation

Gender is known to be a risk factor for ACL injury. Females have twice the risk of males, especially in high school and college sports.[97] Neuromuscular changes during maturation may, in part, explain why there is a noticeable increase in female ACL injuries post-puberty. Hewett et al[36] and Quatman et al[44] found differences in force production and force absorption during the DVJ test. Males increased vertical jump scores by 12.5% with each Tanner stage, while girls had no change in force production.[36] Landing forces decreased in boys but not girls as the matured.[44] Another study by Schmitz and colleagues[89] tested both dynamic knee valgus and muscular strength in young athletes ages 9 to 18 years. The results were somewhat different. Here dynamic knee valgus increased as females matured and decreased as males matured. There was not relationship between muscular strength, measured by distance in a single-leg triple jump, and dynamic knee valgus.[89] More recently, Sigward et al[98] noted that KAM was not significantly different between males and females at pre-puberty. But, the ratio of knee flexion to hip flexion and rates of energy absorption were already lower in females in this first stage. As maturation increased the gender differences in all 3 variables were more apparent.[98] A limitation of these studies is that the presence of secondary sex characteristics was self-reported or reported by parents. Increased neuromuscular control and possibly muscular strength appear to occur in boys between Tanner stages 2 through 5 that are not taking place for females as the grow. This evidence points to the need for training and conditioning programs for females at younger ages than previously thought.

Prediction of Risk of Anterior Cruciate Ligament Injury

The ability to accurately observe or measure a risk factor is only one part of creating an effective screening tool. The second piece is linking the score of the screening test to the occurrence of injury. The presence of a risk factor should increase the likelihood of having a specific injury. Despite researchers' success at being able to isolate and identify the knee valgus position in the laboratory and in field tests, they have been not been able to show that athletes with dynamic valgus injure their ACL at greater rates than those without dynamic valgus. In other words, having positive dynamic valgus doesn't appear to be a predictor of ACL injury.

A study by Hewitt and colleagues[99] in 2005, provides some evidence for the use of the DVJ as an ACL screening test. They conducted a longitudinal cohort study of 205 high school female athletes. Prior to their season, the athletes' biomechanics were analyzed using force plates and 3-D video analysis during the DVJ. Nine ACL injuries occurred in the following season. According to Hewett et al, all 9 athletes displayed dynamic valgus. Those that injured their ACL had significantly greater knee valgus angles at landing, KAM, ground reaction forces, and shorter stance times than the 196 that did not tear their ACL. This study is very limited by the statistical measures used. Unlike most cohort studies, the authors chose not to calculate RR or OR. The fact that the athletes who were injured had measurable dynamic valgus is not enough evidence to conclude that dynamic valgus is a true risk factor. There were likely athletes with dynamic valgus that did not suffer an ACL injury. Unfortunately, this information was not reported.

Recent studies with better methodology have not found any measures of dynamic valgus to be predictive of ACL injury. Nilstad and colleagues[100] assessed multiple physical characteristics of elite female soccer players (N = 173) including BMI, lower extremity strength, dynamic balance, knee valgus during the DVJ, knee joint laxity, and foot pronation. As in the Hewett study, 3-D biomechanical analysis was used to determine the amount of knee valgus in degrees from neutral. The only characteristic that was significantly related to a new injury in the lower extremity was BMI (OR = 1.51, 95% CI 1.21-1.90). The odds of any lower extremity injury were nearly even between those with dynamic valgus and those without (OR = 0.90, 95% CI 0.71-1.15) and quite low for a knee injury (OR = 0.12, 95% CI 0.01-1.30).[100] The algorithm developed by Myers et al[95] to predict KAM from clinical measures and 2-D video analysis was used on 1855 female athletes in a prospective by Goetschius and colleagues.[96] There were 20 confirmed ACL ruptures during the next season. While the risk of injury increased with higher predicted KAM scores, the ORs were not significantly different from those who injured their ACL and those who did not. The LESS has also been tested to see if its scores are predictive of ACL injury. A very large sample (N = 5047) of male and female high school and college athletes was assessed by Smith et al[101] and followed for one season. Again while the odds of suffering an ACL injury increased with higher LESS scores, the ORs were not significantly different from those with lower LESS scores. This was true of both the full sample analysis and of the individual gender analysis.

Possible explanations for the lack of support for dynamic valgus screenings as predictors of ACL injury center around the low frequency of ACL injury, that follow-up is limited to one season, and that the mechanism of injury includes more than just knee valgus. Even the large study by Smith and colleagues only had 28 ACL tears. The smaller number of injured participants limits the power of the statistical analysis when using a case-control method. Each of these studies above only considered the risk of ACL injury in immediate season. Longer follow-up (2 to 4 seasons) may improve the predictive ability of the dynamic valgus tests. Another reasonable conclusion is that the true mechanism of ACL injuries is a combination of factors, both biomechanical and environmental. As suggested by Padua et al,[92] valgus movement alone is not enough to create a shearing force on the ACL. In fact, direct valgus pressure would injure the MCL first. It's more likely that a combination of biomechanical forces (knee valgus, anterior, and rotational loads) is acting on the ACL. Lastly, an athlete with a susceptibility such as dynamic valgus has to encounter a precipitating event. In other words, the at-risk athlete has to be at the wrong place at the wrong time. Other factors besides dynamic knee valgus are involved. For example, the playing surface or conditions, the play occurring, and the aggressiveness of opponents and officiating of the game may contribute.

Need for Corrective Exercise

Dynamic knee valgus may or may not be an actual risk factor for ACL tears, but it is a sign of poor neuromuscular control that can be improved. The root cause of dynamic knee valgus is not completely clear. Its relationship to muscular weakness in the hip abductors and external rotators has been suggested. Cashman[102] reviewed 11 studies that measured the strength of hip abduction and/or external rotation and dynamic knee valgus in healthy active participants. All correlations between FPPA were small to moderate in size. Only 4 studies found a significant relationship between knee valgus and hip weakness; 3 for hip abduction and 1 for external rotation. Cashman concluded that there is some evidence to suggest that dynamic valgus is related to weak lateral and posterior hip muscles.

Resistance training however, has shown to be effective for decreasing dynamic valgus and may reduce the incidence of ACL injuries. Noyes and colleagues report improvements in landing KSD of adolescent female athletes after a 6-week neuromuscular training program.[87] Thirty-nine of the 62 training participants had KSD that were ≤60% of neutral. Post training 23 of the 39 had improved to better than 60%. The exercise program included stretching, plyometric jump training, and weight training for 1 hour, 3 days a week.[87] Similar exercise programs have produced similar results in females in the higher risk sports of soccer,[103] basketball[104] and volleyball,[105] and in pre-pubescent male and female athletes.[37] DiStefanco and colleagues found that the specificity of the training program did not matter. They compared a general training group to a group that received individualized exercises based on their movement deficits. Both groups had similar improvements in LESS scores. However, those with the highest baseline scores had the greatest percentage of improvement.[106] So far, 3 studies have linked neuromuscular training to a lower incidence of ACL injuries. Hewett et al[38] reported a significant decrease in IR per 1000 AE between high school female athletes that completed a plyometric-based program (0.12) and those that were untrained (0.43). The incidence of ACL injury of the trained females was not significantly different than the male comparison group.[38] Noyes and Barber-Westin[107] included these studies along with 5 others that did not find at reduction in ACL injures post neuromuscular training in a systemic review. The authors concluded that there is evidence to support the use of preventive training. The NNT is quite high (ranges from 70 to 98,107) and clinicians should understand the scope on which successful training programs are implemented.

It's unclear if functional movement scores can be improved by physical training. In a recently published CAT, Minthorn et al[108] found 2 out of 3 experimental studies that reported improved FMS scores using post-exercise training. The strongest study was conducted by Bodden et al[109] using martial arts athletes. The researchers tested intervention and control participants at both the mid-point and post the 8-week intervention. The training group had significant increases at 4 weeks and was better than controls at both 4 and 8 weeks.[109] The next study lacked a control group. Kiesel and colleagues[110] put 62 professional football athletes on a 7-week off-season conditioning program that included stretching, trigger point massage, and trunk dynamic balance exercises. It was unclear if these activities were in addition to their normal off-season training or in place of. There was a significant improvement in scores from pre to post and fewer athletes displayed asymmetry after training.[110] The less effective study was conducted by Frost et al[80] using 60 firefighters. Here, the control group had improved scores along with the 2 intervention groups making an accurate comparison difficult. One study has linked corrective core exercise and stretching to a reduction in injuries in firefighters.[79] More evidence is needed to determine if conditioning programs that target the trunk stabilizations, dynamic balance, and/or flexibility can improve FMS scores. Additionally, no study has tested both FMS and dynamic knee valgus to see if a single conditioning program would improve both screening tests.

Bringing it Together

Best practice for medical screening of athletes must include a health history questionnaire, the 12-element CV screening, and the 90-second musculoskeletal screening. Standardization of the PPE is necessary to determine its true efficacy. When chronologically younger athletes are eligible for participation alongside post-pubescent athletes, secondary sexual maturation may assist health care providers in determining physical readiness and can identify lack of maturity as a predictor of injury. Laboratory exercise testing that assesses maximal cardiorespiratory fitness to measure VO_2max and muscular strength using dynamometers can be expensive. Field tests for health and skill related components of fitness are widely used but these scores may not be valid predictors of injury. Dynamic tests, like the FMS and the DVJ, have been developed by clinician's as an alternative and have been linked to risk factors that increase injury risk. In increase in dynamic knee valgus has been noted in post pubescent females (Tanner stage 5). Athletic trainers can use these dynamic measures as baselines, implement corrective exercise programs, and re-asses risk levels post intervention. Improvements to dynamic stability and neuromuscular control will hopefully lead to reduced incidence of injury, especially for post-pubescent females.

Learning Activities

1. Fill out a health history questionnaire (and time how long it takes). Review answers with a parent to determine your accuracy. Copies of the HHQ can be found at:

   - http://www.mcancer.org/files/health-questionnaire.pdf
   - https://www.stlukes.org/uploadedFiles/Patients/Outpatient_Admission_Forms/INTERVENT%20Initial-HHQ.pdf
   - http://myhealthclinicalaska.com/wp-content/uploads/2012/08/health-history-questionnaire.pdf.

2. Make a list of all the reasons why state high school associations should require ECG for all athletes? Now, list all the reasons why they should not.

3. Review the American Academy of Pediatrics Recommendations for participation in competitive sports and identify conditions that would restrict or disqualify an athlete.

4. Conduct these field tests with the class. What were the challenges of testing all in one day?

- FMS
- Push up test
- Curl up test
- Sit and reach
- Vertical jump
- Timed 1-mile run

References

1. Seto C. The pre-participation physical examination: An update. *Clin Sports Med*. 2011:491-501.
2. Armsey T, Hosey R. Medical aspects of sports: Epidemiology of injuries, preparticipation examination, and drugs in sports. *Clin. Sports Med*. 2004 255-279.
3. Sanders B, Blackburn T, Boucher B. Clinical Commentary: Preparticipation screening – The sports physical therapist perspective. *Int J Sports Phys Therapy*. 2013;8:180-193.
4. Seto C, Pendelton M. Preparticipation cardiovascular screening in young athletes: Current guidelines and dilemmas. *Curr Sports Med Rep*. 2009;8:59-64.
5. Levy D, Delaney J. A risk/tolerance approach to the preparticipation examination. *Clin J Sports Med*. 2012;22:309-310.
6. Caine D, Maffulli N, Caine C. Epidemiology of injury in child and adolescent sports injury rates, risk factors, and prevention. *Clin Sports Med*. 2008;27:19-50.
7. Donnelly D, Howard T. Electrocardiography and the preparticipation physical examination: Is it time for routine screening? *Curr Sports Med Rep*. 2006;5:67-73.
8. Rauch C, Phillips G. Adherence to guidelines for cardiovascular screening in current high school preparticipation evaluation forms. *J Pediatr*. 2009;155:584-586.
9. Wingfield K, Matheson G, Meeuwisse W. Preparticipation evaluation: an evidenced-based review. *Clin J Sports Med*. 2004;14:109-122.
10. Carek P, Mainous A. The preparticipation physical examination for athletics: A systematic review of current recommendations. *Brit Med J*. 2003;327:170-173.
11. Mayer F BK, Cassel M, Mueller S, et al. Medical results of preparticipation examination in adolescent athletes. *J Sports Med*. 2012 46:524-530.
12. Robel K. Electronic PPE format dramatically increases complaince. NATA News. 2010;April 26-28.
13. Gomez J, Landry G, Bernhardt D. Critical evaluation of the 2-minute orthopedic screening examination. *Am J Dis Child*. 1993;147:1109-1113.
14. Junge A GK, Feddermann N, Dvorak J Pre-competition orthopedic assessment of international elite football players. *Clin J Sports Med*. 2009;19:316-328.
15. O'Connor F, Johnson J, Chalpin M, Oriscello R, Taylor D. A pilot study of clinical agreement in cardiovascular preparticipation examinations. *Clin J Sports Med*. 2005;15:177-179.
16. Corrado D, Basso C, Pavei A, Michieli P, Schiavon M, Thiene G. Trends in sudden cardiovascular death in young competitive athletes after implementation of a preparticipation screening program. *JAMA*. 2006;296(13):1593-1601.
17. Estes NAM, 3rd, Link MS. Preparticipation athletic screening including an electrocardiogram: an unproven strategy for prevention of sudden cardiac death in the athlete. *Prog Cardiovasc Dis*. 2012;54(5):451-454.
18. Harmon KG, Asif IM, Klossner D, Drezner JA. Incidence of sudden cardiac death in National Collegiate Athletic Association athletes. *Circulation*. 2011;123(15):1594-1600.
19. Sheikh N, Sharma S. Overview of sudden cardiac death in young athletes. *Phys Sportsmed*. 2011;39:22-36.
20. Maron BJ DJ, Haas TS, Tierney DM, Mueller FO. Profile and frequency of sudden death in 1463 young competitive athletes: from a 25 year U.S. national registry, 1980-2005. American Heart Association Scientific Sessions; November 12–15, 2006; Chicago, IL.
21. Steinvil A, Chundadze T, Zeltser D, et al. Mandatory electrocardiographic screening of athletes to reduce their risk for sudden death; proven fact or wishful thinking? *J Am Coll Cardiol*. 2011;57(11):1291-1296.
22. Koch S, Cassel M, Linné K, Mayer F, Scharhag J. ECG and echocardiographic findings in 10-15-year-old elite athletes. *Eur J Prev Cardiol*. 2012;21(6):774-781.
23. Magee C, Kazman J, Haigney M, et al. Reliability and validity of clinician ECG interpretation for athletes. *Ann Noninvasive Electrocardiol*. 2014;19:319-329.

24. Bowerman E, Whatman C, Harris N, Bradshaw E, Karin J. Are maturation, growth and lower extremity alignment associated with overuse injury in elite adolescent ballet dancers? *Phys Therapy Sport*. 2014;15:234-241.

25. Backous D, Farrow J, Friedl K. Assessment of pubertal maturity in boys, using height and grip strength. *J Adolesc Health Care*. 1990 11(6):497-500.

26. Kreipe RE GH. Physical maturity screening for participation in sports. *Pediatrics*. 1985;75(6):1076-1080.

27. Myer GD FK, Divine JG, Wall EJ, Kahanov L, Hewett TE. Longitudinal assessment of noncontact anterior cruciate ligament injury risk factors during maturation in a female athlete: a case report. *J Athl Train*. 2009;44:101-109.

28. Quatman CE FK, Myer GD, Paterno MV, Hewett TE. The effects of gender and maturational status on generalized joint laxity in young athletes. *J Sci Med Sport*. 2008;11:257-263.

29. Malina RM P-RM, Eisenmann JC, Horta L, Rodrigeus J, Miller R. Height, weight, and skeletal maturity of elite Portuguese soccer players aged 11-16. *J Sport Sci*. 2000;18:685-693.

30. Monteilh C KS, Flanders WD, Maisonet M, et al. The timing of maturation and predictors of tanner stage transitions in boys enrolled in a contemporary british cohort. *Paediatr Perinat Epidemiol*. 2010;25:75-87.

31. O'Grady K. Early puberty for girls. The new 'normal' and why we need to be concerned. *Can Womens Health Net*. http://www.cwhn.ca/en/node/39365. Published 2008. Accessed January 9, 2015.

32. Ré A, Bojikian LP, Teixeira CP, Böhme MTS. Relationship between growth, motor performance, chronological age and biological maturation in young male. *Revista Brasileira de Educação Física e Esporte*. 2005;19:153-162.

33. Armstrong N, Welsman J, Kirby B. Submaximal exercise and maturation in 12 year olds. *J Sport Sci*. 1999;17:107-111.

34. Lariviere G LA. Physical maturity in young elite ice hockey players. *Canadian J App Sport Sci*. 1986;11:24.

35. Smits-Engelsman B, Klerks M, Kirby A. Beighton score: a valid measure for generalized hypermobility. *J Pediatr*. 2010;158:119-123.

36. Hewett TE, Myer GD, Ford KR, Slauterbeck JR. Preparticipation physical examination using a box drop vertical jump test in young athletes: the effects of puberty and sex. *Clin J Sport Med*. 2006;16:298-304.

37. Barber-Westin SD, Galloway M, Noyes FR, Corbett G, Walsh C. Assessment of lower limb neuromuscular control in prepubescent athletes. *Am J Sports Med*. 2005;33(12):1853-1860.

38. Hewett TE, Lindenfeld TN, Riccobene JV, Noyes FR. The effect of neuromuscular training on the incidence of knee injury in female athletes: a prospective study. / Effet d'un entrainement neuromusculaire sur l'incidence de blessures au genou chez des athletes feminines. *Am J Sports Med*. 1999;27(6):699-706.

39. Stuart MJ1 SA, Nieva JJ, Rock MG. Injuries in youth ice hockey: a pilot surveillance strategy. *Mayo Clin Proc*. 1995;Apr;70:350-356.

40. Backous D, Friedl K, Smith N, Parr T, Carpine W. Soccer injuries and their relation to physical maturity. *Amer J Disease Child*. 1988;142:839-842.

41. Emery C, Meeuwisse W, Hartmann S. Evaluation of risk factors for injury in adolescent soccer: implementation and validation of an injury surveillance system. *Am J Sports Med*. 2005;33(12):1882-1891.

42. Le Gall F CC, Reilly T Biological maturity and injury in elite youth football. *Scand J Med Sci Sports*. 2007;17(5):564-572.

43. Baxter-Jones A, Maffulli N, Helms P. Low injury rates in elite athletes. *Arch Dis Child*. 1993;68:130-132.

44. Quatman CE, Ford KR, Myer GD, Hewett TE. Maturation leads to gender differences in landing force and vertical jump performance: a longitudinal study. *Am J Sports Med*. 2006;34(5):806-813.

45. Frisch A, Urhausen A, Seil R, Croisier JL, Windal T, Theisen D. Association between preseason functional tests and injuries in youth football: A prospective follow-up. *Scand J Med Sci Sports*. 2011;21(6):e468-e476.

46. Gabbett TJ, Ullah S, Finch CF. Identifying risk factors for contact injury in professional rugby league players – Application of a frailty model for recurrent injury. *J Sci Med Sport*. 2012;15(6):496-504.

47. Gastin PB, Meyer D, Huntsman E, Cook J. Low body mass and aerobic running fitness increase injury risk in elite australian football. *Int J Sports Physiol Perform*. 2014.

48. Lisman P, O'Connor FG, Deuster PA, Knapik JJ. Functional movement screen and aerobic fitness predict injuries in military training. *Med Sci Sports Exerc*. 2013;45:636-643.

49. Poplin GS, Roe DJ, Peate W, Harris RB, Burgess JL. The association of aerobic fitness with injuries in the fire service. *Am J Epidemiol*. 2014;179:149-155.

50. Chomiak J, Junge A, Peterson L, Dvorak J. Severe injuries in football players: influencing factors. Blessures graves chez les joueurs de football: facteurs impliques. *Am J Sports Med*. 2000;28(5 Suppl):S58-s68.

51. Ostenberg A, Roos H. Injury risk factors in female European football. A prospective study of 123 players during one season. *Scand J Med Sci Sports*. 2000;10(5):279.

52. Grant JA, Bedi A, Kurz J, Bancroft R, Gagnier JJ, Miller BS. Ability of preseason body composition and physical fitness to predict the risk of injury in male collegiate hockey players. *Sports Health*. 2015;7:45-51.

53. Riemann BL, Lephart SM. The sensorimotor system, part I: the physiologic basis of functional joint stability. *J Athl Train*. 2002;37:71-79.

54. Dallinga JM, Benjaminse A, Leinmink KAPM. Which screening tools can predict injury to the lower extremities in team sports?: a systematic review. *Sports Med*. 2012;42(9):791-815.

55. Murphy DF, Connolly DAJ, Beynnon BD. Risk factors for lower extremity injury: a review of the literature. *Br J Sports Med.* 2003;37:13.

56. Plisky PJ, Rauh MJ, Kaminski TW, Underwood FB. Star Excursion Balance Test as a predictor of lower extremity injury in high school basketball players. *J Orthop Sports Phys Ther.* 2006;36(12):911-919.

57. Trojian TH, McKeag DB. Single leg balance test to identify risk of ankle sprains. *Br J Sports Med.* 2006;40(7):610-613.

58. Leetun DT, Ireland ML, Willson JD, Ballantyne BT, Davis IMC. Core stability measures as risk factors for lower extremity injury in athletes. *Med Sci Sports Exerc.* 2004;36(6):926-934.

59. Zazulak BT, Hewett TE, Reeves NP, Goldberg B, Cholweicki J. Deficits in neuromuscular control of the trunk predict knee injury risk a prospective biomechanical-epidemiologic study. *Am J Sports Med.* 2007;35(7):1123-1130.

60. Söderman K, Alfredson H, Pietilä T, Werner S. Risk factors for leg injuries in female soccer players: a prospective investigation during one out-door season. *Knee Surg Sports Traumatol Arthrosc.* 2001;9(5):313-321.

61. Cameron M, Adams R, Maher C. Motor control and strength as predictors of hamstring injury in elite players of Australian football. *Phys Ther Sport.* 2003;4:159-166.

62. Kiesel K, Plisky P, Voight M. Can serious injury in professional football be predicted by a preseason functional movement screen? *NAJSPT.* 2007;2:147-158.

63. Kiesel KB, Butler RJ, Plisky PJ. Prediction of injury by limited and asymmetrical fundamental movement patterns in american football players. *J Sport Rehabil.* 2014;23:88-94.

64. Chorba RS, Chorba DJ, Bouillon LE, Overmyer CA, Landis JA. Use of a functional movement screening tool to determine injury risk in female collegiate athletes. *NAJSPT.* 2010;5:47-54.

65. Shojaedin SS, Letafatkar A, Hadadnezhad M, Dehkhoda MR. Relationship between functional movement screening score and history of injury and identifying the predictive value of the FMS for injury. *Int J Contr Saf Promot.* 2014;21:355-360.

66. Knapik JJ, Cosio-Lima LM, Reynolds KL, Shumway RS. Efficacy of functional movement screening for predicting injuries in coast guard cadets. *J Strength Cond Res.* 2014.

67. Butler RJ, Contreras M, Burton LC, Plisky PJ, Goode A, Kiesel K. Modifiable risk factors predict injuries in firefighters during training academies. *Work.* 2013;46:11-17.

68. O'Connor FG, Deuster PA, Davis J, Pappas CG, Knapik JJ. Functional movement screening: predicting injuries in officer candidates. *Med Sci Sports Exerc.* 2011;43(12):2224-2230.

69. Lehr ME, Plisky PJ, Butler RJ, Fink ML, Kiesel KB, Underwood FB. Field-expedient screening and injury risk algorithm categories as predictors of noncontact lower extremity injury. *Scand J Med Sci Sports.* 2013;23:e225-e232.

70. Parchmann CJ, McBride JM. Relationship between functional movement screen and athletic performance. *J Strength Cond Res.* 2011;25(12):3378-3384.

71. Kennedy-Armbruster C, Evans EM, Sexauer L, Peterson J, Wyatt W. Association among functional-movement ability, fatigue, sedentary time, and fitness in 40 years and older active duty military personnel. *Mil Med.* 2013;178(12):1358-1364.

72. Duncan MJ, Stanley M, Wright SL. The association between functional movement and overweight and obesity in British primary school children. *BMC Sports Sci Med Rehabil.* 2013;5:1-8.

73. Okada T, Huxel KC, Nesser TW. Relationship between core stability, functional movement, and performance. *J Strength Cond Res.* 2011;25:252-261.

74. Krumrei K, Flanagan M, Bruner J, Durall C. The accuracy of the functional movement screen to identify individuals with an elevated risk of musculoskeletal injury. *J Sport Rehabil.* 2014;23:360-364.

75. Kraus K, SchÜTz E, Taylor WR, Doyscher R. Efficacy of the functional movement screen: a review. *J Strength Cond Res.* 2014;28(12):3571-3584.

76. Kazman JB, Galecki JM, Lisman P, Deuster PA, O'Connor FG. Factor structure of the functional movement screen in marine officer candidates. *J Strength Cond Res.* 2014;28:672-678.

77. Clifton DR, Harrison BC, Hertel J, Hart JM. Relationship between functional assessments and exercise-related changes during static balance. *J Strength Cond Res.* 2013;27:966-972.

78. Frost DM, Beach TA, Callaghan JP, McGill SM. FMS™ scores change with performers' knowledge of the grading criteria - Are general whole-body movement screens capturing "dysfunction"? *J Strength Cond Res.* 2013.

79. Peate WF, Bates G, Lunda K, Francis S, Bellamy K. Core strength: a new model for injury prediction and prevention. *J Occup Med.* 2007;2:3-3.

80. Frost DM, Beach TAC, Callaghan JP, McGill SM. Using the functional movement screen™ to evaluate the effectiveness of training. *J Strength Cond Res.* 2012;26(6):1620-1630.

81. Maia Pacheco M, Cespedes Teixeira LA, Franchini E, Takito MY. Functional vs. strength training in adults: specific needs define the best intervention. *Int J Sports Phys. Ther.* 2013;8:34-43.

82. Munro A. Anterior cruciate ligament injuries: recognising potentially high-risk athletes. *SportEX Medicine.* 2013(55):7-10.

83. Hewett TE, Ford KR, Hoogenboom BJ, Myer GD. Understanding and preventing acl injuries: current biomechanical and epidemiologic considerations - update 2010. *NAJSPT.* 2010;5:234-251.

84. Myer GD, Brent JL, Ford KR, Hewett TE. Real-time assessment and neuromuscular training feedback techniques to prevent ACL injury in female athletes. *Strength Cond J.* 2011;33:21-35.

85. Hewett TE. Video analysis of trunk and knee motion during non-contact anterior cruciate ligament injury in female athletes: lateral trunk and knee abduction motion are combined components of the injury mechanism. *Br J Sports Med.* 2009;43(6):417-422.

86. Chappell JD, Creighton A, Giuliani C, Yu B, Garrett WE. Kinematics and electromyography of landing preparation in vertical stop-jump risks for noncontact anterior cruciate ligament injury. *Am J Sports Med.* 2007;35:235-241.

87. Noyes FR, Barber-Westin SD, Fleckenstein C, Walsh C, West J. The drop-jump screening test: difference in lower limb control by gender and effect of neuromuscular training in female athletes. *Am J Sports Med.* 2005;33:197-207.

88. Joseph MF, Rahl M, Sheehan J, et al. Timing of lower extremity frontal plane motion differs between female and male athletes during a landing task. *Am J Sports Med.* 2011;39(7):1517-1521.

89. Schmitz RJ, Shultz SJ, Anh-Dung N. Dynamic valgus alignment and functional strength in males and females during maturation. *J Athl Training.* 2009;44:26-32.

90. Harris-Hayes M, Steger-May K, Koh C, Royer NK, Graci V, Salsich GB. Classification of lower extremity movement patterns based on visual assessment: reliability and correlation with 2-dimensional video analysis. *J Athl Training.* 2014;49:304-310.

91. Padua DA, Boling MC, DiStefano LJ, Onate JA, Beutler AI, Marshall SW. Reliability of the landing error scoring system-real time, a clinical assessment tool of jump-landing biomechanics. *J Sport Rehabil.* 2011;20:145-156.

92. Padua DA, Marshall SW, Boling MC, Thigpen CA, Garrett WE, Beutler AI. The landing error scoring system (LESS) is a valid and reliable clinical assessment tool of jump-landing biomechanics: the JUMP-ACL study. *Am J Sport Med.* 2009;37(10):1996-2002.

93. Ugalde V, Brockman C, Bailowitz Z, Pollard CD. Single leg squat test and its relationship to dynamic knee valgus and injury risk screening. *PM R.* 2014;7(3):229-35.

94. Myer GD, Ford KR, Khoury J, Succop P, Hewett TE. Biomechanics laboratory-based prediction algorithm to identify female athletes with high knee loads that increase risk of ACL injury. *Br J Sports Med.* 2010.

95. Myer GD, Ford KR, Hewett TE. New method to identify athletes at high risk of ACL injury using clinic-based measurements and freeware computer analysis. *Br J Sports Med.* 2011;45:238-244.

96. Goetschius J, Smith HC, Vacek PM, et al. Application of a clinic-based algorithm as a tool to identify female athletes at risk for anterior cruciate ligament injury: a prospective cohort study with a nested, matched case-control analysis. *Am J Sports Med.* 2012;40(9):1978-1984.

97. Parkkari J, Pasanen K, Mattila VM, Kannus P, Rimpelä A. The risk for a cruciate ligament injury of the knee in adolescents and young adults: a population-based cohort study of 46 500 people with a 9 year follow-up. *Br J Sports Med.* 2008;42(6):422-426.

98. Sigward SM, Pollard CD, Powers CM. The influence of sex and maturation on landing biomechanics: implications for acl injury. *Scand J Med Sci Sports.* 2012;22:502-509.

99. Hewett TE, Myer GD, Ford KR, et al. Biomechanical measures of neuromuscular control and valgus loading of the knee predict anterior cruciate ligament injury risk in female athletes a prospective study. *Am J Sports Med.* 2005;33:492-501.

100. Nilstad A, Andersen TE, Bahr R, Holme I, Steffen K. Risk factors for lower extremity injuries in elite female soccer players. *Am J Sport Med.* 2014;42:940-948.

101. Smith HC, Johnson RJ, Shultz SJ, et al. A prospective evaluation of the landing error scoring system (less) as a screening tool for anterior cruciate ligament injury risk. *Am J Sport Med.* 2012;40:521-526.

102. Cashman GE. The effect of weak hip abductors or external rotators on knee valgus kinematics in healthy subjects: a systematic review. *J Sport Rehabil.* 2012;21:273-284.

103. Noyes FR, Barber-Westin SD, Tutalo Smith ST, Campbell T. A training program to improve neuromuscular and performance indices in female high school soccer players. *J Strength Cond Res.* 2013;27:340-351.

104. Noyes FR, Barber-Westin SD, Smith ST, Campbell T, Garrison TT. A training program to improve neuromuscular and performance indices in female high school basketball players. *J Strength Cond Res.* 2012;26:709-719.

105. Barber-Westin SD, Smith ST, Campbell T, Noyes FR. The drop-jump video screening test: retention of improvement in neuromuscular control in female volleyball players. *J Strength Cond Res.* 2010;24(11):3055-3062.

106. DiStefano LJ, Padua DA, DiStefano MJ, Marshall SW. Influence of age, sex, technique, and exercise program on movement patterns after an anterior cruciate ligament injury prevention program in youth soccer players. *Am J Sport Med.* 2009;37:495-505.

107. Noyes FR, Barber-Westin SD. Neuromuscular retraining intervention programs: do they reduce noncontact anterior cruciate ligament injury rates in adolescent female athletes? *Arthroscopy.* 2014;30:245-255.

108. Minthorn LM, Fayson SD, Stobierski LM, Welch CE, Anderso BE. The functional movement screen's ability to detect changes in movement patterns after a training intervention. *J Sport Rehabil.* 2014.

109. Bodden JG, Needham RA, Chockalingam N. The effect of an intervention program on functional movement screen test scores in mixed martial arts athletes. *J Strength Cond Res.* 2015;29:219-225.

110. Kiesel K, Plisky P, Butler R. Functional movement test scores improve following a standardized off-season intervention program in professional football players. *Scand J Med Sci Sports*. 2011;21:287-292.

SUGGESTED READINGS

2010 Council on Sports Medicine and Fitness. Preparticipation Physical Evaluation. https://www.aap.org/en-us/about-the-aap/Committees-Councils-Sections/Council-on-sports-medicine-and-fitness/Pages/PPE.aspx.

2014 NATA Position Statement: Preparticipation Physical Examinations and Disqualifications. http://www.nata.org/sites/default/files/Conley.pdf.

2011 ACSM Pre-participation Physical Examinations. https://www.acsm.org/docs/brochures/pre-participation-physical-examinations.pdf.

2005 Consensus Statement of the Study Group of Sport Cardiology of the Working Group of Cardiac Rehabilitation and Exercise Physiology and the Working Group of Myocardial and Pericardial Diseases of the European Society of Cardiology. http://eurheartj.oxfordjournals.org/content/ehj/26/5/516.full.pdf.

Considerations Related to Preparticipation Screening for Cardiovascular Abnormalities in Competitive Athletes: 2007 Update. *Circulation*. 2007;115:1643-1655. http://circ.ahajournals.org/content/115/12/1643.long.

Functional Movement Screening, Part 1 and Part 2. Cook, Burton, Hoogenboom, and Voight. International Journal of Sports Physical Therapy. 2014;9(3,4). http://www.ncbi.nlm.nih.gov/pmc/articles/PMC4060319/, http://www.ncbi.nlm.nih.gov/pmc/articles/PMC4127517/.

11

Prevention Methods

Wanda Swiger, EdD, ATC, CES and Scot A. Ward, MS, ATC

CHAPTER OBJECTIVES

- Describe the risk factors and/or variables that prevention strategies might impact.
- Identify the various procedural and therapeutic prevention strategies thought to reduce sport injury.
- Summarize the basic principles associated with the design, construction, fit, maintenance, and reconditioning of protective equipment, including the rules and regulations established by the associations that govern its use.
- Discuss the advantages and disadvantages of prophylactic taping and bracing, proprioceptive training, and stretching programs as strategies to reduce the incidence of injury.
- Explain how the effectiveness of a prevention strategy can be assessed using clinical outcomes, surveillance, or evaluation data. Recognize the steps to determine effectiveness of various prevention strategies thought to limit sport injury.
- Analyze limitations in current prevention research.

INTRODUCTION

As you may recall from Chapter 1, risk factors are not causes of injury; they are merely associated with it. Some risk factors have a stronger relationship to certain injuries than others. Throughout this text, we have focused on the importance of how known risk factors can be compounded. Furthermore, we have discussed the concept that although some risks are within an individual's control, other factors are not. We previously defined risk factors that are changeable as modifiable. For those who play sports, there may be differences in injury rate between genders,

Adams M, Swiger W.
Epidemiology for Athletic Trainers: Integrating
Evidence-Based Practice (pp 241-267).
© 2016 Taylor & Francis Group.

TABLE 11-1
INTRINSIC FACTORS ASSOCIATED WITH SPORT-RELATED INJURIES[1-4]

• Physical characteristics	• Ligamentous instability
• Age	• Anatomic abnormalities (malalignments)
• Gender	
• Body mass index/somatotype	• Motor abilities
• Previous injury	• Sports-specific skills
• Physical fitness	• Psychological Profile
• Joint mobility	• Motivation
• Muscle tightness, weakness	• Risk taking
	• Coping

TABLE 11-2
EXTRINSIC FACTORS ASSOCIATED WITH SPORT-RELATED INJURIES[1-4]

• Exposure	• Type of playing surface
• Type of sports	• Indoor vs outdoor
• Exposure time	• Weather conditions
• Position in the team	• Time of season
• Level of competition	• Human factors (team mates, opponent, referee, coach, spectators)
• Training	
• Type	• Equipment
• Amount	• Protective equipment
• Frequency	• Playing equipment (eg, racket, stick, etc)
• Intensity	
• Environment	• Footwear, clothing

---

playing positions, and/or between sports. These risk factors can be made better or worse by circumstances, such as playing conditions, rules, and access to protective equipment. The factors associated with sport-related injuries are referred to as intrinsic and extrinsic. These factors have been noted in the literature as predisposing one to injury (Tables 11-1 and 11-2).[1-4]

Prevention interventions focus on limiting these factors and may include some form of therapy or a change in a procedure or policy. For example, rule changes, equipment requirements, and coaching education are procedural, whereas the use of prophylactic bracing or taping or implementing stretching, strength, and conditioning programs are therapeutic. Although many of the prevention strategies in sport are focused on limiting catastrophic injuries, concussion, or musculoskeletal injuries, some interventions have focused on preventing the spread of illness (ie, rules specific to contagious skin lesions; Table 11-3).

TABLE 11-3

RULES PREVENTING ILLNESS TRANSMISSION[5]

CONDITION	RETURN TO PLAY GUIDELINES
Furuncles, carbuncles, impetigo, methicillin-resistant *Staphylococcus aureus*	• No new lesions for at least 48 hrs • Lesions cannot be moist, draining, or exudative • 72-hr minimum antibiotic therapy • Active lesions cannot be covered to allow for participation
Molluscum contagiosum	• Lesions must be removed • Localized lesions must be covered with gas-permeable dressing, underwrap, and stretch tape
Herpes simplex (recurrent)	• No moist lesions, must have firm crust covering • 120-hr minimum antiviral therapy • Active lesions cannot be covered to allow for participation
Herpes simplex (primary)	• Free of systemic symptoms of viral infection (fever, fatigue) • No new lesions for at least 72 hrs • No moist lesions, must have firm crust covering • 120-hr minimum antiviral therapy • Active lesions cannot be covered to allow for participation
Tinea capitis	• 2-wk minimum systemic antifungal therapy
Tinea corporis	• 72-hr minimum topical fungicide therapy • Localized lesions must be covered with gas-permeable dressing, underwrap, and stretch tape

Adapted from Zinder SM, Basler RS, Foley J, Scarlata C, Vasily DB. National Athletic Trainers' Association position statement: skin diseases. *J Athl Train.* 2010;45(4):411-428.

The effect of such programs needs to be evaluated by comparing the rates of injury between athletes who were exposed to the prevention method and those who were not. Some effective injury prevention procedures have been identified and include warm-up sessions, regular systematic training, adequate standard protective equipment, adaptation of rules, and appropriate education by coaches or other trained professionals.[6] But, many other strategies have not been studied or have only a few reports in the literature.

Injury surveillance studies support that injury risk increases with the level of physical contact in the sport; thus, research supports rule changes and protective equipment that reduce this contact or minimize its effect. Strategies designed to prevent sports injuries can be effective. However, many interventions that could measurably alter injury profiles often lack pre- and postintervention data.[7] For example, flexibility or strength training programs are anecdotally reported as effective by coaches and athletic trainers, but few research studies have documented actual changes in injury occurrence. Furthermore, not all rule changes have been effective in reducing injury. Protective equipment designed to reduce specific injuries often distorts the overall effect of injury reduction. For example, the initial design of helmets was to reduce skull injuries and was not to prevent concussions. As we explore topics within this chapter, critically appraise the research for correct identifications of injuries and prevalence and the intrinsic and extrinsic risk factors involved. From this assessment, you will begin to hypothesize what interventions might help reduce sport-related injuries. Finally, visualize how you might monitor the effects of any given intervention to determine its true effect.

POLICY, RULE, AND EQUIPMENT CHANGES

Concussions, spinal cord injury, exertional collapse, heat-related illness, and musculoskeletal injuries have been identified as some of the injuries associated with sport participation. Each injury has established epidemiology data that can help rule makers theorize what changes could be made to reduce the incidence of injury. For example, in ice hockey, spinal cord injuries are related to aggressive checking, particularly from behind and near the ink boards. To reduce this risk, checking rules were changed and are strictly enforced. Since 2011, full-body checking has not been allowed before the U-14 level.[8] Youth lacrosse has also established age-based contact regulations. Interestingly, American Football has long resisted altering rules at the youth level. Policies and rules for all sport become more lax as the level of participation increases from novice to professional. Equipment changes are standardized for most levels of participation, although there are still some instances in which differences exist at the elite level. For example, National Hockey League athletes are only required to wear a half-face shield, whereas amateur ice hockey athletes must wear a full-face shield. The lack of systematic injury data collection, especially at the youth sport level, makes it difficult to determine if these rule changes have had any effect on injuries.

Government Legislation of Sport

In recent years, numerous policies and legislative acts related to concussion have been established. It is unclear whether it is due to the inaction of sport organizations to alter rules or the high visibility of concussions and sudden death in youth sports. Public awareness of the potential effects of head trauma in sport is at an all-time high. These laws are aimed at reducing death and disability of youth athletes through prevention and availability of medical personnel. Most notable are the mandates requiring coach education, no same-day return to play, and clearance by an appropriate health care provider after a concussion.[9,10] These differ from state to state. A summary of state policies can be found at the Korey Stringer Institute website (http://ksi.uconn.edu/high-school-state-policies/concussion-polices/).

There are little data on how these pieces of legislation have influenced the landscape of concussion, but most would argue that, at a minimum, there has been an increased awareness. Epidemiological data concerning time periods before and after these laws will be crucial in understanding their impact and whether athletic trainers and other medical professionals play a role in their effectiveness. One the few studies that has assessed changes to state laws found that high school coaches in Washington state appear to have better concussion knowledge and are receiving more education since the mandate began in 2009.[11] No other studies have quantified outcomes from the legislation. Outcomes have been difficult to quantify due to a lack of overall injury surveillance and the lack of prelegislation data for comparison.

Sport Organization Policies

In addition to legislation, there has also been a flood of policy change in how concussions are managed within athletic associations, school districts, and individual schools. Athletic associations and schools are free to deliver the government mandates in various ways, further complicating the understanding of the laws' impacts. These policies may also influence the number of concussions disclosed and diagnosed because some athletes will view the required time out of sport as too harsh and not report, and not all health care providers are trained to evaluate sport-related concussions. More data are needed to understand which policies are most effective and if any unintended consequences result from such mandates.

Policies and guidelines may also vary from high school to college. High school associations and college regulating bodies often focus on prevention of any sudden death, not just on concussions. Athletic trainers are more likely to be employed at the college level and have standards of care that exceed the school policies. The National Athletic Trainers' Association has produced more than 15 position statements (www.nata.org/position-statements) that establish best practice for clinicians, including Preparticipation Exams, Preventing Sudden Death in Sports, and Managing Disordered Eating. Because these policies are continuously changing, athletic trainers must be aware of legislation, rules, policies, and best practices regarding not just concussion, but any injury or illness.

Rule Changes in Sport

Over the years, rule changes in different sports have affected the incidence of injury. Most notable are those pertaining to spearing (leading with the head into a tackle) in American football. Since the prohibition of spearing in 1976 and the use of the modern helmet, catastrophic head injuries have drastically declined.[12,13] In 2005, the term *intentional* was dropped from the rules. The new definition of spearing is "the use of the helmet (including the face mask) in an attempt to punish an opponent."[10] Furthermore, in 2006, there was emphasis on helmet contact and further defining spearing, face tackling, and butt blocking as illegal actions (http://nccsir.unc.edu/). More recent football rule changes concerning concussion pertain to shortened kick-off distances, prohibition of any head-to-head contact, and increased penalties for fouls. Examples of illegal helmet contact that could result in disqualification include helmet contact against an opponent lying on the ground, helmet contact against an opponent held up by other players, and helmet-to-helmet contact against a defenseless opponent.[10] Research data suggest that since the implementation of these rules, in the National Football League (NFL), the number of concussions has decreased by 13% from 2012 to 2013, with a 23% reduction in concussions caused by helmet-to-helmet contact.[14]

In ice hockey, the most notable rule changes have occurred at the youth level. These rule changes involve reducing head-to-head contact and increasing the age for legal and illegal checking (Bantam level as opposed to the Pee-Wee level).[8] The intent of these changes was to reduce concussion incidence. However, study results are not what one would expect. In a study by Krolikowski et al[17] examining the no-head contact rule, the rate of concussion increased. In Pee Wee, the incident rate ratio was 1.83, and in Bantam, the incident rate ratio was 2.74. In addition, studies found that by not allowing body checking until the Bantam level, the incidence of concussion was lowered in the Pee-Wee level, but there was an overall increase in concussion at the Bantam level. These findings suggest that regardless of when body checking is allowed, that during the initial year when checking is allowed, there will be increased concussion and injury rates.[16]

There have been fewer rule changes in noncollision sports, especially for concussions. Despite many sports not allowing intentional contact, the incidence of concussions in women's ice hockey, basketball, and soccer continues to increase, likely due to increases in awareness. Fair play and following the rules of the game appear to have a large impact on concussion incidence.[17,18] Studies showed an increase in the severity of head impacts on infractions/fouls as compared to legal plays.[19] The incidence of concussions also increases with rule violations compared to appropriate play.[20]

There are additional rule changes for the safety of participants that do not focus on participation but on training practices within their sport. The culture of weight-cutting in wrestling has significantly changed since 1997, when 3 collegiate wrestlers died due to improper weight management.[21] Research has established that there are serious health and performance consequences to rapid, prolonged weight cutting.[22] Citing this evidence, the National Collegiate

Athletic Association (NCAA) placed limits on the amount of weight loss and on methods in which a wrestler is allowed to cut weight. NCAA rule 8.3.3 states that a wrestler cannot wrestle more than one weight class above his or her original weight, that weight classes are set by February 15 (mid-season), and that wrestlers need to follow a prescribed weight loss plan. In addition, the NCAA Weight Management Plan mandates that a wrestler cannot lose more than 1.5% of their body weight per week.[23] NCAA rules are reviewed and updated every 2 years.

EDUCATION EFFORTS

By its nature, epidemiology supports the notion that awareness is a key component of prevention. By identifying risk factors and understanding who is has the greatest risk, researchers are hoping that knowledge will be shared and that injuries will decrease. Primary preventive strategies typically include some educational component. For example, a long-time standard of disease prevention is hand washing. Educating people about the benefits of hand washing and proper methods of hand washing can reduce the frequency of infections. It is also assumed that sport-related injuries can be reduced by educating participants on the risks and proper use of equipment or correct techniques.

The 1976 rule that prohibited spearing in American Football was established because injury data suggested that the mechanism for cervical fractures was axial loading (when a flexed head makes contact with an opponent or the ground).[10] As a result of this information on mechanism of injury and injury incidence data, proper tackling instruction became a focus of coaching in American football. This emphasis, combined with higher equipment standards and improved medical care, appears to have resulted in a 270% reduction in permanent spinal cord injuries. Cervical spinal cord injuries have been the most common catastrophic football injury and the second leading direct cause of death attributable to football. Cantu and Mueller[13] reviewed 25 years of catastrophic neck injuries and found that between 1971 and 1975, the yearly average for spinal cord injuries was 20 in college football. In the past 10 years, that has dropped to 7.2/year.[13] That study also examined the mechanism of injury and variables that increased or decreased risk of injury. Mueller and Colgate[10] also examined the cervical injuries and the mechanisms that increase their risk. A review of injury surveillance findings on mechanism of injury support that there is an increased risk when tackling with the crown of the helmet/head (axial load, slight flexion).[10,13] Coaches at all levels are educated on the need for and methods of how to properly teach tackling. Efforts to ensure head-up tackling continue (www.jonheck.com/hdc/headsupdvd.htm). The improved safety of football in regard to spinal cord injury is evidence that sports injuries can be reduced. These data also provide evidence that change requires multiple components—rules, equipment, and coaching.

Collision sports are not the only ones with a link between poor technique and injury. Faculty mechanics and training are associated with various overuse injuries. All sports and sport skills should be analyzed and examined for associations with injury. Athletic trainers are critically important in identifying these faulty mechanics and educating athletes on correct techniques to reduce less severe overuse injuries. Therefore, athletic trainers must have in depth knowledge of the biomechanics of the sport and the mechanisms of injury. Although most rules changes and education efforts focus on preventing acute traumatic injuries, skill analysis focuses on preventing overuse injuries. Sport injury specialists should take an active role in analyzing sports skill, identifying the various phases of the skill (joint movements, muscle contracting, and identifying how muscles are contracting in each phase of the skill), and creating appropriate conditioning programs that will increase athlete performance and decrease risk of injury.

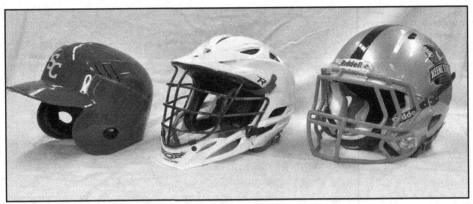

Figure 11-1. Helmet types across sports. (Left to right, baseball [single impact], lacrosse, and football [repetitive blow].)

PROTECTIVE EQUIPMENT

Equipment modifications are one of the most discussed topics in sport-related injury prevention. Recent emphasis on sport safety, especially for youth, involves the addition of new equipment and the improvements to existing equipment. For example, face guards for baseball/softball infielders are a recent addition to that sport's protective equipment, whereas advances in helmet designs for football, men's lacrosse, and ice-hockey continue as manufactures more thoroughly test their products and develop new materials. Generally, as the level of physical contact increases, so does the amount of player equipment. However, some collision sport athletes (rugby and Australian-rules football) wear little protective gear. In addition to helmets, facemasks, shoulder pads, and mouth guards are required equipment for most collision sport positions. Several sports mandate guards to protect against blows to extremities, such as elbow pads in men's lacrosse and shin guards in soccer. Athletes may opt for additional padding to deflect thrown or batted balls. Eye and face protection has improved in collision and contact sports with the addition of eye shields and faceguards. The mouth guard is also standard equipment in many contact sports, such as field hockey, football, ice hockey, and lacrosse. The following sections focus on the evolution and efficacy of the helmets and mouth guards in preventing injury.

Helmets

Helmets are worn in several sports, including American football, men's lacrosse, ice hockey, and downhill skiing. In other sports, helmets are worn based on position (baseball catcher, field hockey goalie), or action occurring (batting; Figures 11-1 and 11-2). The literature supports the use of helmets to prevent impact injuries to the skull.[10,12,13,24] Most modern helmets do an excellent job of preventing skull fractures, and since the introduction of the modern helmet in collision sports, catastrophic head injuries have rapidly declined to very few occurring each year.[10,13,25,26]

The first helmets in American football that offered full skull protection were introduced between 1915 and 1917. Prior designs were essentially harnesses that padded the forehead, crown, and ears. During the 1920s and 1930s, manufacturers began to use thicker leather and elastic suspension so the helmet did not rest directly on the head, allowing for shock absorption. Helmets also evolved away from the flat-top shape to a more of the teardrop shape of the skull (evolution of the helmet and additional equipment changes for football can be found at www.nflevolution.com/home).

In 1939, the John T. Riddell Company of Chicago introduced the plastic shell football helmet. Because plastics and other materials were scarce during World War II, some of Riddell's early

Figure 11-2. Internal padding for single- and repeated-impact helmets.

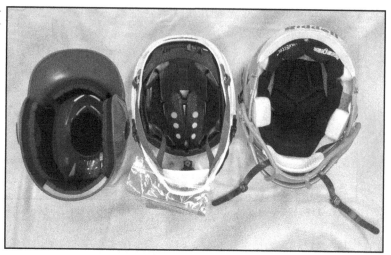

models were not particularly well made and had a high incidence of cracking, so the plastic helmet was banned from the NFL. However, in 1943, all players in the NFL were required to wear some form of head protection. Plastic helmets were reinstated in 1949 after some refinements to the synthetic materials. In the 1950s, helmets were developed with internal padding, and by the 1970s, the helmet design evolved to absorb energy. The first polycarbonate shell, with a harder and slicker surface, was introduced in the late 1980s.[27]

Currently, helmet evaluation and effectiveness in preventing concussion is a topic of research and debate. Studies are mixed as to which helmets are best at preventing concussions.[28,29] The Star-Rating System, one of the most commonly used systems for helmet ratings, only measures impacts directly to the head and does not account for impacts that may occur as the result of a whiplash mechanism. Currently, this system only includes linear forces. However, for the first time, the Star-evaluation system, used in the Virginia Tech Helmet Ratings (Figures 11-3A to 11-3D), have provided consumers with scientific information in a user-friendly manner concerning the safety and value of adult football helmet purchases.[30] Sport injury specialists should be aware of the differences in youth and adult helmets, as well as differences in single-impact (bike and ski helmets) and repeated-impact helmet design. Collision sport helmets typically have a comfort liner, an impact energy attenuating liner, a restraint system, and a shell. Helmets used in motor sport, bicycling, and alpine skiing are designed to attenuate a single impact, meaning that once the helmet has sustained an impact, it must be replaced. Helmets used in ice hockey, football, and lacrosse are designed to withstand multiple impacts over a season of games and practices. The materials used and the design of the helmet differentiate between single- and multiple-impact helmets. Multiple-impact helmets use materials that compress and return to their original dimensions with an outer shell of lightweight plastics and composites for durability and protection. Single-impact helmets use materials that deform or fracture permanently upon impact to dissipate energy.[24]

Beyond helmet design, there have been recent changes at various levels regarding proper fit and securing the equipment. For example, high school rule changes effective during 2006 and 2007 stated that at least a 4-point chinstrap shall be required to secure the helmet, and all mouth guards must be colored, not white or clear.[10] In college football, a player who loses his helmet must come off the field for one play to encourage proper fitting. Most clinicians and experts agree on key elements concerning helmet fit and condition. These include that the helmets be in good condition, fit properly, and be worn properly. Although helmets may dissipate some of the forces transmitted to the brain during a blow, they are most effective at reducing trauma to the skull and will never fully prevent concussion because they cannot prevent brain movement inside of the skull (eg, coup-coutrecoup injury).

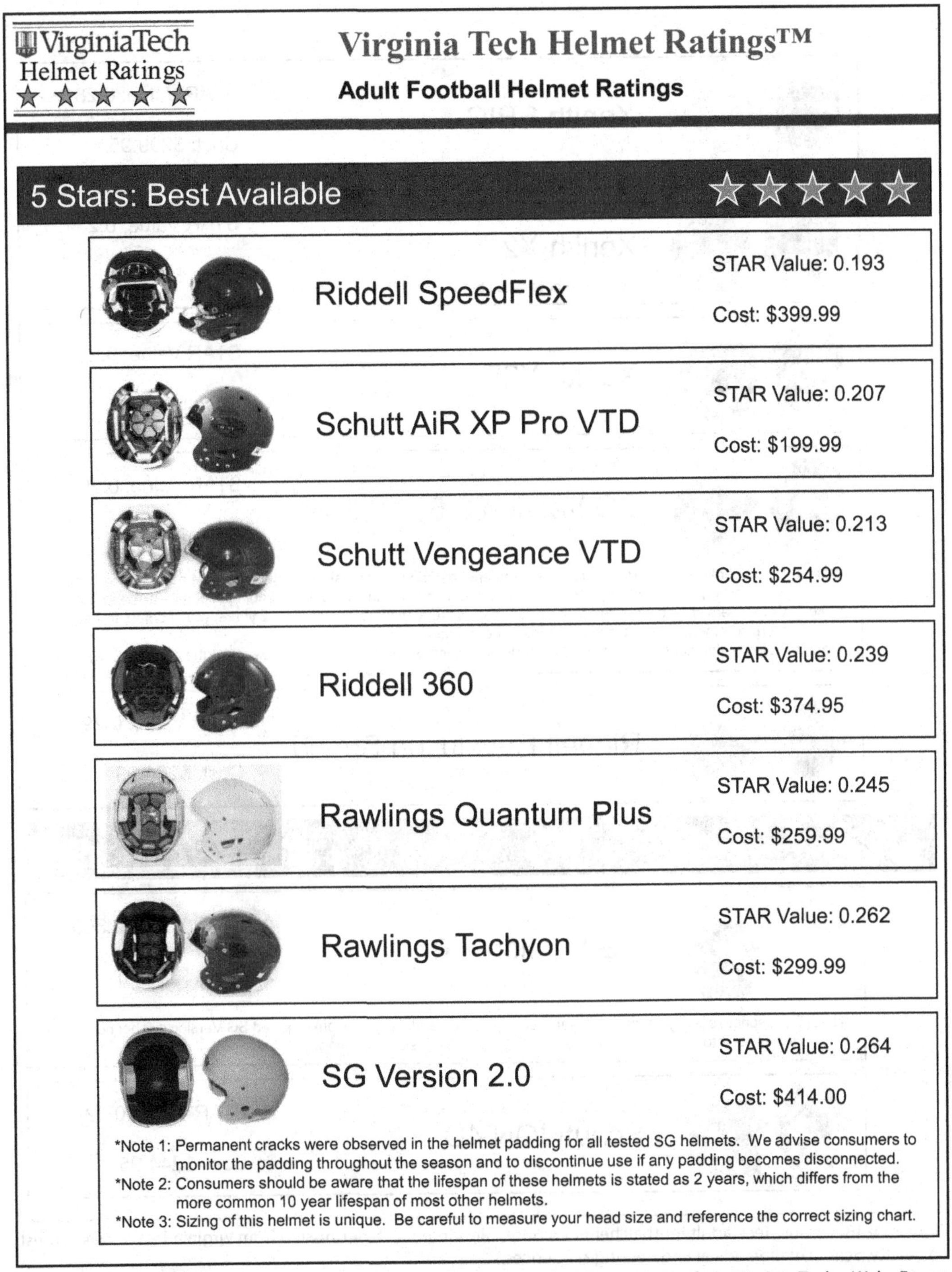

Virginia Tech Helmet Ratings™
Adult Football Helmet Ratings

⎍VirginiaTech
Helmet Ratings
★ ★ ★ ★ ★

5 Stars: Best Available   ☆ ☆ ☆ ☆ ☆

	Riddell SpeedFlex	STAR Value: 0.193 Cost: $399.99
	Schutt AiR XP Pro VTD	STAR Value: 0.207 Cost: $199.99
	Schutt Vengeance VTD	STAR Value: 0.213 Cost: $254.99
	Riddell 360	STAR Value: 0.239 Cost: $374.95
	Rawlings Quantum Plus	STAR Value: 0.245 Cost: $259.99
	Rawlings Tachyon	STAR Value: 0.262 Cost: $299.99
	SG Version 2.0	STAR Value: 0.264 Cost: $414.00

*Note 1: Permanent cracks were observed in the helmet padding for all tested SG helmets. We advise consumers to monitor the padding throughout the season and to discontinue use if any padding becomes disconnected.

*Note 2: Consumers should be aware that the lifespan of these helmets is stated as 2 years, which differs from the more common 10 year lifespan of most other helmets.

*Note 3: Sizing of this helmet is unique. Be careful to measure your head size and reference the correct sizing chart.

Figure 11-3A. Virginia Tech adult football helmet ratings. (Reprinted with permission from Virginia Tech – Wake Forest University, School of Biomedical Engineering & Sciences.)

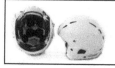

Xenith EPIC

STAR Value: 0.281

Cost: $299.95

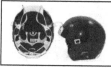

Xenith X2

*Note: Helmets dated before 2013 rated as 3 Stars

STAR Value: 0.284

Cost: $235.00

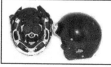

Xenith X2E

STAR Value: 0.285

Cost: $235.00

SG Version 2.5

STAR Value: 0.292

Cost: $414.00

*Note 1: Permanent cracks were observed in the helmet padding for all tested SG helmets. We advise consumers to monitor the padding throughout the season and to discontinue use if any padding becomes disconnected.
*Note 2: Consumers should be aware that the lifespan of these helmets is stated as 2 years, which differs from the more common 10 year lifespan of most other helmets.
*Note 3: Sizing of this helmet is unique. Be careful to measure your head size and reference the correct sizing chart.

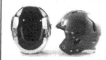

Riddell Revolution Speed

STAR Value: 0.297

Cost: $264.99

4 Stars: Very Good   ★ ★ ★ ★

SG Version 1.0

STAR Value: 0.309

Cost: $398.00

*Note: Retrospective analysis found similar cracking in the padding of previously tested SG Version 1.0 helmets. Please refer to the notes on SG Version 2.0 and SG Version 2.5 ratings.

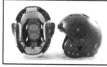

Schutt ION 4D

STAR Value: 0.327

Cost: $244.95

Figure 11-3B. Virginia Tech adult football helmet ratings. (Reprinted with permission from Virginia Tech – Wake Forest University, School of Biomedical Engineering & Sciences.)

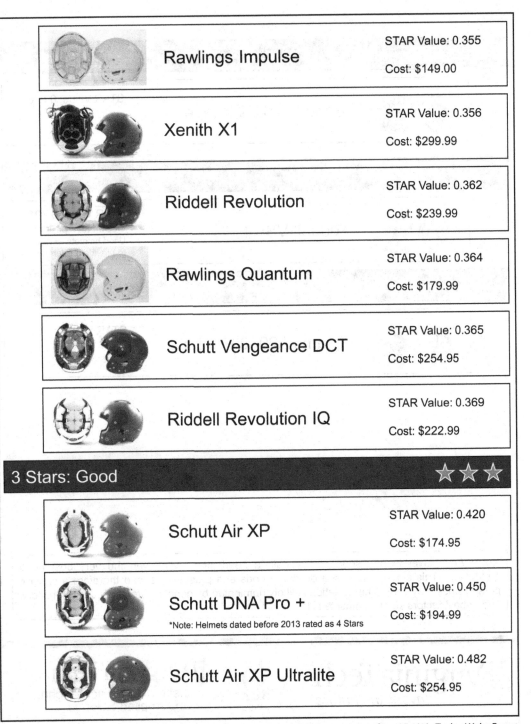

| | STAR Value: 0.355 |
| Rawlings Impulse | Cost: $149.00 |

| | STAR Value: 0.356 |
| Xenith X1 | Cost: $299.99 |

| | STAR Value: 0.362 |
| Riddell Revolution | Cost: $239.99 |

| | STAR Value: 0.364 |
| Rawlings Quantum | Cost: $179.99 |

| | STAR Value: 0.365 |
| Schutt Vengeance DCT | Cost: $254.95 |

| | STAR Value: 0.369 |
| Riddell Revolution IQ | Cost: $222.99 |

3 Stars: Good ★★★

| | STAR Value: 0.420 |
| Schutt Air XP | Cost: $174.95 |

| | STAR Value: 0.450 |
| Schutt DNA Pro +
*Note: Helmets dated before 2013 rated as 4 Stars | Cost: $194.99 |

| | STAR Value: 0.482 |
| Schutt Air XP Ultralite | Cost: $254.95 |

Figure 11-3C. Virginia Tech adult football helmet ratings. (Reprinted with permission from Virginia Tech – Wake Forest University, School of Biomedical Engineering & Sciences.)

2 Stars: Adequate

Schutt Air Advantage

STAR Value: 0.678

Cost: $159.99

1 Star: Marginal

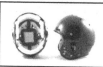
Riddell VSR4

STAR Value: 0.791
Cost: Not Applicable
Used helmets were tested
to provide a reference

NR: Not Recommended

Adams A2000 Pro Elite

STAR Value: 1.700

Cost: $199.95

Note: Any player in any sport can sustain a head injury with even the very best head protection. This analysis is based on data trends and probabilities, and therefore a specific person's risk may vary. This variation is likely dominated by genetic differences, health history, and impact factors such as muscle activation.

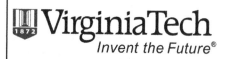

Figure 11-3D. Virginia Tech adult football helmet ratings. (Reprinted with permission from Virginia Tech – Wake Forest University, School of Biomedical Engineering & Sciences.)

Mouth Guards

One-third of all dental injuries each year are sports related.[31] During a single athletic season, athletes have a 1-in-10 chance of a facial or dental injury.[32] Anywhere from 10% to 61% of athletes have experienced at least 1 orofacial injury during their participation in sports.[33] The American Dental Association reported that an athlete is 60 times more likely to suffer dental injuries when not wearing a mouth guard.[34] Since mouth guards have been made mandatory in football, face and mouth injuries have dropped from 50% of all injuries to less than 0.5%.[35] The National Federation of State High School Associations currently mandates the use of mouth guards in football, field hockey, ice hockey, lacrosse, and wrestling (for wrestlers wearing braces; www.nfhs.org/sports-resource-content/position-statement-and-recommendations-for-mouthguard-use-in-sports/).

Originally developed in 1890, mouth guards were developed to decrease lip lacerations in boxing. They were first seen in the United States in 1916 and became mandatory for boxing in the 1930s. Initially, they were made from gutta percha, a natural polymer that is chemically the same as rubber. Modern mouth guards use an array of synthetic materials. A dentist developed the first reusable mouth guard in the 1930s.[33] Mouth guards became mandatory for United States high School football in 1962 and for NCAA College football in 1973.[35] Mouth guards are now the most common form of protective equipment worn by high school athletes.[36]

A mouth guard is considered "a resilient device or appliance placed inside the mouth to reduce mouth injuries, particularly to teeth and surrounding structures."[33] There are several types of mouth guards. Stock mouth guards are found in stores, are ready to wear, and are not fitted to the teeth. Boil and bite guards are heated and partially molded to the teeth during cooling. This is the most common type seen in sport. Custom made guards require an impression of the patient's teeth, and the guard is made from the cast molding. Single or multiple layers of polyvinyl acetate or polyethylene are heated and pressed over the cast to form a more rigid and better fitting guard. Athletes can modify one of these to a cut-off that has no posterior tooth coverage.[37] Each type of mouth guard has advantages and disadvantages. Stock mouth guards are inexpensive and ready to wear. However, they provide minimal protection, are uncomfortable, inhibit speech, and may interfere with breathing because of their lack of fitting. Boil and bite mouth guards are easily obtainable, relatively inexpensive, and provide more protection than stock guards. The negatives are that they are still bulky, ill fitting, and lose their shape after multiple uses. Custom-made mouth guards are the highest quality and are the most comfortable to wear. The custom fit allows for easy breathing and better speaking. They permanently retain their shape. The major disadvantage is cost, ranging from $150 to $200, and fitting may require multiple trips to the dentist.[38] According to Patrick et al[37] and Greasley and Karet,[38] the following criteria should apply to mouth guards to ensure protection; however, these are typically seen in custom-fit mouth guards only:

- They should enclose the maxillary teeth to the end of the second molars and should be 3 mm thick on the outward-facing surface, 2 mm on the biting surface, and 1 mm on the inner surface of the tooth.

- The labial flange of the mouth guard should extend to within 2 mm of the border between the gingiva and the cheek.

- The palatal flange of the mouth guard should extend about 10 mm above the gum line.

- The edge of the labial flange should be rounded in cross section, whereas the palatal edge should be tapered.

- When a maxillary guard is constructed, it should be articulated against the matching mandibular model for optimum comfort.

Controversy surrounds the notion that mouth guards can prevent concussions. Historical research reported that mouth guards were effective protection from concussive blows.[39,40] Initially, the claim came from an anecdotal report by Stenger et al[39] in 1964, who said that the use of mouth guards appeared to have abolished symptoms of vertigo, tinnitus, transient numbness, and tingling in a college football year over a single season. This article had almost no statistical analysis and, thus, insufficient support for its conclusion. Hickey et al[40] measured intracranial pressure in cadaver skulls during simulated blows to the head with and without mouth guards in place. The authors reported less intracranial pressure when mouth guards were used. This article became the primary support for the notion that mouth guards prevent concussions despite several limitations. Hickey et al[40] assumed that concussions were due to linear blows and that higher intracranial pressure was an indication of brain trauma. Neither are actually indicative. They used a cadaver skull and its fixation so that it remained stationary and did not simulate actual concussive blows in living athletes. All forces were applied directly to the chin rather than from angles or to the cranium. A more recent supporter of mouth guards for concussion prevention is Winters[41] in 2001, who designed a study similar to that performed by Hickey et al[40] using a fabricated skull. The hypothesis was that mouth guards, when properly fitted, increase the time and distance involved in the acceleration of the head during an upward blow to the mandible, meaning that the forces would be spread out over a longer time and space. They measured the separation distance that occurs at the head of the condyle and the base of the skull and the time it took to reach peak separation. The conclusion was that a thicker posterior mouth guard would reduce the forces on the brain and, thereby, decrease concussions.[40] Again, the fixation, linear chin blow, and nonhuman model limit the value of their results.

Knapik et al[33] reviewed the literature in 2007 to determine what evidence existed to support the claims that mouth guards were likely to reduce the risk of concussion. A total of 69 studies were found that provided quantitative data on mouth guard use and injury. Fourteen studies met the review criteria requiring data on users and nonusers. However, the methodological quality scores were poor, especially for research published before the 1980s. Despite these issues, Knapick[33] indicated that the risk of an orofacial sports injury was 1.6 to 1.9 times higher when a mouth guard was not worn. However, the evidence that mouth guards protect against concussion was inconsistent, and no conclusion regarding the effectiveness of mouth guards in preventing concussion was determined. Two recent studies looked specifically at mouth guards and preventing concussion. Marshall et al[42] investigated the injury rates of rugby players to determine if mouth guards lowered the risk of concussions. In a sport in which players are largely unprotected from impact forces, 65% percent of the 304 participants reported using mouth guards (teeth/mouth/jaw injury: mouth guard users = 0.45/1000 athlete-exposures [AEs]; nonusers = 0.61/1000 AEs [P = .73]; concussion: mouth guard users = 2.12/1000 AEs; nonusers = 0.91/1000 AEs [P = .16]; relative risk [RR] = 1.62; 95% confidence interval [CI], 0.50, 5.25). The authors concluded that the current measures taken in rugby to reduce risk of injury are limited and may increase the chance of concussion.[42] Labella et al[43] investigated 50 Division I basketball teams for injury rates of dental injuries and concussion in mouth guard users and nonusers (dental injury: mouth guard users = 0.12/1000 AEs; mouth guard nonusers = 0.67/1000 AEs [P = .02]; dental referrals: mouth guard users = 0/1000 AEs; mouth guard nonusers = 0.72/1000 AEs [P < .01]; concussions: mouth guard users = 0.35/1000 AEs, mouth guard nonusers = 0.55/1000 AEs [P = .25]). Although the dental injuries appear to be lower in mouth guard users, the incident of concussion is inconclusive.

It is the authors' opinion that the current literature does not support mouth guard use for prevention of concussions. Early studies were based on anecdotal evidence and assumptions about how to measure brain injury. Other studies have had serious validity issues. Others show an increase in concussions with mouth guard use. There appears to be a significant lack of evidence to support the use of mouth guards to protect against concussions.

CLINICAL PREVENTION METHODS

The risk of acute and chronic injury in sport has been documented. Musculoskeletal injuries of the upper extremity seem to plague overhead athletes, whereas lower extremity injuries are more common in sports that involve running, cutting, and jumping. The high incidence of ankle sprains in contact and noncontact sport and the negative consequence for future sport participation call for preventive measures. In an attempt to prevent ankle sprains, prophylactic taping, braces, specially designed shoes, and proprioceptive training have been implemented. Balance and coordination training are common components of intervention programs for the prevention and treatment of acute lateral ankle sprains and chronic ankle instability.[44] Flexibility has been presented as one of the primary etiological factors associated with injury and, specifically, with musculotendinous strains, the most frequent athletic related injury.[45,46] Anecdotally, stretching has been promoted before athletic activity as a method of improving joint range of motion (ROM), muscle flexibility, improving performance, and preventing injury.[45,46] However, its effects on performance and injury prevention are not clear. The next section reviews the literature to determine the effectiveness of these measures.

Prophylactic Ankle Bracing and Taping

The ankle joint is one of the most frequently injured sites for individuals who participate in recreational or competitive athletics. Garrick and Requa[47] reviewed injuries treated in a sports medicine clinic over a 6.5-year period and determined that 25% of 12,681 injuries were to the ankle and foot. Ankle sprains accounted for approximately 85% of the injuries to this region. Most ankle sprains result from a stress on an inverted and plantarflexed (supinated) foot that damages the lateral ligaments. Individuals who sustain ankle sprains demonstrate high recurrence rates and disability and may develop chronic pain or chronic ankle instability.[48]

In theory, prophylactic taping has an effect by reducing ROM of plantarflexion and inversion of the ankle. However, research has shown that this restricting effect is lost after periods of exercise.[49] This loss of effect does not occur when using a brace. Taping can be applied individually similar to braces, but the use of braces is more cost effective.[50] Recent research strengthens the idea that taping and bracing act more by improving neuromuscular feedback than by restricting the ROM. Most evidence supports the prophylactic effects of the use of external support or balance/coordination training in the prevention of first-time and recurrent sprains.[51]

There is historical evidence for use of prophylactic taping and bracing. A 1973 study of intramural college basketball players found a higher rate of ankle injury in untaped than taped participants (injury rate [IR] = 14.7 vs 32.8/1000 games) over 2 years.[52] Ankle taping was more effective in those with a history of ankle sprains than in those without a prior ankle injury. The IR for those previously injured with tape was 16.4/1000 games and 55.3/1000 games for previously injured, untaped participants.[52] Surve et al[53] determined that a semirigid stirrup orthosis significantly reduced the incidence of ankle sprains in soccer players with previous ankle sprains. The study reported an incidence of ankle sprains in male soccer players with a history of injury while wearing a semirigid stirrup orthosis as 0.46/1000 playing-hours. This was significantly lower than the previously injured control group without external support of 1.16/1000 playing-hours. The reported incidence of participants without history of injury while wearing a semirigid stirrup orthosis was 0.97/1000 playing-hours compared to a control group without external support of 0.92/1000 playing-hours.[53] Sitler et al[54] evaluated the effect of a semirigid ankle brace in a 2-year randomized, clinical trial of 1601 intramural basketball players at West Point. The injury rate was significantly lower in the braced group (1.6 sprains/1000 AEs), whereas the unbraced control group had 5.2 sprains/1000 AEs. The study concluded that the risk of sustaining an ankle injury was 3 times greater for the control subjects not wearing an ankle stabilizer.[54]

More recently, McGuine et al[55] examined the effectiveness of lace-up ankle braces on first-time and recurrent ankle injuries in a group of high school basketball players. A key objective of this study was to determine whether using lace-up ankle braces reduces the number and severity of acute first-time ankle injuries. The study recruited 1460 players (720 in the control group and 740 in the braced group). Seventy-eight ankle sprains and fractures were sustained by the control group, and 27 ankle injuries occurred in the braced group out of 112,439 total exposures. The overall incidence of acute ankle injury per 1000 exposures was lower in the braced group (IR = 0.47/1000 AEs; 95% CI, 0.30, 0.74) than in the control group (IR = 1.41; 95% CI, 1.05, 1.89). McGuine et al[48] defined first event acute ankle sprain as the first acute ankle sprain that occurred after the study began. Results for this study used this term. There were 75 first-event acute ankle injuries in the control group compared with 26 in the braced group (hazard ratio [HR] = 0.32; 95% CI, 0.20, 0.52; P <.001). First-time acute ankle injuries occurred 68% less often in braced athletes than in controls. For players who reported a previous ankle injury, the incidence of acute ankle injury was lower in the braced group (IR = 0.83/1000 AEs; 95% CI, 0.37, 1.84) than in the control group (IR = 1.79; 95% CI, 0.98, 3.27), and first-event acute ankle injuries occurred about 60% less often in braced athletes than in controls (HR = 0.39; 95% CI, 0.17, 0.90; P = .028). For players who did not report a previous ankle injury, the incidence of a first-event acute ankle injury was lower in the braced group (IR = 0.40; 95% CI, 0.23, 0.70) than in the control group (IR = 1.35; 95% CI, 1.00, 1.81), and first-event acute ankle injuries occurred 70% less often in braced athletes than in controls (HR = 0.30; 95% CI, 0.17, 0.52; P <.001). Therefore, McGuine et al[55] concluded that lace-up ankle braces reduce the incidence of injury in basketball athletes with and without a history of ankle injury.

McGuine et al[56] continued examining the effectiveness of lace-up ankle braces on first-time and recurrent ankle injuries in a group of high school football players. A total of 2081 athletes (control, n = 1088; braced, n = 993) had 125,419 football exposures, resulting in 95 first-event acute ankle injuries (control, 68; braced, 27). The incidence of ankle injury per 1000 exposures was significantly lower for the braced group (0.48) than for the control group (1.12). The RR of sustaining of an ankle injury in the braced group was 0.435 (95% CI, 0.281, 0.674). The incidence of an acute ankle injury was reduced in the braced group by 70% for players who reported a previous ankle injury and 57% for players with no previous ankle injury. Overall, using a lace-up ankle brace reduced the incidence of acute ankle injuries by 61% in high school football players.

Olmsted et al[50] investigated the works of Garrick and Requa,[47] Sitler at al,[54] and Surve et al[53] to determine numbers needed to treat (NNT). NNT can provide the clinical usefulness of an intervention by producing estimates of the number of treatments to prevent 1 injury occurrence. In collegiate intramural basketball players, the prevention of 1 ankle sprain required the taping of 26 athletes with a history of ankle sprain and 143 with no prior history. In a military academy intramural basketball program, prevention of 1 sprain required bracing of 18 athletes with a history of ankle sprain and 39 with no history. Ankle bracing in competitive soccer players produced an NNT of 5 athletes with a history of previous sprain and 57 with no prior injury.[50] McGuine et al[56] also produced the NNT for each of their studies (14.5 for the basketball athletes and 28.3 for the football athletes). It can be considered that a high school team of 60 football players that 1 to 3 ankle injuries can be avoided during the season depending on the athletes' prior histories.

A final review by Parkkari et al[7] summarized prevention programs and their effectiveness. The review identified 16 randomized controlled trials (RCTs) that have been published on prevention of sports injuries from 1970 to 2000. Four of these studies examined ankle stabilizers and provided high-quality evidence that use of semirigid ankle stabilizers reduces the risk of ankle sprains, especially among those with previous ankle instability problems. Recurrent ankle sprains can be prevented by ankle supports (ie, semirigid orthoses) in high-risk sporting activities, such as soccer and basketball.[52-55,57]

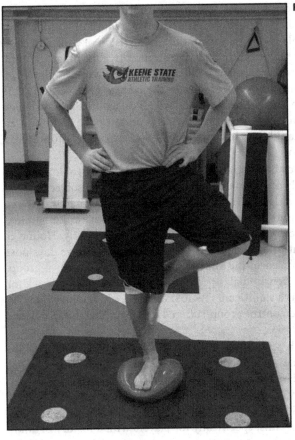

Figure 11-4. Proprioceptive training.

In the 2013 National Athletic Trainers' Assocation position statement titled "Conservative Management and Prevention of Ankle Sprains in Athletes,"[48] the use of prophylactic bracing and taping was supported for those with a history of ankle injury. Athletes with previous ankle sprains who braced or taped the ankle had approximately 70% fewer ankle injuries than athletes without prophylactic support. Participants who had a previous history of ankle sprains had a reduction in the incidence of ankle sprains when wearing a semirigid brace. However, in athletes with no history of ankle injuries, there was no difference in the incidence of ankle sprains between the control and braced groups.

These results demonstrate a benefit in ankle taping[52] and semirigid[54,55] and lace-up[55,56] ankle bracing as beneficial in reducing the incidence of acute ankle injuries. This protective effect was observed in players with and with no history of ankle injury. Wearing ankle braces may be a cost-effective injury prevention strategy compared to ankle taping. But, there are other intervention options available to reduce the incidence of ankle sprains.

Prevention Through Proprioceptive Training

As early as 1965, Freeman[58] hypothesized that balance and coordination training could reduce the proprioceptive deficits associated with ligamentous injury to the ankle. Proprioception refers to the inborn kinesthetic awareness of body posture, including movement.[44,57] Proprioceptive training typically involves activities in a single-limb stance that challenge the person's ability to maintain balance. Balance training programs have used balance boards, foam pads, and dynamic hopping activities while performing functional sport activities, such as throwing, catching, and dribbling on one leg. Ankle balance training is a unique method because it stimulates multiple planes of ankle movement on a weight-bearing foot (Figure 11-4).[44]

Several studies have examined the effectiveness of these training programs. Parkkari et al[7] identified 4 RCTs that indicated that the general injury rate can be reduced by ankle disk training.[44,59-61] Mohammadi[59] used 80 male soccer players in the first division of a men's league with previous inversion sprains. Intervention options included proprioceptive training, strength training, orthosis, and no intervention/control group. The incidence of ankle sprains in players of the proprioception training group was significantly lower than in the control group (RR = 0.13; 95% CI, 0.003, 0.93; P = .02). The strength and orthotic groups were not significantly different from the control group. Therefore, Mohammadi[59] determined that proprioceptive training was an effective strategy in reducing the rate of ankle sprains among male soccer players who suffered ankle sprain compared with no intervention.

Tropp[62] investigated the effect of balance board training on the incidence of ankle injuries. In a 6-month prospective, randomized study of 439 male soccer players, 5% of the subjects in the balance board training group sustained an ankle sprain. That was significantly less than the 17% of players who sustained ankle sprains in the control group. For subjects with previous ankle sprains, 2% of the ankle disk group and 25% of the control group sustained injury. Similarly, Holme et al[63] studied 92 recreational athletes without prior complaints of ankle instability. Five days post sport-related injury, each participant was placed in the ankle balance training or control group. The treatment group participated in comprehensive balance training exercises twice per week for 12 months. The authors found that there was a significant (P < .05) difference in reinjury rate (7% in the training group), whereas 29% in the control group suffered reinjury. The ankle balance training group had a reduced reinjury risk.[63]

Wester et al[64] examined 48 patients with acute ankle sprains. They determined that balance board training for 12 weeks for 15 minutes/day, was effective in reducing the number of recurrent ankle injury. Twenty-five percent of the balance training group compared to 54% of the control group had recurrent ankle sprains. Similarly, Verhagen et al[60] followed Dutch Division II and III volleyball players and found use of a proprioceptive balance board program during the 36-week season to be effective for preventing ankle sprains, specifically for players with a history of ankle sprains. Significantly fewer ankle sprains in the intervention group were found compared to a control group (risk difference = 0.4/1000 playing-hours; 95% CI, 0.1, 0.7).

In a 2008 systematic review, McKeon and Hertel[44] found several positive outcomes from ankle proprioceptive training. Three articles met the inclusion criteria to answer the question, "Can prophylactic balance training reduce the risk of sustaining a lateral ankle sprain?" RR reduction (RRR) of sustaining an ankle sprain ranged from 20% to 60% after balance and coordination training. Of the 8 comparisons within the articles, half had a 95% CI that went below zero. The NNT point estimates for the various comparisons ranged from 12 to 44 NNT-benefit. But, the 95% CI's point estimates ranged from 6 NNT-benefit to 10 NNT-harm, indicating uncertainty as to the nature of the preventive effect of the balance training to prevent lateral ankle sprain.[44] Two articles met the inclusion criteria to answer the question, "Can balance and coordination training improve treatment outcomes associated with acute ankle sprains?" Their review revealed point estimates of 54% to 76% RRR of sustaining recurrent ankle sprain after undergoing balance training following an acute ankle sprain. The 95% CIs for the RRR did not cross zero and ranged from 0 to 94. The NNT analysis revealed that in order to prevent one recurrent ankle sprain, 4 to 5 patients recovering from acute ankle sprains would need to complete the rehabilitation training, with 95% CIs around these point measures ranging from 2 to 17 NNT-benefit.[44] This demonstrates that balance training can greatly decrease the risk of recurrent ankle sprains. These researchers concluded that prophylactic balance and coordination training substantially reduced the risk of ankle sprains in athletes, with a greater effect seen in those with a history of sprain.[44]

Many studies have documented that balance board training will reduce the risk of ankle sprains in athletes with a history of an ankle sprain. The efficacy of a balance board training program as the primary intervention for the prevention of sprains in athletes with healthy ankles remains to be determined.[60,61] In a randomized, intervention trial, McGuine and Keene[61] set out to determine if a program of balance training, implemented in the preseason and maintained throughout the season, would reduce the risk of ankle sprains in high school athletes. The ankle sprain IR was significantly lower for the intervention subjects (1.13/1000 AEs) compared to (1.87/1000 AEs) in the control group. Furthermore, it appears that athletes with a previous history of ankle sprain preforming the intervention program cut their risk of another ankle sprain in half (RR = 0.56). These results suggest that a balance training program, implemented throughout a sports season, will reduce the rate of ankle sprains in previously uninjured and injured athletes, although the greatest benefit is seen in previously injured athletes.[61]

Although the evidence appears in favor of proprioception training, many questions remain. The number of ankle sprains was reduced when these training programs were used. However, the reason for the reduction is largely unknown.[48] Kaminski et al[48] stated that no evidence suggests that improving ROM or strength should be considered strategies to prevent ankle injury. However, indirectly, ROM and strength deficits have been identified in those with a history of ankle injury, and ankle muscle strength is improved with balance training. Strength deficits and imbalances may play a role in vulnerable positioning of the foot during athletics, adding to the risk of ankle injury.[48] Verhagen et al[60] also supported the notion that proprioceptive function at the ankle joint is reduced after injury and can lead to the increased risk of reinjury. Because impaired proprioceptive function is restored with balance training, this might suggest that they identified a rehabilitative effect and not a preventive effect. This is supported by Verhagen et al[65] which summarizes that balance training appears to reduce the risk of ankle sprains in athletes suffering from recurrent sprains. To truly identify these primary effects, any subject with a history of ankle sprain would need to be eliminated from the study. In addition, the duration, frequency, and length of the training programs reported a range from 10 minutes to 1 hour/session, repeated 1 to 7 times/week, and performed over a 3- to 12-month period. So, the optimal training protocol is still in question.

From these reviews, balance and coordination training is an effective intervention to reduce the incidence and recurrence of ankle sprains. In addition, the longer these programs are implemented, the greater the effect.[44] Based on the evidence presented, one can recommend the use of balance and coordination training to prevent ankle sprains, especially in those with a history of ankle injury.

Preventing Musculotendinous Injury

A muscle strain, the partial or complete tear of the muscle-tendon unit, is a common sport-related injury. Hamstring strains are common injuries in kicking and sprinting sports in which sudden acceleration is required.[66] In theory, the purposes of stretching before an athletic event are to ensure sufficient ROM in the joints to perform the activity optimally and to decrease muscle stiffness or increase muscle flexibility. Stretching is therefore intended to affect performance and injury risk.[67] Stretching might improve, have no effect on, or impair performance. Similarly, stretching might decrease, have no effect on, or increase injury risk. Sports such as American football, soccer, and track have a high incidence of hamstring injuries. These injuries can be significant and force lengthy rehabilitation times and are subject to reinjury. The effectiveness of stretching to prevent hamstring injuries is the focus of the following review.

Cross and Worrell[46] compared the number of lower extremity muscle strains in a season of college football after introducing a static stretching program to the number of strains in the previous nonintervention season. The static stretching intervention consisted of 3 stretches held for 15 seconds each for each muscle group of the lower extremity. The number of muscle strains was significantly lower for the intervention season. Specifically, muscle strains were reduced by 48.8% (from 43 to 21 injuries).

Although not specifically evaluating the hamstring muscle group, Pope et al[68] studied 1583 male Australian army recruits randomly assigned to stretching or control groups. Both

Figure 11-5. Hamstring lowers (Nordic ski exercise).

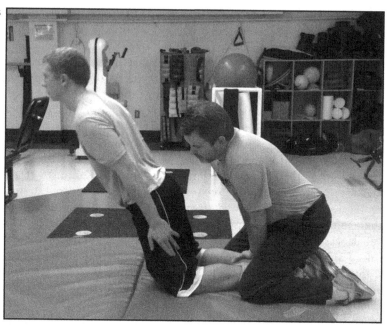

groups performed warm-up activities prior to physical training. The stretching group performed one 20-second static stretch for 6 lower extremity muscle groups, whereas the control group did not stretch. Over a 12-week period of training, there were a total of 333 lower extremity injuries, including 214 soft tissue injuries. There were 158 injuries to the stretch group and 175 to the control group. The HR of the nonstretching group (0.95) was similar to the HR of the stretching group (1.00), essentially indicating no difference in IRs between the groups. The pre-exercise stretching protocol did not produce a clinically useful reduction in injury risk.[68]

Arnason et al[66] tested the effect of eccentric strength training and flexibility training on the incidence of hamstring strains in soccer. The authors previously determined an IR of 3.0 to 4.1/1000 hours of competition and 0.4 to 0.5/1000 hours of training.[66,69] Hamstring strains and player exposure were recorded during 4 consecutive soccer seasons for elite soccer teams from Iceland and Norway. The first 2 seasons provided the baseline hamstring injury data. In the next seasons, athletes participated in a prevention program that consisted of warm-up stretching, flexibility training, and/or eccentric strength training. The warm-up stretches were done in pairs using the contract-relax method of proprioceptive neuromuscular facilitation stretching and occurred before any sprinting or shooting exercises prior to every training session and game. The flexibility training program was performed after training 3 times/week and used similar partner contract-relax stretches. The eccentric strength training program was prescribed for the Icelandic teams during both seasons and for the Norwegian teams during one season. The eccentric program was based on the Nordic hamstring lowers exercise (www.richmondphysiotherapyclinic.com.au/physiotherapy/research/hamstring-strengthening-and-prevention-of-injury) (Figure 11-5). The authors[66] discovered no significant difference in the incidence of hamstring strains between the teams that did and did not follow the flexibility intervention program (IR = 0.54 ± 0.12 vs 0.35 ± 0.10; RR = 1.53; 95% CI, 0.76, 3.08; P = .22). Also, no difference was found in the incidence of hamstring strains between the intervention group and all teams from the previous year (IR = 0.54 ± 0.12 vs 0.52 ± 0.09; RR: 1.03, 0.59 to 1.79; P = .91), nor between the 2 seasons for the intervention group only (IR = 0.54 ± 0.12 vs 0.61 ± 0.18; RR: 0.89, 0.42 to 1.85; P = .75). With regard to the eccentric training program, the overall incidence of hamstring strains was 65% lower among the teams that used the program compared with the teams that did not use the program (IR = 0.22 ± 0.06 vs 0.62 ± 0.05; RR: 0.35; 95% CI, 0.19, 0.62; P = .001).[62] It was determined that stretching during warm-up and flexibility training of the hamstrings group had no effect on the incidence of hamstring strains. Interestingly, the main finding of the study was that eccentric strength training with Nordic hamstring lowers combined with warm-up stretching seems to be effective in preventing hamstring strains in soccer.[66] This is supported by Shrier's[70] review that found beneficial effects when stretching was used in combination with other interventions. Three of the 4 articles that showed a positive effect incorporated other elements, such as a warm-up or rehabilitation exercise. Therefore, it is impossible to determine which intervention is responsible for the decreased IR.

Active, dynamic, passive, and/or proprioceptive neuromuscular facilitation stretching treatment to improve flexibility have been used by coaches, strength coaches, athletic trainers, and physical therapists for many years. Yet, there are mixed results to the question of whether stretching reduces muscle strain injury. Authors report that preparticipation stretching in addition to warm-up will have no impact on injury risk.[67] Others declare there is some evidence to indicate that preparticipation stretching reduces muscle injuries[46] and decreases risk of muscle strains.[67] More state that stretching programs do not produce clinically useful reduction in IR[61] and no effect on the incidence of hamstring strains.[66] Reduced flexibility is one of many risk factors involved in musculotendinous injuries. Lower hamstring injuries appear to be the result of combined interventions with stretching, such as warm-up,[70] strength training, and eccentric strength training.[66] A common limitation is the inability to isolate the effect of stretching alone. There are a limited number of RCTs to study whether stretching reduces the risk or incidence of hamstring stains. The ideal randomized trial would include the following 4 groups: (1) a group performing stretching alone, (2) a group performing warm-up alone, (3) a group performing stretching plus warm-up, and (4) a group performing neither.[67]

One of the first RCTs published implemented a multifactorial prevention program on soccer players.[71] Because this study included several prevention strategies, it created limitations to the study that precluded it from determining which component of the prevention program was effective and which components were not effective at all. However, with regard to stretching, studies failed to show any positive effect of stretching on individual injury risk.[66,68-70,72]

Discussion

Rules, policy, and legislation have been developed to decrease injury incidence in sport. Some rules were determined based on epidemiological data and an understanding of the mechanism of injury, whereas others were generated by public awareness and have not been well studied. Depending on the level of sport (youth, high school, college, or professional), rules for safe play are reviewed annually or biannually. Fair play appears to have a positive impact on decreasing injury incidence.[14,17-19] Although some of these policies and legislations may have decreased injury rates,[11-13] others have not.[15,16]

Protective equipment is required for many sports and recommended for others. Typically, noncontact sports do not have equipment rules. Manufacturers are more focused on establishing the effectiveness of their products; thus, more research is being conducted on different types of equipment. Minimum standards and certification for sport equipment has also improved. The National Operating Committee on Standards for Athletic Equipment certifies all helmets, faceguards, and headwear prior to retail distribution. However, a literature review found some equipment to be effective in decreasing injuries, such as dental, facial, or skull injuries,[33,35,36] but they lack evidence for influencing concussion.[25,26,39,41] Sports injury specialists need to continue to identify when mandates on sports equipment were required and then analyze pre- and postinjury surveillance data to determine the efficacy of equipment decreasing injury.

Athletic trainers should be aware of products marketed under the premise of concussion or injury prevention. Many of these products have not been extensively studied through independent research. Therefore, there are little empirical data on the prevention capabilities of these products

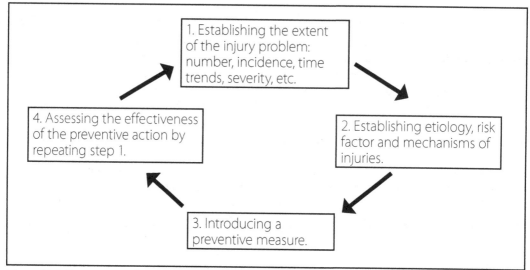

Figure 11-6. The sequence of prevention of sports injuries.[66]

concerning their abilities to reduce the risk of sustaining a concussion or other sport-related injury. Sports medicine professionals should understand the mechanics of these products and carefully consider their ability to prevent injury based on the known mechanisms and etiologies of injury. They are often asked if these products work.

Most preventive strategies suggested in the literature come from descriptive research and have not been derived from risk factors that have been substantiated as injury predictors through longitudinal or experimental research. Valid and reliable measurement of exposures must include exact information about the population at risk and exposure time.[73] The true efficacy of a preventive strategy can be best evaluated through a well-planned, randomized trial. In nonrandomized studies, samples who use protective equipment and those who do not creates a bias. However, studies using carefully supervised, prospective, longitudinal cohorts lead to a more valid comparison of IR, but they are usually focused on small groups of athletes. A prospective approach that follows a large group of participants through various exposures allows for better comparisons but may include more inaccuracies on classification of injuries. Studies using passive methods of data collection can cover a large number of severe injuries rather well, and based on these studies, it is possible to define the risk profiles of different types of sports. Consequently, the case-control studies (retrospective longitudinal cohorts) and cohort studies, when interpreted correctly, may provide important clues for injury prevention (Figure 11-6).[72]

BRINGING IT TOGETHER

Athletic trainers should identify interventions commonly used in sport prevention and determine if these techniques are effective in preventing injuries. Questions focus on the nature of the injury, the intervention applied, and how to measure the outcome. The first step in the process is to establish IRs and injury mechanisms. The next step is to evaluate the risk factors and opportunities to modify them. The third step is to implement the intervention. In research terms, an RCT has the highest level of evidence. In order for outcomes to be determined, postinjury rates must then be established and compared to the preintervention rates. Many variables might contribute to whether a prevention strategy is effective. For example, in educational or training programs, the duration of the intervention is a variable. Current research has identified some

TABLE 11-4 PROPHYLACTIC DEVICES—COMPLETE THE CHART			
PROPHYLACTIC DEVICE	**SPORT COMMONLY USED**	**POSITION**	**POSSIBLE INJURY BEING PREVENTED**
Lateral knee stabilizers	Football	Linemen	Knee injuries

effective interventions. But, common limitations include nonrandomized groups, a lack of pre- and postinjury rates, and attempts to determine an intervention's effect on a risk factor rather than the IR. Unlike general health epidemiology, which has a long history of research on prevention, sport epidemiology continues to need additional research to support preventive strategies.

LEARNING ACTIVITIES

1. Investigate the differences between high school (www.nfhs.org) and college (http://www.ncaa.org/championships/playing-rules?division=d1) equipment mandates for your favorite sport (Table 11-4).

   a. Are there more or less requirements as players age?

   b. Are there gender differences in equipment or rules?

2. Review the NFL football rules changes timeline (http://www.steelerfury.com/drupal/?q=node/3). Which changes in the last 20 years do you think have had the most effect on athlete safety? Identify which sports have age- or gender-specific rules (as noted earlier in ice hockey and checking), and hypothesize why those requirements are in place (eg, injury prevention of concussion, sudden death, or musculoskeletal injuries) (Table 11-5).

3. Create one sport-related rule (any sport) that might reduce the incidence of an injury, and explain the rationale behind the rule change. Provide evidence that supports the rule change.

4. A certified athletic trainer is caring for the college women's basketball and men's baseball teams. What are all of the considerations that she or he must make when addressing prevention of musculoskeletal injury of the players on each team? What are some prevention tools and techniques that might be implemented? Contrast these choices with teams of varying age, gender, and sport.

5. Investigate other common interventions for high-risk vs overuse injuries and determine their effectiveness.

TABLE 11-5 FAIR PLAY RULES AND INJURIES—COMPLETE THE CHART				
SPORT	SPORT TYPE	RULE	CONSEQUENCE OF FOUL PLAY	POSSIBLE RESULTANT INJURY
Soccer	Contact	Studs-up tackle	Yellow or red card	Lower-extremity injury to opponent

- Plyometric training and neuromuscular training for anterior cruciate ligament or hamstring injury
- Patellofemoral injuries and vastus medialis oblique training
- Rotator cuff injuries and rotator cuff strength training or periscapular strengthening.

REFERENCES

1. Van Mechelen W. Aetiology and Prevention of Running Injuries [dissertation]. Amsterdam, The Netherlands: Free University of Amsterdam; 1992.
2. Taimela S, Kujala UM, Osterman K. Intrinsic risk factors and athletic injuries. *Sports Med.* 1990;9(4):205-215.
3. Lysens RJ, de Weerdt W, Nieuwboer A. Factors associated with injury proneness. *Sports Med.* 1991;12(5):281-289.
4. Maffulli N, Wong J, Almekinders LC. Types and epidemiology of tendinopathy. *Clin Sports Med.* 2003;22(4):675-692.
5. Zinder SM, Basler RS, Foley J, Scarlata C, Vasily DB. National Athletic Trainers' Association position statement: skin diseases. *J Athl Train.* 2010;45(4):411-428.
6. Backx FJ, Beijer HJ, Bol E, Erich WB. Injuries in persons and high-risk sports. A longitudinal study in 1818 school children. *Am J Sports Med.* 1991;19(2):124-130.
7. Parkkari J, Kujala UM, Kannus P. Is it possible to prevent sports injuries? Review of controlled clinical trials and recommendations for future work. *Sports Med.* 2001;31(14):985-995.

8. USA Hockey. 2013-17 Official Rules of Ice Hockey. http://assets.ngin.com/attachments/document/0042/4244/2013-17_USAH_Rulebook.pdf. Published 2013. Accessed October 21, 2015.

9. Tomei KL, Doe C, Prestigiacomo CJ, Gandhi CD. Comparative analysis of state-level concussion legislation and review of current practices in concussion. *Neurosurg Focus.* 2012;33(6):E11:1-9.

10. Mueller FO, Colgate B. Annual Survey of Football Injury Research, 1931-2012. http://nccsir.unc.edu/files/2014/05/2011FBAnnual.pdf. Published February, 2012. Accessed December 2, 2015.

11. Chrisman SP, Schiff MA, Chung SK, Herring SA, Rivara FP. Implementation of concussion legislation and extent of concussion education for athletes, parents, and coaches in Washington State. *Am J Sports Med.* 2014;42(5):1190-1196.

12. Mueller FO, Blyth CS. North Carolina high school football injury study: equipment and prevention. *J Sports Med.* 1974;2(1):1-10.

13. Cantu RC, Mueller FO. Catastrophic spine injuries in American football, 1977-2001. *Neurosurgery.* 2003;53(2):358-362.

14. Associated Press. NFL: 13 percent fewer concussions. http://espn.go.com/nfl/story/_/id/10377147/nfl-says-13-percent-fewer-concussions-season Published January 30, 2014. Accessed April 11, 2014.

15. Krolikowski M, Black A, Kang J, Emery C. Did "zero tolerance for head contact" rule enforcement change the risk of game related concussions in youth ice hockey players? *Br J Sports Med.* 2014;48(7):621-622.

16. Emery CA, Kang J, Shrier I, et al. Risk of injury associated with body checking among youth ice hockey players. *JAMA.* 2010;303(22):2265-2272.

17. Lincoln AE, Caswell SV, Almquist JL, Dunn RE, Norris JB, Hinton RY. Trends in concussion incidence in high school sports: a prospective 11-year study. *Am J Sports Med.* 2011;39(5):958-963.

18. Marar M, McIlvain NM, Fields SK, Comstock RD. Epidemiology of concussions among United States high school athletes in 20 sports. *Am J Sports Med.* 2012;40(4):747-755.

19. Mihalik JP, Greenwald RM, Blackburn JT, Cantu RC, Marshall SW, Guskiewicz KM. Effect of infraction type on head impact severity in youth ice hockey. *Med Sci Sports Exerc.* 2010;42(8):1431-1438.

20. Emery CA, Kang J, Schneider KJ, Meeuwisse WH. Risk of injury and concussion associated with team performance and penalty minutes in competitive youth ice hockey. *Br J Sports Med.* 2011;45(16):1289-1293.

21. Bubb RG, Smith T. 2010 and 2011 NCAA Wrestling Rules and Interpretations. Indianapolis, Indiana: NCAA; 2009. http://www.ncaapublications.com/productdownloads/WR11.pdf. Accessed October 8, 2015.

22. Rosenfeld V. Weight loss in wrestling: current state of science. NCAA Health and Safety Sport Science Institute. http://www.ncaa.org/health-and-safety/sport-science-institute/weight-loss-wrestling-current-state-science. Published September 11, 2014. Accessed November 2014.

23. Beaschler, R. *2013-2014 and 2014-2015 NCAA Wrestling Rules and Interpretations.* Indianapolis, IN: The National Collegiate Athletic Association: July 2013.

24. McIntosh AS. Helmets and head protection for the athlete as a means to prevent injury. *Int SportsMed J.* 2003;4(1):1-9.

25. Weaver NL, Mueller FO, Kalsbeek WD, Bowling JM. The north carolina high school athletic injury study: design and methodology. *Med Sci Sports Exerc.* 1999;31(1):176-182.

26. Boden BP, Tacchetti RL, Cantu RC, Knowles SB, Mueller FO. Catastrophic head injuries in high school and college football players. *Am J Sports Med.* 2007;35(7):1075-1081.

27. National Football League. History of the NFL football helmet. http://www.nfl.com/news/story/0ap1000000095139/article/history-of-the-nfl-football-helmet. Published November 14, 2012. Accessed November 2014.

28. Rowson S, Duma SM. Development of the STAR evaluation system for football helmets: integrating player head impact exposure and risk of concussion. *Ann Biomed Eng.* 2011;39(8):2130-2140.

29. Collins M, Lovell MR, Iverson GL, Ide T, Maroon J. Examining concussion rates and return to play in high school football players wearing newer helmet technology: a three-year prospective cohort study. *Neurosurgery.* 2006;58(2):275-286.

30. Virginia Tech Department of Biomedical Engineering and Mechanics. Virginia tech helmet ratings. http://www.beam.vt.edu/helmet/donate.php. Accessed on January 30, 2015.

31. Berry D, Miller M. Athletic mouth guards and their role in injury prevention. *Athl Ther Today.* 2001;6(5):52-56.

32. Woodmansey KF. Athletic mouth guards prevent orofacial injuries. *J Am Coll Health.* 1997;45(4):179-182.

33. Knapik JJ, Marshall SW, Lee RB, et al. Mouth guards in sport activities: history, physical properties and injury prevention effectiveness. *Sports Med.* 2007;37(2):117-144.

34. Hopkins R. Mouth guards: essential athletic gear. *Hughston Health Alert.* http://www.hughston.com/Userfiles/Health-Alerts/vol19no4.pdf. Fall 2007;19(4):4. Accessed on March 17, 2014.

35. Newsome PH. The role of the mouthguard in the prevention of sports-related dental injuries. *Int Sportmed J.* 2003;4(1):1-7.

36. Francis KT, Brasher J. Physiological effects of wearing mouth guards. *Br J Sports Med.* 1991;25(4):227-231.

37. Patrick DG, Van Noort R, Found MS. Scale of protection and the various types of sports mouthguard. *Br J Sports Med.* 2005;39(5):278-281.

38. Greasley A, Karet B. Towards the development of a standard test procedure for mouth guard assessment. *Br J Sports Med.* 1997;31(1):31-35.

39. Stenger JM, Lawson EA, Wright JM, Ricketts J. Mouthguards: protection against shock to the head, neck and teeth. *J Am Dent Assoc.* 1964;69:273-281.

40. Hickey JC, Morris AL, Carlson LD, Seward TE. The relation of mouth protectors to cranial pressure and deformation. *J Am Dent Assoc.* 1967;74(4):735-740.

41. Winters JE Sr. Commentary: role of properly fitted mouth guards in prevention of sport-related concussion. *J Athl Train.* 2001;36(3):339-341.

42. Marshall SW, Loomis DP, Waller AE, et al. Evaluation of protective equipment for prevention of injuries in rugby union. *Int J Epidemiol.* 2005;34(1):113-118.

43. Labella CR, Smith BW, Sigurdsson A. Effect of mouthguards on dental injuries and concussions in college basketball. *Med Sci Sports Exerc.* 2002;34(1):41-44.

44. McKeon PO, Hertel J. Systematic review of postural control and lateral ankle instability, part II: is balance training clinically effective? *J Athl Train.* 2008;43(3):305-315.

45. Weldon SM, Hill RH. The efficacy of stretching for prevention of exercise-related injury: a systematic review of the literature. *Man Ther.* 2003;8(3):141-150.

46. Cross KM, Worrell TW. Effects of a static stretching program on the incidence of lower extremity musculotendinous strains. *J Athl Train.* 1999;34(1):11-14.

47. Garrick JG, Requa RK. Epidemiology of foot and ankle injuries in sports. *Clin Sports Med.* 1988;7(1):29-36.

48. Kaminski TW, Hertal J, Amendola N, et al. National Athletic Trainers' Association position statement: conservative management and prevention of ankle sprains in athletes. *J Athl Train.* 2013;48(4):528-545.

49. Gross MT, Lapp AK, Davis JM. Comparison of Swede-O-Universal ankle support and Aircast Sport-Stirrup orthoses and ankle tape in restricting eversion-inversion before and after exercise. *J Orthop Sport Phys Ther.* 1991;13(1):11-19.

50. Olmsted LC, Vela LI, Denegar CR, Hertel J. Prophylactic ankle taping and bracing: a numbers-needed-to-treat and cost-benefit analysis. *J Athl Train.* 2004;39(1):95-100.

51. McKeon PO, Mattacola CG. Interventions for the prevention of first time and recurrent ankle sprains. *Clin Sports Med.* 2008;27(3):371-382.

52. Garrick JG, Requa RK. Role of external support in the prevention of ankle sprains. *Med Sci Sports.* 1973;5(3):200-203.

53. Surve I, Schwellnus MP, Noakes T, Lombard C. A fivefold reduction in the incidence of recurrent ankle sprains in soccer players using the Sport-Stirrup orthosis. *Am J Sports Med.* 1994;22(5):601-606.

54. Sitler M, Ryan J, Wheeler B, et al. The efficacy of a semirigid ankle stabilizer to reduce acute ankle injuries in basketball. A randomized clinical study at West Point. *Am J Sports Med.* 1994;22(4):454-461.

55. McGuine TA, Brooks A, Hetzel S. The effect of lace-up ankle braces on injury rates in high school basketball players. *Am J Sports Med.* 2011;39(9):1840-1848.

56. McGuine TJ, Hetzel S, Wilson J, Brooks, A. The effect of lace-up ankle braces on injury rates in high school football players. *Am J Sports Med.* 2012;40(1):49-57.

57. Mickel TJ, Bottoni CR, Tsuji G, Chang K, Baum L, Tokushige KA. Prophylactic bracing versus taping for the prevention of ankle sprains in high school athletes: a prospective, randomized trial. *J Foot Ankle Surg.* 2006;45(6):360-365.

58. Freeman MA. Instability of the foot after injuries to the lateral ligament of the ankle. *J Bone Joint Surg Br.* 1965;47(4):669-677.

59. Mohammadi F. Comparison of 3 preventive methods to reduce the recurrence of ankle inversion sprains in male soccer players. *Am J Sports Med.* 2007;35(6):922-926.

60. Verhagen E, van der Beek A, Twisk J, Bouter L, Bahr R, van Mechelen W. The effect of a proprioceptive balance board training program for the prevention of ankle sprains. *Am J Sports Med.* 2004;32(6):1385-1395.

61. McGuine TA, Keene JS. The effect of a balance training program on the risk of ankle sprains in high school athletes. *Am J Sports Med.* 2006;34(7):1103-1111.

62. Tropp H, Askling C, Gillquist J. Prevention of ankle sprains. *Am J Sports Med.* 1985;13(4):259-262.

63. Holme E, Magnusson SP, Becher K, Bieler T, Aagaard P, Kjaer M. The effect of supervised rehabilitation on strength, postural sway, position sense and re-injury risk after acute ankle ligament sprain. *Scand J Med Sci Sports.* 1999;9(2):104-109.

64. Wester JU, Jespersen SM, Nielsen KD, Neumann L. Wobble board training after partial sprains of the lateral ligaments of the ankle: a prospective randomized study. *J Orthop Sports Phys Ther.* 1996;23(5):332-336.

65. Verhagen EA, van Mechelen W, de Vente W. The effect of preventative measures on the incidence of ankle sprains. *Clin J Sport Med.* 2000;10(4):291-296.

66. Arnason A, Anderson TE, Holme I, Engebretsen L, Bahr R. Prevention of hamstring strains in elite soccer: an intervention study. *Scand J Med Sci Sports.* 2008;18(1):40-48.

67. McHugh MP, Cosgrave CH. To stretch or not to stretch: the role of stretching in injury prevention and performance. *Scand J Med Sci Sports.* 2010;20(2):169-181.

68. Pope RP, Herbert RD, Kirwan JD, Graham BJ. A randomized trial of preexercise stretching for prevention of lower-limb injury. *Med Sci Sports Exerc.* 2000;32(2):271-277.

69. Arnason A, Sigurdsson SB, Gudmundsson A, Holme I, Engebretsen L, Bahr R. Risk factors for injuries in football. *Am J Sports Med.* 2004;32(1 suppl):5S-16S.

70. Shrier I. Stretching before exercise does not reduce the risk of local muscle injury: a critical review of the clinical and basic science literature. *Clin J Sport Med.* 1999;9(4):221-227.

71. Ekstrand J, Gillquist J, Liljedahl SO. Prevention of soccer injuries. Supervision by doctor and physiotherapist. *Am J Sports Med.* 1983;11(3):116-120.

72. Van Mechelen W, Hlobil H, Kemper HC, Voorn WJ, de Jongh HR. Prevention of running injuries by warm-up, cool-down, and stretching exercises. *Am J Sports Med.* 1993;21(5):711-719.

73. Caine CG, Caine DJ, Lindner KJ. The epidemiological approach to sports injuries. In: Caine DJ, Caine CG, Lindner KJ, eds. *Epidemiology of Sports Injuries.* Champaign, IL: Human Kinetics; 1996:1-13.

Financial Disclosures

Dr. Melanie Adams has no financial or proprietary interest in the materials presented herein.

Mr. William M. Adams has no financial or proprietary interest in the materials presented herein.

Dr. Thomas Cappaert has no financial or proprietary interest in the materials presented herein.

Dr. Ashley S. Long has no financial or proprietary interest in the materials presented herein.

Dr. Brendon P. McDermott has no financial or proprietary interest in the materials presented herein.

Dr. Johna K. Register-Mihalik has current research funding from the CDC/NCIPC, the National Operating Committee for Standards on Athletic Equipment.

Dr. Wanda Swiger has no financial or proprietary interest in the materials presented herein.

Dr. Jeffrey Timmer has no financial or proprietary interest in the materials presented herein.

Mr. Scot A. Ward has no financial or proprietary interest in the materials presented herein.

Index

ACL (anterior cruciate ligament) injuries, 56, 59, 149, 154–158, 220–221, 227–234

ACSM (American College of Sports Medicine), 25, 27, 29, 31, 208

activities of daily living (ADLs), 22

adaptations to physical activity, 24–26

adolescent growth spurts, 138–139, 142, 192, 220–221

AE (athlete-exposure), 53, 56, 72–73, 77

aerobic exercise. See cardiovascular fitness/ aerobic exercise

age as a risk factor for injuries, 151–153, 158, 220–221

AHA (American Heart Association), 25, 26–27, 121–122, 210, 214–215

alcohol abuse, 170–172, 182–183, 185–186. See also substance abuse

alpha (α), 47–48

Alzheimer's disease, 7, 14–16, 23, 175–176, 195

amenorrhea, 139, 141–142, 219

American Academy of Pediatrics Council on Sports Medicine and Fitness, 142, 208

American College of Sports Medicine (ACSM), 25, 27, 29, 31, 208

American Heart Association (AHA), 25, 26–27, 121–122, 210, 214–215

American Medical Association, 70, 208

American Medical Society for Sports Medicine, 142

amphetamines, 184–185

analysis of covariance, 61–62

analysis of variance (ANOVA), 47–48

ankle injuries, prevention of, 255–259

annual prevalence, 53

anorexia nervosa, 172–173, 187–189

ANOVA (analysis of variance), 47–48

anterior cruciate ligament (ACL) injuries, 56, 59, 149, 154–158, 220–221, 227–234

anxiety disorders, 170, 176–177

apolipoprotein E (APOE), 15–16

Appropriate Medical Coverage of Inter-collegiate Athletics (AMCIA), 78

atherosclerosis, 8–9, 26

athlete-exposure (AE), 53, 56, 72–73, 77

athletic heart, 121

athletic trainers, role of, 45, 66
    concussion, 108, 114, 261–262
    epidemiology statistics, 52, 59
    injury prevention, 246, 261–262
    injury surveillance systems, 73, 75–76, 78
    mental health, 168, 186, 192, 196
    policies, awareness of, 245
    sudden death in sport, 120, 122, 124, 126, 131–132

attributable risk, 57–58

average (mean), 45–49

Balance Error Scoring System, 113

balance testing, 113, 223

balance training, 25, 257–259

bar graphs, 49–51

Beighton Joint Laxity Scale, 219–220

bias and errors in research, 59–62, 94–95

binge drinking, 170–171, 182–183, 185–186

binge eating disorder, 172–173, 187–189

bipolar disorder, 170

blinded studies, 94

BMI (body mass index), 23

body composition, 23, 26

brain injuries. See concussion; head injuries, catastrophic

breast cancer, 31

bulimia nervosa, 172–173, 187–189

cancer, 7, 13–14, 23, 30–31

cardiac output, 25

cardiometabolic benefits of exercise, 26

cardiorespiratory endurance, 22

cardiorespiratory fitness testing, 221–222

cardiovascular disease (CVD), 7–9, 12, 23, 25–26, 28–33

cardiovascular fitness/aerobic exercise, 23
    adaptations of body to, 24–26
    health benefits of, 22, 27–33, 194
    importance of, 22, 34

cardiovascular screening, 121–122, 214–216

case reports, 43–44, 91

case-control studies, 57, 91

catastrophic injuries. See sudden death in sport

CATs (critically appraised topics), 98

cause-and-effect (causal) relationship, 42–43, 90, 95–96

Center for Injury Research and Policy-Reporting Information Online, 74

Centers for Disease Control and Prevention (CDC), 6, 76

cerebrovascular disease, 7, 9–11

cervical spine injuries, 127–129, 246

CHD (coronary heart disease), 7–8, 26, 28–30, 32–33

cholesterol, high. *See* high cholesterol

chronic bronchitis, 11–12

chronic lower respiratory infections, 7, 11–13

chronic obstructive pulmonary disease (COPD), 11–13

chronic traumatic encephalopathy (CTE), 108, 181, 195

CINAHL database, 87

clinical decision making, 42, 97–98

clinical tests, validity of, 53–55

Cochrane Library database, 87

cohort studies. *See* longitudinal cohort studies

colon cancer, 31

commotio cordis, 120

comorbidity, definition of, 12

computerized searching, 87–89

concussion, 77, 220
  assessment protocols, 111–114
  definition of, 106, 109
  depression and, 108, 180–181
  epidemiological studies, barriers to, 109–110
  incidence of, 106–109, 146–147
  mechanism and pathophysiology, 110–111, 195
  overview, 105–106
  position and consensus statements, 114
  prevention of, 244–245, 248, 253–254, 261–262
  questions and activities, 114–115
  recovery from, 108–110
  recurrent injuries, 110, 129
  risk factors for, 111
  symptom scale, 112

confounding variables, 61–62, 95

construct validity, 59

contact injuries, 67

coordination training, 25, 257–259

COPD (chronic obstructive pulmonary disease), 11–13

coronary heart disease (CHD), 7–8, 26, 28–30, 32–33

correlational studies, 42, 43–44, 90, 92

criterion validity, 59

Critical Appraisal Worksheets, 90, 100–102

critically appraised topics (CATs), 98

cross-sectional studies, 42, 43–44, 47, 91

CTE (chronic traumatic encephalopathy), 108, 181, 195

curvilinear relationships, 51–52

CVD. *See* cardiovascular disease (CVD)

data, types of, 45

databases for sports medicine, 73–74, 87

death, premature, reduced risk of, 24, 27–28, 34

death, sports-related. *See* sudden death in sport

death in U.S., leading causes of, 6–16

degree of injury, 69

dependent variables or outcomes, 42–43, 61

depression, 23
  comorbidities, 178–180
  concussion and, 108, 180–181
  diagnosis/symptoms of, 168, 169, 178
  protective role of physical activity, 35, 178, 194
  risk factors for, 178
  stress response and, 175–176, 178–179, 195
  symptoms of, 169, 178

descriptive statistics, 45–47

descriptive studies, 42–44, 90, 92

diabetes mellitus, 7, 11–12, 23, 26, 32

Diagnostic and Statistical Manual (DSM), 168

disordered eating, 189

dose-gradient relationship, 32, 50, 96

dose-response relationship, 29, 50–51

double-blinded studies, 43, 94

driving while impaired (DWI), 185

drug testing, 186

drug use. *See* substance abuse

DSM (Diagnostic and Statistical Manual), 168

duration of activity, 153

dynamic stability tests, 223, 225–227

dynamic valgus testing, 227–233

dysthymia, 169

EAP (emergency action plan), 122, 130–132

eating disorders
  in athletes, 177, 187–193
  disordered eating continuum, 188
  in general population, 172–174
  health consequences of, 190
  key behaviors of, 173–174
  risk factors for, 172, 174, 190–192

screening and treatment, 192–193
types of, 172–173, 187
eating disorders not otherwise specified
(EDNOS), 172–173, 188
EBM (evidence-based medicine), 83
EBP. *See* evidence-based practice (EBP)
echocardiograms, 121–122
EDNOS (eating disorders not otherwise
specified), 172–173, 188
education, as prevention strategy, 246
effect size, 58
EHS (exertional heat stroke), 124–126
electrocardiograms (ECG, EKG), 121–122,
215–216
emergency action plan (EAP), 122, 130–132
emphysema, 11–12
environments, and risk factors, 5
epidemiology
basic concepts of, 3–5
leading causes of death in the U.S., 6–16
questions and activities, 16–17
sport, 5–6
epidemiology, definition of, 3
epidemiology statistics
bias and errors in research, 59–62, 94–95
clinical tests, validity of, 53–55
incidence and prevalence of injuries, 53,
71–73
learning activities, 62–63
overview, 4, 52
predicting risk, 55–58, 71–73
treatment, effect of, 58–59
equipment changes, 76–77, 247–254, 261
ergogenic substances, 150, 184–185, 187
etiology, definition of, 8
evidence pyramid, 43–44, 87–88
evidence-based medicine (EBM), 83
evidence-based practice (EBP), 87
applying evidence to clinical situations,
97–98
conducting searches, 87–89
Critical Appraisal Worksheets, 90, 100–102
critically evaluating evidence, 89–96, 100–
102
developing clinical questions, 84–86
evaluating effectiveness of clinical practice,
98–99
learning activities, 99
overview, 83–84
exercise, definition of, 22. *See also* physical
activity

exertional heat stroke (EHS), 124–126
exertional sickling, 122–124
experimental studies, 43–44, 47, 90–91, 93
extrinsic factors associated with injuries, 242

face validity, 59
false negative, 54
false positive, 54
fatalities. *See* sudden death in sport
female athlete triad syndrome, 141–142
50th percentile, 46
fitness, and sexual maturity, 219
fitness, components of, 22–23. *See also* physical
activity
fitness and dynamic movement testing,
221–234
flexibility, 22–23, 25, 223, 225, 260–261
functional movement screening (FMS), 223,
225–227

GAD (generalized anxiety disorder), 176–177
game injuries, 67, 140–141, 144–145, 149
gender differences, 6, 12–13, 111, 139, 141–143,
149, 154–157. *See also* specific illness;
injury
generalized anxiety disorder (GAD), 176–177
government legislation of sport, 208, 210,
217–218, 244
graphs, 49–52
grip strength, 219, 224
growth spurts, 138–139, 142, 192, 220–221

hamstring injuries, prevention of, 259–261
Hawthorne effect, 60, 95
HCM (hypertrophic cardiomyopathy), 120–121,
215
HDL-C (high-density lipoprotein cholesterol),
26, 32–33
head injuries, catastrophic, 126–129. *See also*
concussion
health benefits of physical activity, 23–33, 35,
194–195
health disparities, 5, 6, 12–13. *See also* specific
illness; injury
Health History Questionnaire, 211–212
heart disease. *See* cardiovascular disease (CVD)
heart rate (HR), 25, 26–27
heat-related deaths. *See* exertional heat stroke
(EHS)
helmets, 109, 127, 247–252
hemorrhagic strokes, 9–10

high blood pressure. *See* hypertension
high cholesterol, 7–9, 26, 32–33
high-density lipoprotein cholesterol (HDL-C), 26, 32–33
Hill's Criteria for Causation, 95–96
history of epidemiology, 4
hyperlipidemia, 32–33
hypertension, 7–9, 11, 12, 23, 26, 31
hypertrophic cardiomyopathy (HCM), 120–121, 215

incidence, 3, 53, 71–73
incidence proportion (IP), 72
incidence rate (IR), 71–73
independent variables, 42–43
infectious diseases, 4
inferential statistics, 47–48
injury, definitions of, 68–69
injury, location of, 69–70
injury, mechanism of, 67–68
injury, severity of, 69
injury, time frame for, 67
injury classification systems, 70–71
injury risk, acceptable levels of, 77
injury surveillance systems (ISS)
    basic components of, 66–71
    epidemiology definitions and calculations, 71–73
    issues with data collection, 75–76
    outcomes of, 76–78
    overview, 65–66
    questions and activities, 79–80
    research databases and collection agencies, 73–74
insomnia, 179
internal validity, 60–62
interval data, 45
intima, 8–9
intratester reliability, 59–60, 94–95
intrinsic factors associated with injuries, 242
inverse relationships, 51–52
IP (incidence proportion), 72
IR (incidence rate), 71–73
ischemic strokes, 9–10

Jenner, Edward, 4
John Henry effect, 95
joint laxity, 149, 156, 219–220

King-Devick test, 114
knee abduction moment (KAM), 229, 232

LDLs (low-density lipoproteins), 8–9, 26
learning effect, 60, 95
LESS (landing error scoring system), 229–231
life expectancy in U.S., 6, 34
lifetime prevalence, 53
lightning fatalities, 130–132
line graphs, 50–52
linear relationships, 51
literature reviews, 43–44
location of injury, 69–70
longitudinal cohort studies, 5, 43–44, 47, 91
low-density lipoproteins (LDLs), 8–9, 26
lower respiratory infections, 7, 11–13
lumen, 8–9

Marfan syndrome, 120, 211, 214
marijuana, 183–184, 185
maximal oxygen consumption (VO2max), 24–25, 27, 50, 221
mean (average), 45–49
mechanism of injury, 67–68
median, 45–47
medical screenings. *See* pre-activity screenings
medical staffing and coverage, 78
mental health. *See also* anxiety disorders; depression; eating disorders; substance abuse
    athletic trainers, role of, 168, 186, 192, 196
    classification of concerns, 168
    learning activities, 196–197
    mental health professionals, 168–169
    overview, 167–168, 195–196
    physical activity, benefits of, 35, 176, 178, 194–195
    prevalence of conditions in general population, 169–174
    stress response, 174–176, 178–179, 194–195
    terminology and measurement, 168
MET (metabolic equivalent of task), 28
meta-analyses, 44, 91, 102
minorities, 5, 6, 12–13. *See also* specific illness; injury
mode, 46–47
mood disorders, 169–170
motor vehicle deaths, 185
mouth guards, 253–254

muscular fitness tests, 222–225
muscular strength and endurance, 22, 26. *See also* strength and resistance training
musculoskeletal examination, 212–214
musculoskeletal injuries
    ACL injuries, 56, 59, 149, 154–158, 220–221, 227–234
    activity-specific motions, 159–161
    age as a risk factor for, 151–153, 158
    incidence of, 138–151
    overview, 137–138
    prevention of, 157, 159, 233–234, 255–261
    questions and activities, 161
    rotator cuff injuries, 157–159

narrative reviews, 43–44
NATA. *See* National Athletic Trainers' Association (NATA)
National Association for Intercollegiate Athletics (NAIA), 208, 210
National Athletic Injury/Illness Reporting System (NAIRS), 70, 73
National Athletic Trainers' Association (NATA), 44, 78, 106, 108–109, 114, 125, 130, 143, 168, 174, 187, 192–193, 208, 212, 245, 257
National Center for Catastrophic Sport Injury Research, 74
National Collegiate Athletic Association Injury Surveillance System (NCAA ISS), 72, 74–76, 143
National Collegiate Athletic Association (NCAA), 65, 69, 76–77, 120, 123–126, 143–148, 168, 174, 182–186, 193, 208, 210, 212, 245–246
National Physical Activity Guidelines, 25
neuroplasticity, 176
NNT (numbers needed to treat), 58–59
nominal data, 45
noncontact injuries, 67
nonexperimental studies, 43–44, 47, 50–51
nonparametric data, 45–46
numbers needed to treat (NNT), 58–59

obesity, definition of, 23
odds ratio (OR), 56–57
older adults
    injuries in, 152–153, 158
    physical activity, benefits of, 22, 33, 194–195

one-tail tests, 48
Orchard Sports Injury Classification System (OSICS), 70
ordinal data, 45
overhead activity injuries, 160–161
overload, 23–24
overtraining syndrome, 142, 180
overuse injuries, 67, 138, 142, 149, 152, 160, 246

parametric statistics, 45–46
participant fatigue, 60, 95
patient values and preferences, 97–98
Pearson correlation, 47
PEDro database, 87
performance anxiety, 177
performance-enhancing drugs, 150, 184–185, 187
physical activity
    concepts of, 21–23
    epidemiological research, impact of, 34
    health benefits of, 23–33, 35, 194–195
    importance of, 35–36
    physical activity guidelines
        ACSM/AHA recommendations, 24–25
        evolution of, 26–27
        key studies related to, 27–33
        promotion of, 34–35
        questions and activities, 36
        volume of, 29–30
Physical Activity Guidelines for Americans, 24–25
physical examinations. *See* pre-activity screenings
physical fitness, components of, 22–23
physical fitness testing, 221–234
physical maturity. *See* Tanner Maturation Scale
PICO (Patient(s), Intervention, Comparison, Outcomes) format for clinical questions, 84–89
placebos, 94, 95
playing surface, 67–68, 150
policy changes, 244–245, 261. *See also* rule changes
POMS (Pubertal Maturational Observational Scale), 218
position papers, 44, 90
posture, 22–23
practice injuries, 67, 140–141, 144–145, 149

pre-activity screenings
  fitness and dynamic movement testing,
      221–234
  learning activities, 234–235
  overview, 207–208
  pre-participation physical examinations
      (PPEs)
    administration of, 210–221
    effectiveness of, 210
    goals of, 208–209
    sudden death in sport, 121–125, 129
prevalence, 3, 53, 71
prevention strategies. *See also* pre-activity
      screenings
  concussion, 244–245, 248, 253–254, 261–262
  eating disorders, 192–193
  education efforts, 246
  equipment changes, 76–77, 247–254, 261
  injury surveillance systems and, 77–78
  learning activities, 263–264
  musculoskeletal injuries, 157, 159, 233–234,
      255–261
  overview, 241–244
  policies and legislation, 244–245, 261
  predicting risk, 55–58, 71–73
  research, limitations of, 243, 262
  rule changes, 76–77, 127, 129, 245–246, 261
  substance abuse, 186–187
  sudden death in sport, 121–124, 126, 129,
      130–132, 246
prognostic factors, 55, 58
prophylactic ankle bracing and taping, 255–257
proprioceptive training, 257–259
protective equipment, 76–77, 247–254, 261
Pubertal Maturational Observational Scale
      (POMS), 218
public health, 4
PubMed database, 87

qualitative data, 45
quality of life, 195
quantitative data, 45
quartiles, 47
quasiexperimental studies, 43–44
questions and learning activities
  concussions, 114–115
  epidemiology, 16–17
  epidemiology statistics, 62–63
  evidence-based practice, 99
  injury surveillance systems, 79–80
  mental health, 196–197

musculoskeletal injuries, 161
physical activity, 36
pre-activity screenings, 234–235
prevention methods, 263–264
sudden death in sport, 132–133

racial/ethnic disparities, 5, 6, 12–13. *See also*
      specific illness; injury
randomized, controlled trials (RCTs), 43–44,
      87, 91, 102
range of motion (ROM), 22–23, 223
ratio data, 45
RCTs (randomized, controlled trials), 43–44,
      87, 91, 102
recurrent injuries, 67, 72, 110, 129, 258–259
relative risk (RR), 55–56
reliability, 59–62, 94–95
reportable injuries, 68–69
research databases, 73–74, 87
research study design, 42–44, 59–62, 90–96
resistance training. *See* strength and resistance
      training
retrospective longitudinal cohort studies, 57
return to play (RTP), 108–109, 193
review questions. *See* questions and learning
      activities
risk, acceptable levels of, 77
risk, predicting, 55–58, 71–73
risk factors, 4–5, 55, 58. *See also* pre-activity
      screenings; prevention strategies;
      specific injury
ROM (range of motion), 22–23, 223
rotator cuff injuries, 157–159
RR (relative risk), 55–56
rule changes, 76–77, 127, 129, 245–246, 261
rules preventing illness transmissions, 243
runner's high, 194
running injuries, 160

SAC (Standardized Assessment of Concussion),
      113
sample bias, 60, 94
SCAT-3 (Sport Concussion Assessment Tool),
      113–114
SCD (sudden cardiac death), 120–122, 215–216
screenings. *See* pre-activity screenings
SD (standard deviation), 45, 47–49
SEBT (Star Excursion Balance Test), 223
self-efficacy, 35
self-reported data, 61
sensitivity, 53–55

severity of injury, 69

sexual maturation, 217–221, 231–232

sexually transmitted infections (STIs), 185–186

shoulder injuries, 160–161, 146–147. *See also* rotator cuff injuries

sickle cell trait, 122–124, 212

Single Leg Balance (SLB) test, 223

skeletal age, 219

SMDCS (Sports Medicine Diagnostic Coding System), 70–71

smoking, 5, 14, 183–184

SnNOut acronym, 54

Snow, John, 4

social anxiety, 176–177

social desirability, 60–61

spearing, 127, 129, 245, 246

specificity, 53–55, 96

spine injuries, catastrophic, 126–129, 246

sport classification, 67

Sport Concussion Assessment Tool (SCAT-3), 113–114

sport organization policies, 244–245

sport selection, 77

sport specialization, 139, 142, 192

SPORTDiscus database, 87

sports, as physical activity, 22

sports epidemiology, 5–6

Sports Medicine Diagnostic Coding System (SMDCS), 70–71

sport-specific injury rates, 139–141, 144–149. *See also* specific injury

SpPin (Specific, Positive, In), 55

standard deviation (SD), 45, 47–49

Standardized Assessment of Concussion (SAC), 113

Star Excursion Balance Test (SEBT), 223

state anxiety, 177

state policies, 208, 210, 217–218, 244

statistical concepts. *See also* epidemiology statistics

   evidence, levels of, 43–44, 87–88, 90

   overview, 41

   relationships between variables, 42–43, 95–96

   Strength of Recommendation Taxonomy, 44

   understanding data and results, 45–52

statistical significance, 47–49, 58, 95

statistical symbols, 49

steroid use, 150, 184–185

STIs (sexually transmitted infections), 185–186

strength and resistance training, 23–24, 25, 26, 30–31, 34, 233, 260–261

Strength of Recommendation Taxonomy, 44

strength tests, 222–225

stress response, 174–176, 178–179, 194–195

stress-injury model, 194

stretching, 259–261

stroke, 9–11, 23

stroke volume, 25

substance abuse

   alcohol, 170–172, 182–183

   depression and, 178–179

   ergogenic substances, 150, 184–185, 187

   prevalence of, 170–172, 181–186

   prevention programs, 186–187

   tobacco and marijuana, 5, 14, 183–184

sudden cardiac death (SCD), 120–122, 215–216

sudden death in sport, 71, 74

   exertional heat stroke (EHS), 124–126

   exertional sickling, 122–124

   head and spine injuries, 126–129, 245, 246

   lightning strikes, 130–132

   overview, 119–120

   questions and activities, 132–133

   sudden cardiac death (SCD), 120–122, 215–216

suicide, 172, 178

surveillance studies, 3. *See also* injury surveillance systems (ISS)

survey data, 61

systematic reviews, 44, 87, 91, 102

Tanner Maturation Scale, 217–221, 231–232

thrombus, 8

TIA (transient ischemic attack), 9–11

time frame for injury, 67

tobacco. *See* smoking

training injuries, 67, 140–141, 144–145, 149

trait anxiety, 177

transient ischemic attack (TIA), 9–11

traumatic injuries, 67

treatment, effect of, 58–59, 98

true negative, 54

true positive, 54

tumors, 13

two-tailed tests, 48

United States Consumer Product Commission
        National Electronic Injury Surveillance
        System (NEISS), 74
U.S., lack of physical activity in, 34
U.S., leading causes of death in, 6–16
U.S., life expectancy in, 6, 34

validity, 59–62, 94
variables, relationship between, 42–43, 95–96
Venn diagram, 88–89
Vestibular Oculomotor Screening, 114
Virginia Tech Helmet Ratings, 249–252
volume of physical activity, 29–30

weight loss, 33, 50–51
white papers, 87

Printed in the United States
by Baker & Taylor Publisher Services

Printed in the United States
by Baker & Taylor Publisher Services